Manual of
Childhood Infections

SECOND EDITION

ii

Commissioning editor: Deborah Russell
Development assistant: Samantha Tooby
Project manager: Rolla Couchman
Production manager: Helen Sofio

Manual of Childhood Infections

SECOND EDITION

E Graham Davies MA FRCP FRCPCH
Consultant Paediatrician/Immunologist,
Great Ormond Street Hospital, London, UK

David A C Elliman FRCPCH DCH
Consultant in Community Child Health,
St George's Healthcare NHS Trust, and Honorary Senior Lecturer in Child Health,
St George's Hospital Medical School, London, UK

C Anthony Hart MBBS BSc PhD FRCPCH FRCPath
Professor and Honorary Consultant in Medical Microbiology, Department of
Medical Microbiology and Genitourinary Medicine, Medical School,
University of Liverpool, Liverpool, UK

Angus Nicoll MSc FRCP FFPHM FRPCH
Director, Public Health Laboratory Service
Communicable Disease Surveillance Centre, London, UK

Peter T Rudd MD FRCPCH
Consultant Paediatrician and Honorary Senior Lecturer, Children's Centre,
Royal United Hospital, and Senior Lecturer, University of Bath, Bath, UK

*For the Royal College of Paediatrics
and Child Health*

W. B. SAUNDERS

LONDON • EDINBURGH • NEW YORK • PHILADELPHIA • ST LOUIS • SYDNEY • TORONTO 2001

WB SAUNDERS
An imprint of Harcourt Publishers Limited

iv © Royal College of Paediatrics and Child Health 2001

[K] is a registered trademark of Harcourt Publishers Limited

The right of E Graham Davies, David A C Elliman, C Anthony Hart, Angus
Nicoll and Peter T Rudd to be identified as authors of this work has been
asserted by them in accordance with the Copyright, Designs and Patents
Act 1988.

First edition published 1996
Reprinted in 1998
Second edition published 2001

ISBN 0 7020 2626 3

British Library Cataloguing in Publication Data
A catalogue record for this book is available from the British Library

Library of Congress Cataloging in Publication Data
A catalog record for this book is available from the Library of Congress

Note
Medical knowledge is constantly changing. As new information becomes available,
changes in treatment, procedures, equipment and the use of drugs become necessary. The editors and the publishers have taken care to ensure that the information
given in this text is accurate and up to date. However, readers are strongly advised
to confirm that the information, especially with regard to drug usage, complies with
the latest legislation and standards of practice.

Existing UK nomenclature is changing to the system of Recommended International
Nonproprietary Names (rINNs). Until the UK names are no longer in use, these more
familiar names are used in this book in preference to rINNs, details of which may be
obtained from the British National Formulary.

Printed in China

Table of contents

Part Two: Specific infections

vi

Part Three: Appendices

Additional contributors

Barbara Bannister MSc FRCP   **ix**
Consultant in Infectious and Tropical Diseases, Department of Infectious
and Tropical Diseases, Royal Free Hospital, London, UK

Nicola Barrett PhD CBiol Mbiol
Formerly Principal Scientist (Epidemiology),
Communicable Diseases Surveillance Centre, London, UK

Robert Booy MD MBBS(Hons) FRACP FRCPCH
Professor and Head of Child Health, Department of Child Health, St
Bartholomews and Royal London School of Medicine and Dentistry,
London, UK

Andrew J Cant MD BSc FRCP FRCPCH
Consultant Paediatrician, Paediatric Immunology and Infectious Diseases
Unit, Newcastle General Hospital, Newcastle-upon-Tyne, UK

J Brian S Coulter BA MD FRCPI FRCPCH DCH
Senior Lecturer in Tropical Paediatrics, Liverpool School of Tropical
Medicine, Liverpool, UK

Rami Dhillon MRCP MRCPCH
Consultant Paediatric Cardiologist, Birmingham Children's Hospital,
Birmingham, UK

Brendan Drumm MD FRCPC FRCPI FRCPCH
Professor of Paediatrics, University College Dublin, Our Lady's Hospital
for Sick Children, Dublin, Republic of Ireland

Adam Finn MA PhD FRCP FRCPCH
Senior Lecturer in Immunology and Infectious Disease, Children's
Hospital NHS Trust, Sheffield Institute for Vaccine Studies, University of
Sheffield, Sheffield, UK

Diana Gibb MD FRCPCH
Senior Lecturer in Infectious Diseases and Honorary Consultant
Paediatrician, MRC Clinical Trials Unit, University College London
Medical School, London, UK

Lyda P Jadresic MD FRCPCH MBBS
Consultant Paediatrician, Department of Paediatrics, Gloucester Royal
Hospital, Gloucester, UK

Vas Novelli MB FRACP FRCP FRCPCH
Consultant in Paediatric Infections Diseases, Great Ormond Street
Hospital for Sick Children, London, UK

James Y Paton MD FRCP(Glas) FRCPCH BSc MBChB(Hons) DCH
Senior Lecturer in Paediatric Respiratory Disease and Consultant
Paediatrician, Department of Child Health, Royal Hospital of Sick
Children, Glasgow, UK

Tom Rogers MA MSc FRCPI FRCPath
Professor of Bacteriology, Department of Infectious Diseases, Imperial
School of Medicine, Hammersmith Hospital, London, UK

Michael Sharland MBBSc MD FRCPCH MRCP DTMH
Consultant in Paediatric Infectious Disease, Paediatric Infectious
Diseases Unit, St George's Hospital, London, UK

Alistair Thomson MD DRCOG DCH FRCP FRCPCH
Consultant Paediatrician, Mid-Cheshire Hospitals NHS Trust, Crewe, UK

E Jane Tizard MBBS FRCP FRCPCH
Consultant Paediatric Nephrologist, Children's Renal Unit, Richard Bright
Kidney Unit, Southmead Hospital, Bristol, UK

Jenny C Tyrrell DM FRCPCH
Consultant Paediatrician, Children's Centre, Royal United Hospital,
Bath, UK

Acknowledgements

The Editors also wish to acknowledge the following persons and institutions who made invaluable contributions to the book in various ways:

Dr Bob Adak
Miss Annabel Attridge
Dr Norman Begg
Dr Liz Boxhall
Dr Moyra Brett
Dr Sandy Calvert
Ms Bernadette Carroll
Mrs Penny Cooper
Mr Ian Costello
Miss Lisa Forsyth
Prof Richard Gilbert
Dr Rob George
Dr Paul Heath
Mr Doug Henderson
Ms Anitra Jones
Dr Ian Jones
Mrs Carol Joseph

Ms Deidre Kells
Mrs Clare Kelly
Dr Gil Lea
Dr Jim McLaughlan
Dr Elizabeth Miller
Dr Elizabeth Mitchell
Dr Philip Mortimer
Ms Lisa Newton
Dr Mary Ramsay
Dr David Salisbury
Dr Mark Taylor
Ms Rosemary Tucker
Dr Paul Van Buynder
Dr Jane Watkeys
Dr John Watson
Ms Joanne White
Ms Penny Whiting

British Paediatric Surveillance Unit of the Royal College of Paediatrics and Child Health

Central Public Health Laboratory, London

Department of Health, London

Department of Health and Social Services, Northern Ireland

General Register Office for Scotland

Information and Statistics Division, Common Services Agency, Scotland

Office for National Statistics

Public Health Laboratory Service Communicable Disease Surveillance Centre

Public Health Laboratory Service Malaria Reference Laboratory, London

Scottish Centre for Infection and Environmental Health

Foreword

In the 1960s and 1970s improved living standards and hygienic conditions, together with successful immunisation campaigns, led to the reduction or even disappearance of many traditional communicable diseases. Simultaneously, the clinical course of many bacterial infections has become milder and long-term sequelae rarities with the use of effective antimicrobials. These facts are familiar to every layman and politician.

However more recently there are clear signs that the problems caused by infectious diseases have increased during the last two decades, not decreased as everybody expected. New infections have emerged and some old infections have re-emerged, some of these with the added dangers of antimicrobial resistance. Infections remain a major cause of mortality and morbidity at the global level. Acute respiratory infections alone cause an estimated 4.3 million deaths annually, and diarrhoeal diseases an additional 3.1 million deaths. Paediatric infections account for the majority of these deaths. However paediatric infections are equally important in industrialised countries, accounting for numbers of hospital and primary-care consultations that are disproportionate to the actual numbers of children. The economical consequences of acute infections are also remarkable. Recent estimates are that annual costs of intestinal infections in the USA was $23 billion and that of sexually transmitted infections and HIV $8 billion. The public health threat and vast economical burden associated with nosocomial infections have only recently been realised, especially in the context of rising numbers of immunocompromised children, those with HIV infection, others with neoplastic diagnoses under treatment, chronic conditions such as renal impairments, etc.

Every clinician, irrespective of speciality, meets infections in his or her everyday practice. However this is especially true with paediatricians. Infections are the leading cause for outpatient visits in children. They can pose particularly difficult challenges to paediatricians working in hospitals and intensive care units.

Some of the challenges in the infectious disease field have changed. Prevention of certain classical communicable diseases has succeeded so well that they do not deserve so much of our attention. But then the focus moves towards other problems: severe infections in the immuno-compromised host, treatment problems due to antimicrobial resistance, or prevention of common childhood infections like otitis or pneumonia. One potentially very important area for research is the interplay between microbes and host defence mechanisms. Rapidly-growing evidence even suggests that infections are associated with many chronic 'non-communicable' diseases. For example, childhood infection with *Helicobacter pylori* seems to cause later peptic ulceration in the upper gastrointestinal tract. If such associations are true, and especially if they are shown to represent causal relationships, diseases like juvenile diabetes or arteriosclerosis may in the future be treated with antimicrobials or prevented with vaccines.

Rapid progress in basic science, especially in genetics, molecular biology and immunology, has provided new means to the clinical use. In order to take full advantage of the development in diagnostic and therapeutic methods, clinicians need to keep themselves well-trained and well informed. For that purpose we need updated and revised editions of good manuals and textbooks. That is why I particularly welcome this new and updated edition of the Royal College of Paediatrics and Child Health *Manual of Childhood Infections*. I commend it to all clinicians. More important than to have a new edition is to read it, and even more important still is to use your new knowledge in practice.

Juhani Eskola MD
Research Professor, National Public Health Institute, Finland
Former President, European Society for Paediatric Infectious Diseases

What's new in the Year 2001 edition?

Following an external review of the first edition, carried out by Professor Simon Kroll of Imperial College, London, all sections of the manual have been revised and updated. The changes are too many to list exhaustively but they include the following.

Account has been taken of new authoritative guidance on management of possible contacts of patients with proven or suspected meningococcal infection; management and treatment of tuberculosis in children, screening for hepatitis B, HIV and syphilis in pregnancy so as to minimise the risk of mother-to-child transmission, new treatments for HIV prevention in childhood and the latest thinking on minimising the risk of mother-to-child transmission of HIV. (In the UK this followed a report of the Inter-collegiate Working Party on reducing mother-to-child transmission published by the Royal College of Paediatrics and Child Health with the other medical and nursing colleges.) Particular attention has been paid to the evidence underlying periods of communicability for individual conditions and advice on exclusion from schools and nurseries, which was the subject of an evidence-based review undertaken by Dr Martin Richardson (St George's Hospital, London and Joint Royal College of Paediatrics and Child Health and Public Health Laboratory Service Fellow). The section on Immunisation of the Immunocompromised Child takes into account the thinking of a Working Party of RCPCH members.

In addition this edition also sees a number of important innovations. There are eight colour plates of important rashes, new sections on Emerging and Re-emerging Infections, Antibiotic Resistance, The Child with an Implant Infection (paediatric infections associated with long-lines, shunts, etc.), The Child with an Enlarged Lymph Node and The Injured Child. Sections have been added on new important infections – *Ehrlichia*, Hepatitis G, Rickettsia – as well as streptococcal and pneumococcal infection (the omission of which in the first edition was an oversight). The section on Infection Control in the Community contains specific guidance on managing needlestick injuries and animal and human bites, as well as on preventing infections of children in schools and nurseries and on farm visits.

Graham Davies
David Elliman
Tony Hart
Angus Nicoll
Peter Rudd

January 2001

Surveillance of paediatric infections

Routine surveillance of infections in children is an essential function. It detects outbreaks and epidemics, reveals new infections and conditions and monitors the progress of vaccination and screening programmes. Clinicians make important and essential contributions through statutory notifications (see Notifiable Diseases 2000, p 480), reporting by routine and reference laboratories and reporting through the British Paediatric Surveillance Unit (BPSU) (a unit of the Royal College of Paediatrics and Child Health).

Certain conditions should be reported to the BPSU by consultant paediatricians in the UK and the Republic of Ireland. This is important so as to achieve the aim of the BPSU, which is to facilitate research into uncommon disorders for the advancement of knowledge and improvement of prevention, treatment and service planning. All reporting is voluntary and confidential. Those conditions currently reportable (2000) are highlighted in Part One and listed below. Normally, reports are made by ticking the orange card that is sent to all consultant paediatricians every month. If consultants do not receive these, if they are not certain if a particular case has been reported or if they wish further details of the BPSU scheme, they should contact the Surveillance Unit Scientific Co-ordinator at the Royal College of Paediatrics and Child Health (020 7307 5600). The Unit is the result of a collaboration between the Royal College of Paediatrics and Child Health, the Public Health Laboratory Service, the Institute of Child Health, London, and other interested bodies.

Similar paediatric surveillance units function in Australia, Canada, Germany, Malaysia, the Netherlands, New Zealand, Papua New Guinea and Switzerland and these are linked into a network, the International Network of Paediatric Surveillance Units (INoPSU).

Currently reportable infections and infection-related conditions (year 2000): AIDS and HIV in children, congenital rubella syndrome, hepatitis C, encephalitis in young children (aged 2 months to 3 years), invasive *Haemophilus influenzae* infection, haemolytic uraemic syndrome (*Escherichia coli* O157 infection), progressive intellectual and neurological deterioration (including variant Creutzfeldt–Jakob disease) and subacute sclerosing panencephalitis.

REFERENCES

1. Hall SM, Nicoll A (1998) The British Paediatric Surveillance Unit – a pioneering method for investigating the less common disorders of childhood. *Child Care, Health and Development* **24**: 129–143.

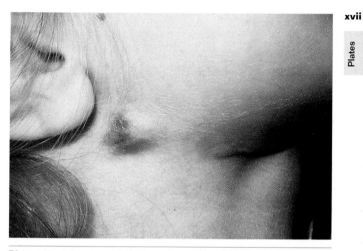

Plate 1 Non tuberculous (atypical) mycobacterial lymphadermitis with involvement of the overlying skin (see p 43 and p 364)

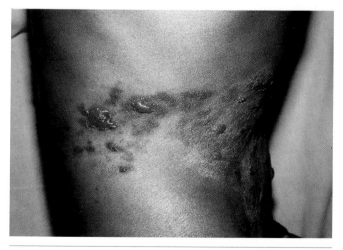

Plate 2 Herpes zoster – shingles (see p 241)

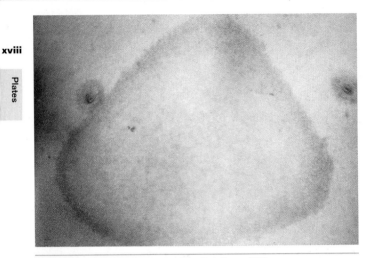

Plate 3 Tinea corporis – ringworm of the body (see p 257)

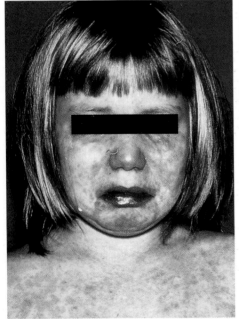

Plate 4 Florid ampicillin-induced rash in a child with infectious mononucleosis (see p 267)

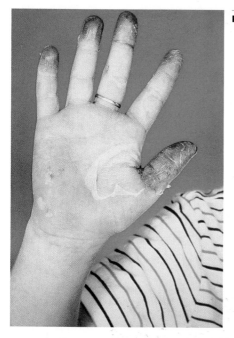

Plate 5 Characteristic desquamation in convalescent phase of Kawasaki disease (see p 328)

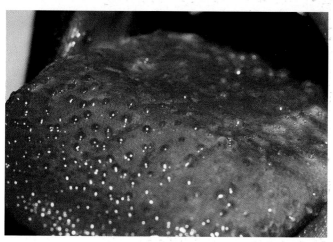

Plate 6 Red strawberry tongue in scarlet fever. See Streptococcal infections (p 413)

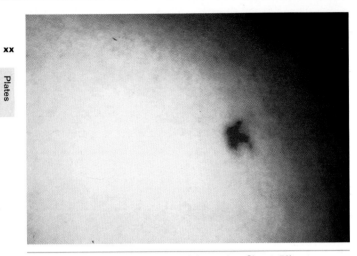

Plate 7 Purpuric lesion in meningococcal disease (see Chapter 78)

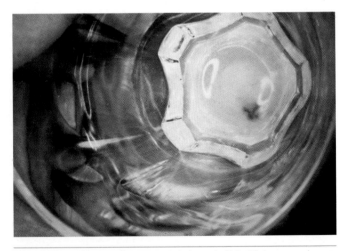

Plate 8 The tumbler test. Same purpuric lesion as in Plate 6 being pressed upon by a glass tumbler. Note that blanching does not occur (see p 352)

Part One: General

Part One: General

1 Emerging and re-emerging infections

In the 1960s and early 1970s the official medical view of infections was optimistic. Fuelled by the success of antibiotics and vaccines and some long-term secular declines in infections such as tuberculosis, there was an impression that infections were becoming less important to human health – 'Medicine, particularly the practice of controlling infectious disease, has made tremendous progress during the twentieth century. Diseases like tuberculosis, once great scourges, have been controlled.' Truer pictures are well captured by Zinsser: 'Infectious disease is one of the great tragedies of living things, the struggle for existence between two different forms of life – incessantly the pitiless war goes on without quarter or armistice, a nationalism of species against species', or McNeill: 'Ingenuity, knowledge and organisation alter but cannot cancel humans' vulnerability to invasion by parasitic forms of life. Infectious disease, which antedated the emergence of humankind, will last as long as humanity itself, and will surely remain, as it has been hitherto, one of the fundamental parameters and determinants of human history.' The past three decades have seen the emergence of many infections and their consequent diseases and the re-emergence of others, which affect children as much as they do adults (Table 1.1). These are infections and diseases that have either newly appeared in the population, such as HIV, *Escherichia coli* O157, *Vibrio cholerae* 0139 and multiply drug-resistant tuberculosis worldwide, new variant Creutzfeldt–Jakob disease in the UK; those that have reappeared, such as tuberculosis worldwide and diphtheria in the states of the former USSR; those that have rapidly increased in incidence, such as food poisoning in the UK; those that are increasing their geographical range, such as dengue fever; and those that are newly recognised, such as hepatitis C, hantavirus and human herpes virus 6, 7 and 8. The final group are simply explained by increasing human scientific knowledge, recognising that much of what was previously 'non-A non-B hepatitis' was in fact caused by hepatitis C (the diversity of which suggests that it is in fact an older virus than the earlier-discovered hepatitis A and B). The forces underlying these changes are various (Table 1.2); they include economic and ecological factors, changes in human behaviour, increasing international travel and commerce, technological advances and changes in industrial and farming practices, microbiological adaptation and change and, in some instances, breakdown in public health measures.

Table 1.1 Diseases important to child and adolescent health: major aetiological agents identified since 1973 (adapted from: CDC Staff 1997 *Emerging Infectious Diseases*, 1: 3)

Year of report	Agent	Disease
1973	Rotavirus	Major cause of infantile diarrhoea worldwide
1975	Parvovirus B19	Fifth disease; aplastic crisis in haemolytic anaemia
1976	*Cryptosporidium parvum*	Acute enterocolitis
1977	Ebola virus	Ebola haemorrhagic fever
1977	*Legionella pneumophila*	Legionnaires' disease
1977	Hantaan virus	Haemorrhagic fever with renal syndrome (HFRS)
1977	*Campylobacter* spp.	Enteric pathogens distributed globally
1980	Human T-cell lymphotrophic virus-1 (HTLV 1)	T-cell lymphoma; leukaemia
1981	*Staphylococcus* toxin	Toxic shock syndrome associated with tampon use
1982	*Escherichia coli* O157: H7	Haemorrhagic colitis; haemolytic uraemic syndrome
1982	HTLV-II	Hairy cell leukaemia
1982	*Borrelia burgdorferi*	Lyme disease
1983	Human immunodeficiency virus (HIV)	HIV disease, including AIDS
1983	*Helicobacter pylori*	Peptic ulcers
1988	Human herpes virus-6 (HHV-6)	Exanthem subitum and encephalitis
1989	*Ehrlichia chaffeensis*	Human ehrlichiosis
1989	Hepatitis C	Parenterally transmitted non-A, non-B hepatitis
1990	Human herpes virus-7 (HHV-7)	Exanthem subitum and encephalitis
1991	Guanarito virus	Venezuelan haemorrhagic fever
1992	*Vibrio cholerae* O139	New strain associated with epidemic cholera
1992	*Bartonella* (= *Rochalimaea*) *henselae*	Cat-scratch disease; bacillary angiomatosis
1993	Hantavirus isolates	Hantavirus pulmonary syndrome
1994	Sabia virus	Brazilian haemorrhagic fever
1995	Human herpes virus-8 (HHV-8)	Kaposi's sarcoma
1997	BSE agent (a prion)	Variant Creutzfeldt–Jakob disease

Table 1.2 Factors in infectious disease emergence and re-emergence relevant to child and adolescent health

Factor	Examples of specific factors	Examples of disease
Ecological changes (including those due to economic development and land use)	Agriculture: dams, changes in water ecosystems; deforestation/reforestation; flood/drought; famine, climate changes	Schistosomiasis (dams); Rift Valley fever (dams, irrigation); Argentine haemorrhagic fever (agriculture); Hantaan–Korean haemorrhagic fever (agriculture); hantavirus pulmonary syndrome, south-western USA, 1993 (weather anomalies)
Human demographics, behaviour	Societal changes and events: population growth and migration (movement from rural areas to cities); war or civil conflict; urban decay; sexual behaviour; intravenous drug use; preference for 'fast foods'; use of high-density facilities	Introduction of HIV; spread of dengue; spread of HIV and other sexually transmitted diseases; meningococcal disease; cholera; increases in food poisoning (*Salmonella enteritidis, Campylobacter*)
International travel and commerce	Worldwide movement of goods and people: air travel	'Airport' malaria; dissemination of mosquito vectors; rat-borne hantaviruses; antibiotic-resistant gonorrhoea; introduction of cholera into South America; dissemination of *V. cholerae* 0139
Technology and industry	Globalisation of food supplies; changes in food processing and packaging; organ or tissue transplantation; drugs causing immunosuppression; widespread use of antibiotics	Haemolytic uraemic syndrome (*E. coli* O157 contamination of hamburger meat); *S. agona* in kosher snacks; transfusion-associated hepatitis (hepatitis B, C); opportunistic infections in immunosuppressed patients; Creutzfeldt–Jakob disease from contaminated batches of human growth hormone (medical technology)
Microbial adaptation and change	Microbial evolution, response to selection in environment	Antibiotic-resistant bacteria (multiply resistant *Mycobacterium tuberculosis*); 'antigenic drift' in influenza virus; zidovudine-resistant HIV
Breakdown in public health measures	Curtailment or reduction in prevention programmes; inadequate sanitation and vector control measures; immunisation myths	Whooping cough in the UK; resurgence of tuberculosis in the USA; cholera in refugee camps in Africa; resurgence of diphtheria in the former Soviet Union; measles in Ireland (Dublin)

Antibiotics are produced from microorganisms, which, by definition, must be resistant to their action. Thus antibiotic resistance genes and mechanisms were present prior to the antibiotic era. The use of antibiotics in human and veterinary medicine, in farming, agriculture and aquaculture has speeded up evolution by exerting a selection pressure in which resistant bacteria have an advantage.

Nowadays there is concern that we might be approaching the end of the antibiotic era because of increasing resistance and a slowing of production of new classes of antimicrobials (Table 2.1). We are not at this stage yet but what is not clear is whether stopping or limiting the use of antibiotics will reverse or limit the trend.

Table 2.1 The antibiotic era

Year	Agent	Source	Discoverer
1929	Penicillin	*Penicillium notatum*	Fleming
1935	Sulphonamides	Synthetic	Domagk
1941	Purified benzyl penicillin	*Penicillium notatum*	Florey and Chain
1944	Streptomycin	*Streptomyces griseus*	Waksman
1944	Tetracycline	*Streptomyces aureofaciens*	Duggar
1945	Cephalosporins	*Cephalosporium acremonium*	Brotzu
1947	Chloramphenicol	*Streptomyces venezuelae*	Ehrlich
1952	Erythromycin	*Streptomyces erythreus*	McGuire
1956	Vancomycin	*Amycolatopsis orientalis*	McCormick
1956	Trimethoprim	Synthetic	Hitchings
1957	6–amino penicillanoic acid nucleus	Purified	Rolinson
1959	Metronidazole	Synthetic	Cosar
1962	Nalidixic acid	Synthetic	Lescher
1962	Fusidic acid	*Fusidium coccineum*	Godtfredsen
1964	Gentamicin	*Micromonospora* spp.	Weinstein
1965	Rifampicin	*Streptomyces mediterranei*	Bergamini
1971	Mupirocin	*Pseudomonas fluorescens*	Fuller
1978	Aztreonam	*Chromobacter violaceum*	Sykes
1984	Fluoroquinolones	Synthetic	Various
1987	Oxazolidinones	Synthetic	Various

LABORATORY ASSESSMENT OF RESISTANCE

It must be recognised that antibiotic resistance is not an absolute. Most bacteria will be susceptible to most antimicrobials, providing a high enough concentration is applied. Clinical resistance is linked to the concentration of an antibiotic that can be safely achieved at an infected site. This varies by site; for example, antimicrobials such as trimethoprim, ampicillin or cephradine are excreted in very large amounts in urine and resistant bacteria will have very high minimum inhibitory concentrations (MICs). In contrast, antibiotics such as penicillin penetrate poorly into cerebrospinal fluid and a small increase in MIC (from 0.01 mg/L to 0.2 mg/L in *Streptococcus pneumoniae*) renders bacteria clinically resistant. Interestingly, such a rise in MIC does not prevent successful penicillin therapy of pneumococcal pneumonia.

The laboratory assessment of sensitivity or resistance tries to take into account the above variables. It is assessed with varying degrees of sophistication, from simple disc diffusion methods to breakpoints, to measurement of MICs and in some cases MBCs (minimum bactericidal concentrations). The breakpoint method is being increasingly applied and involves setting a concentration of antibiotic below which bacteria are considered sensitive and above which resistant. Agar plates containing the antibiotic at the breakpoint concentration are prepared and a set number of bacteria (c. 10^5 cfu) is applied as spots to the plate. If growth occurs the bacterium is called clinically resistant. These breakpoints are derived by taking into account pharmacokinetic data on peak concentrations, half-lives and tissue penetration. In fact, there is little direct clinical evidence that if patients are treated with an antibiotic to which the infecting bacterium is resistant then treatment will fail. The only evidence available is when there are marginal rises in MIC such as penicillin treatment failures in meningitis with intermediately resistant pneumococci and fluoroquinolone treatment failure in typhoid fever due to nalidixic-acid-resistant *Salmonella typhi*.

DEVELOPMENT AND GENETICS OF RESISTANCE

Some bacteria are intrinsically resistant to an antibiotic, usually because they do not possess the target for the agent. An example of this is that all Gram-positive bacteria are resistant to polymyxin B because they do not possess an outer membrane, which in Gram-negative bacteria contains lipopolysaccharide. In a susceptible population of bacteria there will always be a minority that are less susceptible to an antibiotic and if antibiotic levels are not sufficiently high then this minority population will multiply as the more susceptible bacteria die. This phenomenon applies in the case of the recently described vancomycin-resistant MRSA (methicillin-resistant *Staphylococcus aureus*). Bacteria multiply very rapidly (some, under optimal conditions, have a doubling time of 20 minutes). As they replicate random mutations occur, which on occasion affect antibiotic susceptibility. Under antibiotic selection (and sometimes even in its absence), the mutated gene would be stably inherited by daughter bacteria (vertical transmission). In addition, it is now apparent that bacteria can acquire resistance genes from other species and genera (horizontal transmission). Most bacteria have a single large DNA loop as their chromosome but many also contain extrachromosomal DNA called plasmids. Antibiotic resistance genes can be situated on the chromosome, on the plasmid or both.

Plasmids are extrachromosomal loops of supercoiled DNA thought originally to have been derived from bacterial viruses (bacteriophages). These can carry antibiotic resistance, metabolic and pathogenicity genes.

Transposons are small sequences of DNA encoding only a few genes (often resistance genes) that have inverted repeats or insertion sequences at each end. These can be excised from one DNA chain (chromosome or plasmid) and reinserted into another. Sequential addition of transposons is a mechanism by which multiple resistance plasmids can evolve.

Integrons are larger sequences of DNA, which may encode resistance to several antibiotics; they can be mobilised (excised) from the chromosome of one bacterium, transferred to another bacterium and undergo site-specific recombination into its chromosome or plasmids.

Plasmids may be transferred horizontally by conjugation or transduction and in the laboratory by transformation. Conjugation is the most frequently used method and involves a sex pilus (hollow protein spike) joining the mating bacteria. Plasmid DNA passes through the tube to the recipient, which stably inherits it. This process is used extensively by Gram-negative bacteria. Transduction involves transfer of DNA by bacteriophages and is important in the transfer of plasmids between staphylococci. Transformation is exchange of naked DNA between bacteria. It is of clinical importance in *Streptococcus pneumoniae*, *Haemophilus influenzae* and *Neisseria* spp. For example, penicillin-resistant pneumococci appear to have produced penicillin-binding protein genes that are mosaics derived from two or more bacteria and do not have high affinity for penicillin.

MECHANISMS

There are four major mechanisms by which antibiotic resistance is mediated.

- **Altered target site**. The fluoroquinolones exert their antibacterial effect by inhibiting the enzymes (DNA gyrase) that coil DNA and are essential for chromosomal replication. Resistant mutants have produced an enzyme with greatly diminished ability to bind the fluoroquinolone. Trimethoprim-resistant *E. coli* produces a dihydrofolate reductase enzyme that is no longer inhibitable by the antimicrobial.
- **Bypass pathway**. In this, bacteria produce an alternative enzyme or pathway that is not inhibited by the antimicrobial. A prime example is in methicillin-resistant *S. aureus*, which is resistant to all β-lactam antibiotics. In this a new penicillin-binding protein (PBP-2a) is produced in addition to the normal PBPs. This is under the control of the *mecA* gene and, because PBP-2a is not inhibited by β-lactams, including flucloxacillin, peptidoglycan synthesis can continue and the bacterium survives and thrives. Some enterococci produce an alternative pentapeptide (the peptide part of peptidoglycan) that no longer binds vancomycin, thus rendering them vancomycin-resistant.
- **Decreased uptake**. Most antimicrobials must enter the bacterial cell to cause damage. Bacteria have evolved mechanisms that prevent ingress of the drug or increase its efflux. The aminoglycosides are taken into bacteria by ATP-dependent carriers. The aminoglycoside-modifying enzymes phosphorylate, adenylate or acetylate the agent as

it is taken across bacterial membrane by the carrier, and causes them to block the pathway. Some bacteria that possess the *tetA* gene actively pump out any tetracycline that gains intracellular access. A recently discovered, more worrying, mechanism is encoded by the *mar* (multiple antibiotic resistance) locus. Mutations in this locus cause two- to fourfold increases in resistance to a range of different antimicrobials by preventing synthesis of a pore in the bacterial membrane and thus entry of the drugs.

- **Enzymatic destruction or modification**. The best examples of this mechanism are the β-lactamases that open the β-lactam ring and inactivate penicillins, cephalosporins, monobactams and penems. No β-lactam is immune to the activity of one or more β-lactamase and as new β-lactams are produced resistance follows quickly. Some strains of resistant *H. influenzae*, for example, produce an enzyme that acetylates chloramphenicol and prevents it from binding to its target.

It is not uncommon for bacteria to use more than one mechanism to produce increased resistance to particular antimicrobials.

ANTIVIRAL RESISTANCE

The numbers and range of antiviral drugs available are much less than for antibacterials. Nevertheless there are already problems of antiviral resistance. Most often this occurs by mutation leading to alterations in, or even complete loss of, genes encoding target enzymes. Resistance to almost every antiviral can be selected by serial passage of the virus in the presence of the antiviral. However development of antiviral resistance among isolates of herpes simplex virus (HSV), hepatitis B virus (HBV) and human immunodeficiency virus (HIV) has had the greatest clinical impact.

HSV Aciclovir (ACV) is phosphorylated intracellularly to the mono-, then the di- and finally the triphosphate and only then does it have antiviral activity by inhibiting the viral DNA polymerase. The conversion to the monophosphate occurs only in virus-infected cells and is mediated by the viral thymidine kinase (TK). The most frequent mechanism of ACV resistance is by HSV becoming TK-deficient (TK⁻ mutants). These arise by non-sense, frameshift or mis-sense mutations. Problems arise particularly in immunoincompetent patients (usually AIDS or bone marrow transplant (BMT) recipients), who are receiving long-term ACV prophylaxis. For example, up to 18% of HSV isolates from BMT recipients are ACV-resistant and up to 4% from AIDS patients. Such TK⁻ mutants exhibit much lower neurovirulence. TK⁻ mutants also do not show cross-resistance to foscarnet, which acts directly on the viral DNA polymerase. However, there are some mutants that are resistant to ACV by alteration in the DNA polymerase such that its affinity for ACV triphosphate is very low. Such mutations also give rise to cross-resistance to foscarnet.

HBV Both lamivudine (3TC) and famciclovir have been used to decrease hepatitis B viral load or to prevent HBV infection in newly transplanted livers in chronic carriers. Both drugs target HBV DNA polymerase (which also has reverse transcriptase activity). *Pol* mutations have arisen quite readily that impart resistance to lamivudine and/or famciclovir.

HIV HIV has a single-stranded RNA genome that must be copied several times (including via a reverse transcriptase step to proviral DNA) during its replicative cycle. Along with most single-stranded RNA viruses, the genome replication does not include proofreading so a multitude of point mutations arise. It is estimated that the mutation rate is approximately 1 in 1000. Use of reverse transcriptase (RT) inhibitors or protease inhibitors will of course select for resistant mutants. Resistance to nucleoside RT inhibitors is selected relatively slowly compared to the non-nucleotide RT inhibitors. For example, there are about 15 point mutations (giving rise to amino acid substitutions) described that give resistance to nucleoside analogues but over 20 to the non-nucleosides. Acquisition of zidovudine resistance mutations does not necessarily impart cross-resistance to other nucleoside analogues. Indeed, monotherapy with lamivudine selects for a mutation at amino acid position 184 that resensitises the virus to zidovudine (if resistance was due to a substitution at position 70). At least 27 point mutations in the protease gene have been described that give resistance to the protease inhibitors. Combination therapy or highly active antiretroviral therapy (HAART), in which nucleoside and non-nucleoside RT inhibitors and protease inhibitors are combined, should slow the development of resistance.

3 Congenital infections

This section summarises the major congenital infections. Most are discussed in more detail in Part Two. The presentation of these infections is varied, from acute illness in the case of herpes simplex or streptococcal infections to silent disease for most cases of cytomegalovirus infection. For many the signs are nonspecific and congenital infection should always be considered as a possible diagnosis in the sick neonate. The diagnosis will depend on appropriate use of laboratory tests. One such commonly performed investigation is the TORCH screen (toxoplasmosis, rubella, herpes and cytomegalovirus serology). This investigation is expensive and has been used rather indiscriminately in the past. It is not indicated for the small-for-dates baby where this is the only abnormality.

Table 3.1 Summary of congenital infections (These include infections transmitted from the mother to the fetus or newborn infant; further details are given in the individual disease sections)

Organism/disease	Investigation and management in pregnancy if suspected in the mother	Investigation and management in the newborn	Refer to Chapter no.
Chlamydia trachomatis	Treat parents/partners with tetracycline or azithromycin after diagnosis of neonatal/infant infection.	Rapid. Immunofluorescent test on eye swab, or nasopharyngeal aspirate (NPA). PCR is more sensitive. Oral erythromycin alone for 14 days.	43
Cytomegalovirus (CMV)	Rarely diagnosed. Screening not considered useful at present.	Throat swab, blood or urine for culture and/or PCR. CMV-specific IgM. Symptomatic treatment. Audiology early.	47
Enterovirus	No action if in early pregnancy.	Serology and culture. Symptomatic treatment and intravenous immunoglobulin. Isolate from other infants.	50
Hepatitis B (HBV)	HBsAg test; if positive, test for HBe antigen/ antibody. Test and immunise partner when indicated.	Management determined by maternal status. For HBsAg positive, HBe antibody positive – immunise only. For HBe antibody negative – immunise and give HB immune globulin	64
Hepatitis C (HCV)	Perinatal transmission occurs at an estimated rate of 5% or less. Risk of transmission increases if there is coexisting HIV infection. Screening not considered useful.	Serology (persisting seropositivity) and RT-PCR. No evidence that HCV is transmitted in breast milk.	65
Herpes simplex virus infection (HSV)	Screening not considered useful. Greatest risk in primary infection. No indication for serial cervical swabs where history of infection. May consider caesarean section in presence of lesions and labour less than 4 hours.	Electron microscopy of lesions. Appropriate cultures. Aciclovir for definite or suspected infection.	68

3 Congenital infections

Table 3.1 continued

Organism/disease	Investigation and management in pregnancy if suspected in the mother	Investigation and management in the newborn	Refer to Chapter no.
Human immuno-deficiency virus infection (HIV)	Screening all women every pregnancy. Serology. Consider AZT perhaps with other antiretrovirals during later pregnancy and labour. Offer LSCS.	Isolation unnecessary. Extreme care with body fluids. Do not breast feed. Consider AZT for first few weeks.	23
HTLV-1	Very rare except in south Japan, South America and Caribbean. Cause of some T-cell lymphomas.	Perinatal spread – blood and breast milk known to occur.	–
Listeria monocytogenes	Blood culture. Cervical swabs. Ampicillin 4–6/day in acute infection.	Blood culture, lumbar puncture, surface swabs. Ampicillin plus gentamicin.	74
Measles	Serology. Only if acute infection is suspected.	Very rare. Serology.	77
Mumps	Serology. Only if acute infection is suspected. Termination is not indicated.	Very rare. Serology.	79
Mycobacterium tuberculosis/ tuberculosis (TB)	If suspected, positive tuberculin test (where no previous BCG) + positive chest X-ray. Needs treatment.	Tuberculin test not indicated. For mother with active TB give isoniazid (INAH) and BCG to infant. Infant with TB – INAH and rifampicin.	105
Neisseria gonorrhoeae/ gonorrhoea	Culture. Ampicillin/benzylpenicillin or cefotaxime if β-lactamase producer.	Culture of conjunctival pus. Topical treatment and benzylpenicillin or cefotaxime IV for 7 days. If infected mother, asymptomatic baby, give single dose of cefotaxime.	55
Human papilloma virus	Virology (PCR)	Very unusual for this to be present at birth. Incubation period several months.	107

Parvovirus	Serology–cordocentesis. May require transfusion for hydrops.	Parvovirus IgM. Symptomatic treatment.	83
Rubella	Screen all women for antibodies to rubella in every pregnancy. Serology: anti-IgG and IgM. Counsel for possible termination following infection before 18 weeks gestation.	Symptomatic. Audiology. Serology.	94
Streptococcus agalactiae (group B streptococcus)	Cervical swab. Urine culture. Ampicillin 2 g 4-hourly where amniotic fluid is shown to be colonised. Screen a mother when previous morbidity/mortality from group B streptococcus. Case for routine screening of pregnant women and prophylactic treatment in the UK has not yet been made, but is standard practice in USA.	Appropriate cultures. Benzylpenicillin/ampicillin/ cefotaxime IV.	99
Toxoplasma gondii/ toxoplasmosis	Screening not considered useful in the UK. If acute infection suspected, serology on mother. Cordocentesis for fetal serology. Spiramycin until definite fetal infection confirmed. Then pyrimethamine, sulphadiazine and folinic acid, alternating with spiramycin.	Serology. Pyrimethamine, sulphadiazine and folinic acid, alternating with spiramycin.	104
Treponema pallidum/ syphilis	Treponemal serology. FTA antibody test. Screen all women in every pregnancy and refer those found positive to genitourinary medicine for evaluation and consideration of treatment with benzylpenicillin	Benzylpenicillin	100
Varicella/chickenpox	Varicella serology. If seronegative and contact, give varicella-zoster immunoglobulin (VZIG). Termination not indicated. Aciclovir for acute infection.	VZIG essential when maternal infection 7 days before to 7 days after delivery. VZIG not indicated at other times or for exposure to infection in neonatal period. Aciclovir for infection acquired perinatally.	42

Key: AZT = zidovudine; BCG = bacillus Calmette–Guérin; EM = electron microscopy; HBsAg = hepatitis B surface antigen; Ig = immunoglobulin; IV = intravenously; LSCS = lower segment caesarian section; PCR = polymerase chain reaction test; RT = reverse transcriptase.

4 Neonatal infection

INTRODUCTION

Immaturity of host defence mechanisms makes neonates very susceptible to a whole variety of microbial pathogens. This susceptibility is found
in term as well as preterm infants. However it is generally true that the
more premature the baby the greater the risk, particularly as prematurity
increases the need for 'invasive' intensive care, which further compromises the host defences and also is associated with reduced transfer of
maternal immunoglobulin G across the placenta. Small-for-gestational-age
babies have additional deficiencies in their immune defences and are
especially vulnerable to infection.

Neonates not only have a higher incidence of infections but when
infected they become more rapidly and more seriously ill. For this reason
it is often necessary to treat with antibiotics at the earliest suspicion of
infection.

BACTERIAL SEPSIS

It is useful to divide this into two types:

- **Early onset infection** is that producing symptoms at birth (the
  infection is established in the baby while in the uterus) or within the
  first 48 hours of life. The infection often follows a fulminant course and
  mortality is high despite antibiotic treatment. The organisms responsible come from the maternal genital tract and the species involved are
  relatively few. These are, in order of frequency:
    - Group B streptococcus (*S. agalactiae*)
    - *Escherichia coli*
    - Others, including other streptococci, *Haemophilus* spp. and anae-
      robes
    - *Listeria monocytogenes*.
- **Late onset infection** has its onset after 48 hours of age. The
  responsible organism may have been acquired from the mother's genital tract or from the postnatal environment. Infection at this stage may
  be fulminant but more often has an insidious onset and is more likely
  to be focal in nature, e.g. meningitis. The list of possible causative
  organisms includes those responsible for early-onset sepsis plus a
  large number of possible 'opportunist' pathogens, including:
    - coagulase-negative staphylococci
    - *Staphylococcus aureus*
    - group D streptococci (enterococci)
    - *Streptococcus pneumoniae*
    - *Klebsiella/Enterobacter* species
    - *Pseudomonas aeruginosa*
    - *Candida* spp.

SUSPECTING THE DIAGNOSIS

Early-onset sepsis – risk factors

Maternal
- Unexplained premature rupture of the membranes and/or premature labour (group B streptococcus and *Listeria* infection in particular may promote premature labour)
- Maternal fever
- Unexplained fetal distress
- Prolonged rupture (> 24 hours) of the fetal membranes
- Meconium staining of the liquor in a premature infant (consider especially *Listeria*)
- History of previous baby in the family suffering group B streptococcal sepsis and maternal swabs again positive

Baby
- Unexplained birth asphyxia
- Respiratory distress (the radiographic appearance of pneumonia may be indistinguishable from hyaline membrane disease)
- Poor circulatory status (low BP, cold peripheries)
- Unexplained metabolic acidosis
- Unexplained hypoglycaemia
- Unexplained neutropenia (neutrophil count < 1000/mm^3)
- Rash (consider *Listeria*)
- Hepatosplenomegaly
- Jaundice

Late-onset sepsis

This has to be considered as a differential diagnosis for any untoward event that befalls the baby. Such events include:
- Bradycardia and apnoea
- Poor feeding/vomiting/increasing gastric aspirates/abdominal distension
- Irritability
- Convulsions
- Increasing jaundice
- Increasing respiratory distress
- For ventilated babies:
    - Unexplained increased ventilatory requirements
    - Increased volume and 'purulence' of endotracheal secretions
    - Increased shadowing on chest X-ray
- Unexplained increase or rapid decrease in neutrophil and/or platelet counts
- Signs/symptoms of necrotising enterocolitis (see below)
- Signs of focal inflammation such as periumbilical cellulitis, infected drip site, etc.

INVESTIGATIONS

Early-onset sepsis

Blood culture This is the most important test. A minimum of 0.5 mL per blood culture bottle should be taken. Take from a peripheral vein, ideally by 'clean' venepuncture using a 'closed system' rather than by the broken needle technique. Peripheral arterial samples are also suitable but are difficult because of the need to use a 'no touch' technique. Samples from a freshly sited umbilical artery catheter taken by the person siting the catheter, while still under aseptic precautions, are acceptable. *Note*: In symptomatic babies antibiotics should not be delayed. Therefore venous blood cultures should be taken and the first dose of antibiotics given before UAC insertion is attempted (other bloods can wait).

Full blood count including differential white cell count.

Deep ear swab Take using a swab passed through a sterile speculum. The idea of this is to obtain cultures from a site that reflects amniotic fluid infection in utero but has not come into direct contact with the birth canal during delivery. There is no point in taking this swab if more than 6 hours has elapsed since birth (by then the external auditory canal will have become colonised).

Maternal cultures including high vaginal swab, blood cultures and placental cultures.

Chest X-ray to look for pneumonia or other pulmonary cause of the clinical deterioration (though different pathologies are not always readily distinguishable).

Lumbar puncture This is performed to determine whether meningitis is part of the sepsis. This will have a bearing on the length of treatment and future prognosis. However it is not essential to do this before commencing antibiotics and in an unstable baby it can be delayed. Confirmation of the presence and cause of meningitis can often be made on a post-antibiotic sample using antigen detection tests.

Swabs of any focal site of inflammation – septic spots, etc. (unusual in early-onset infection).

Other tests needed to help in the management of the 'septic' baby include analysis of urea and electrolytes, creatinine, glucose, bilirubin, coagulation screen, group and save serum. 'Routine' surface swabs do not contribute to the diagnosis of neonatal sepsis. It is, however, normal practice to perform these on babies transferred from other hospitals if part of a hospital's policy for surveillance for MRSA. Urine cultures are unnecessary in early-onset sepsis unless there are particular reasons to suspect a urological abnormality.

Late-onset sepsis

Routine surveillance cultures of stool and pharyngeal flora performed on infants in neonatal intensive care units have little value in predicting the cause of subsequent sepsis. They may be useful in monitoring trends in predominant colonising bacterial strains and antibiotic-resistant strains. In ventilated infants there may be some benefit in regular routine culture of endotracheal secretions as a predictor of cause of subsequent pneumonic episodes, although good evidence confirming their value is lacking.

In suspected late-onset sepsis, before starting antibiotics the following tests should be performed:

- **Blood cultures** – see notes under 'Investigations: early-onset sepsis'.
- **Full blood count** including differential.
- **Suprapubic or clean catch urine** (see below), but do not delay antibiotics if infant is sick.
- **Chest X-ray.**
- **Endotracheal tube secretions** (in ventilated babies) – usually culture only; microscopy is rarely helpful.
- **Lumbar puncture** – not always necessary (e.g. in ventilated babies with suspected chest infections). However, a low threshold is needed for doing this test. Can be deferred in a very sick baby with an unstable condition.
- **Swabs from sites of inflammation**, e.g. inflamed umbilicus, infected drip site, etc. 'Routine' surface swabs are not necessary.

TREATMENT

In general it is necessary to treat on suspicion – antibiotics can be stopped after 48 hours if cultures are negative.

General treatment of severe sepsis

In addition to antibiotics infants may need the following support:

- **Ventilation**: Consider early.
- **Circulation**: Plasma expanders and inotropes.
- **Haematological**: Blood and platelets. In addition, fresh frozen plasma is used for coagulation disturbance. White cell infusions are very rarely used. If profound neutropenia occurs, especially with disseminated intravascular coagulation (DIC), consider a single volume exchange transfusion. Recombinant granulocyte colony stimulating factor is a promising new adjuvant therapy for enhancing neutrophil numbers and function in neonatal sepsis and currently under investigation.
- **Immunological**: Fresh frozen plasma provides immunoglobulin and complement factors as well as clotting factors. Intravenous immunoglobulin infusion may also provide benefit in some types of neonatal sepsis.
- **Renal**: Sepsis is often associated with renal impairment. Plasma creatinine should be monitored and antibiotic levels carefully monitored.
- **Gut and nutrition**: The intestine usually stops working in severe sepsis and enteral feeding should therefore be stopped. Consider early institution of total parenteral nutrition (TPN) but the precise constitution of TPN needs careful judging as the babies will be catabolic and unable to handle large nitrogen loads.
- **Hepatic**: Liver dysfunction, especially conjugated hyperbilirubinaemia, is common in sepsis. Give prophylactic vitamin K.

Antibiotic treatment of early-onset sepsis

Treatment of mother

If there is reason to suspect in utero infection of the baby, ask obstetricians to take a cervical swab and blood cultures from mother and start intravenous ampicillin. Encourage early delivery.

Treatment of the baby

Babies should be screened and put on antibiotics. Penicillin and gentamicin is a standard combination to use at this stage but some units may prefer other regimens, including the use of third-generation cephalosporins (but see below).

Any symptomatic newborn baby should be admitted to the neonatal unit for treatment and monitoring. Since the symptoms of infection may mimic most neonatal problems, most babies admitted to a neonatal unit are given antibiotics.

If *Listeria* infection is suspected use ampicillin and gentamicin. Suspicion of *Listeria* should be aroused by any of the following:

- Maternal influenza-like febrile illness preceding the onset of labour, especially if there has been spontaneous premature rupture of the membranes
- Meconium staining of the liquor in a premature baby (unusual in normal circumstances)
- Baby ill with rash (usually sparse papular eruption) and/or hepatosplenomegaly
- Gram-positive rods seen in cerebrospinal fluid.

Penicillin covers 90% of *Listeria* isolates. Ampicillin covers 100% but is not used routinely because listeriosis is rare and excessive use of this antibiotic would lead to increased antibiotic resistance in the bacterial flora in the unit – ultimately complicating the treatment of late-onset sepsis.

Some units use third-generation cephalosporins (cefotaxime or ceftazidime) in early-onset sepsis. However such a policy has a number of disadvantages:

- It provides no cover against *Listeria*
- Evidence suggests that excessive use of these agents empirically in the neonatal intensive care setting leads to the emergence of resistant organisms. This lessens the usefulness of these agents for treating proven late-onset sepsis.

This last objection is less relevant outside neonatal special/intensive care units.

Antibiotic treatment of late-onset sepsis

The baby's recent microbiological results should be reviewed, looking particularly for antibiotic-resistant isolates. In ventilated babies, there may be routine endotracheal secretion culture results available. Choice of antibiotics for late-onset sepsis should therefore take into account the most recent microbiological data. One cannot assume that the bacteria isolated on screening cultures are the cause of the presumed sepsis but it is sensible to cover for them.

If there is nothing specific to guide antibiotic choice then azlocillin and gentamicin is a reasonable empirical choice. With the increasing emergence of coagulase-negative staphylococci as the cause of late-onset sepsis, combinations such as vancomycin (or teicoplanin) and ceftazidime are increasingly used. This is not recommended as an empirical device (because of concern over emerging resistance to both components). If intra-abdominal sepsis, e.g. NEC or post-surgical sepsis is suspected, metronidazole should be added. Flucloxacillin is added if bone, soft tissue or superficial sepsis is present. If antibiotic-resistant bacteria are identified other combinations such as ceftazidime and gentamicin or a β-lactam antibiotic and amikacin can be used (Table 4.1).

If meningitis is suspected, ampicillin and ceftazidime (for babies undergoing neonatal intensive care) or ampicillin and cefotaxime (other babies) should be used.

Vancomycin (or teicoplanin) is used if coagulase-negative staphylococci have been isolated. Vancomycin and gentamicin have additive toxicity and the combination should be avoided if at all possible. If Gram-negative cover is required with vancomycin, ceftazidime or ciprofloxacin can be used.

Once a significant bacterial isolate and its sensitivities have been obtained antibiotic treatment should be rationalised (Table 4.2).

Monitoring the response to therapy

It cannot be assumed that the antibiotics will always clear the infection. While the baby remains unwell, especially if there are positive blood cultures, or if there is a central venous or umbilical arterial line in place, further sets of blood cultures should be taken daily. Persistent positive blood cultures may suggest:

Table 4.1 Common antibiotics and combinations

1. Penicillin + gentamicin	Early-onset sepsis
2. Azlocillin + gentamicin	Late-onset sepsis
3. Vancomycin/teicoplanin + ceftazidime	Late-onset sepsis with suspected coagulase-negative staphylococcus
4. Vancomycin/teicoplanin + ciprofloxacin	As 3 but with previous resistant Gram-negative isolates
5. Ceftazidime + gentamicin	Late-onset sepsis with resistant bacteria
6. Azlocillin/ceftazidime + amikacin	As 5
7. Azlocillin + gentamicin + flucloxacillin	Late-onset sepsis with focal superficial infection
8. Cefotaxime/ceftazidime + ampicillin (± gentamicin)	Empirical treatment of neonatal meningitis
9. Metronidazole + combination 2, 5 or 6	Intra-abdominal and/or postsurgical sepsis, necrotising enterocolitis
10. Meropenem	Reserve for resistant strains
11. Trimethoprim	Prophylaxis against urinary tract infections
12. Erythromycin	Chlamydial and mycoplasmal infections

Table 4.2 Best antibiotics for given organisms

Organism	Antibiotic
Group A streptococcus	Penicillin
Group B streptococcus	Penicillin (+ gentamicin initially)
Group D streptococcus*	Ampicillin + gentamicin
	Vancomycin/teicoplanin
Streptococcus pneumoniae	Penicillin
Staphylococcus aureus	Flucloxacillin ± gentamicin (+ sodium fusidate for deep infection)
Methicillin-resistant Staphylococcus aureus	Vancomycin/teicoplanin
Coagulase-negative staphylococcus	Vancomycin/teicoplanin
Listeria monocytogenes	Ampicillin (+ gentamicin initially)
Escherichia coli*	Cefotaxime
Klebsiella/Enterobacter spp.*	Cefotaxime
Pseudomonas aeruginosa*	Azlocillin + gentamicin (or ceftazidime)
Bacteroides spp.	Metronidazole
Haemophilus influenzae	Cefotaxime

* **Resistance may be a problem; review antibiotics when culture results available.**

- inadequate antibiotic levels or regimen
- resistant organism
- focal infection – abscess/osteomyelitis/endocarditis
- line infection.

Alteration of therapy and/or further investigation (ultrasound/skeletal X-rays/echocardiogram) may be indicated. Vascular lines will probably need to be removed and the length of the treatment course extended in those with a slow microbiological response.

Length of treatment

This will depend on a number of variables – type of organism, clinical response, etc. Some general guidelines are:

- Antibiotics started on possibility of infection but subsequently no clinical evidence of infection and cultures are all negative – 48 hours
- Antibiotics started on suspicion, cultures negative but clinically believed to have been infected and responded to antibiotics – 5 days
- Pneumonia on chest X-ray but cultures negative – 7 days
- Positive blood cultures – negative CSF – 10 days from last positive blood culture
- Positive CSF – depends on organism: see *Meningitis* below
- Deep-seated fungal infections, osteomyelitis, endocarditis and deep abscesses not surgically drained require several weeks of antibiotic therapy – seek advice.

Prevention

Recent evidence from the USA suggests that intrapartum antibiotic prophylaxis for high-risk mothers reduces the incidence of early-onset group B streptococcal disease (see Chapter 99, p. 416 and further reading).

FUNGAL SEPSIS

Invasive fungal sepsis, usually due to *Candida* species, though still a relatively unusual problem in neonates may be increasing in frequency. It can occur relatively early on in life (and even be congenital) but more commonly it complicates the management of long-standing patients who have been very sick and received a lot of broad-spectrum antibiotics and/or steroid treatment.

The diagnosis is suspected on similar grounds to other forms of neonatal sepsis. Absence of a history of previous superficial fungal infection does not rule it out.

Tests for fungal sepsis include blood cultures (arterial cultures are considered more likely to be positive than venous although there is no sound evidence to support this) and suprapubic urine, looking specifically for yeasts on microscopy (bag urine specimens are of no use in this situation). Endotracheal secretions should be cultured in ventilated infants and, because of the possibility of associated fungal meningitis, a lumbar puncture should be performed. *Candida* antigen tests can be performed on serum but it is unlikely that the results will be available sufficiently quickly to influence the decision to treat and, in any case, false-negative results do occur. Nevertheless, a positive result may be useful in confirming the diagnosis.

Treatment

Intravenous amphotericin B and 5-flucytosine (5FC) is standard therapy. The latter is important because of its ability to penetrate well into central nervous system and renal tissues, both being relatively common sites of involvement in neonatal fungal sepsis.

Amphotericin B is potentially toxic, although it is generally better tolerated in neonates than in older individuals. Occasionally, acute systemic reactions – pyrexia, tachycardia, hypotension – may occur and for this reason it is usual to give a test dose of 0.1 mg/kg before starting therapy in earnest. The need for building up the dosage over a number of days has been questioned as it delays the achievement of full therapeutic dosage. However this should remain the usual practice except in cases of overwhelming infection. A reasonable starting dose (to follow on from the test dose) is 0.3 mg/kg, making a total first day dosage of 0.4 mg/kg. The dose is increased by 0.25 mg/kg each day to a maximum of 1.0 mg/kg although, if a good response is achieved, it is often possible to stop the escalation short of this maximum dose thus reducing the incidence of side-effects. Occasionally in very severe infections daily doses of up to 1.5 mg/kg can be given. Blood levels are not helpful. The drug should be given in special pH-tested 5% dextrose and cannot be mixed with other drugs (even electrolytes). Fluid volumes may be a problem.

The main toxicity problem affects renal function. Hypokalaemia (due to renal leak) is very common (try to keep ahead with K^+ supplements). If this cannot be controlled by potassium supplementation then amiloride treatment usually helps. Rising urea and creatinine may occur and necessitate a dosage reduction. Other potentially nephrotoxic drugs such as aminoglycosides and vancomycin should be avoided if possible.

Prolonged treatment is usually needed. Once clinical response has been achieved, alternate-day amphotericin (same dose as daily) may be given as this reduces toxicity.

Liposomal amphotericin produces much less nephrotoxicity. This preparation should be used in infants who show or develop renal problems or who are otherwise intolerant of conventional amphotericin. There are also available various lipid-complexed amphotericin preparations. These offer reduced toxicity compared to conventional amphotericin and reduced cost compared to the liposomal preparation but there is limited experience of their use in neonates.

5-flucytosine may cause bone-marrow suppression. Blood levels should be monitored, aiming to keep levels below 100 µg/mL. Dosage should be reduced if there is renal impairment. 5FC is well absorbed and enteral administration can be employed after initial response has been obtained.

Fluconazole has been used successfully to treat neonatal candidal sepsis. However, there is relatively limited experience and acquired drug resistance of *C. albicans* or inherent resistance of certain other *Candida* species may be a problem.

Prevention

Babies at high risk for fungal infection should be given prophylactic nystatin, ideally split half and half oral and nasogastric. All cases of superficial candidiasis should be treated vigorously with topical antifungals. Where persistent problems occur consideration should be given to using prophylactic fluconazole.

SPECIFIC INFECTIONS

MENINGITIS

The peak incidence of meningitis occurs in the neonatal period. It can occur as an apparently focal infection (usually in late-onset sepsis) or as part of a multisystem process with septicaemia. In this age group the clinical signs are very nonspecific and there should therefore be a very low threshold for performing a lumbar puncture (LP).

Contraindications to lumbar puncture

- Baby too sick – especially with cardiorespiratory instability. Treat with antibiotics anyway and perform deferred LP when condition improves.
- Severe coagulopathy or thrombocytopenia. Consider deferred LP with FFP/platelet cover.

- Known noncommunicating hydrocephalus (usually following an earlier intraventricular haemorrhage). In this situation an intraventricular tap can be performed instead.

N.B. In contrast to other age groups, raised intracranial pressure is not per se a contraindication to LP in neonates.

Treatment

Antibiotics

- Empirical (unknown organism): Use ampicillin plus a third-generation cephalosporin (ceftazidime on NICU, otherwise cefotaxime). Gentamicin may also be added to enhance Gram-negative bacillary cover. Try to rationalise treatment when cause identified.
  Organism known:
  - **group B streptococcus** – benzylpenicillin (initially with gentamicin) × 14 days
  - **Listeria** – ampicillin + gentamicin × 14 days followed by ampicillin alone for a further 7 days
  - **Gram-negative bacilli** – cephalosporin + gentamicin × 21 days (minimum; depends on sensitivity of organism); will usually need repeat LPs ± CSF bactericidal levels (N.B. Intraventricular/intrathecal antibiotics are of no added benefit)
  - **coagulase-negative staphylococcus** (usually as a complication of a ventriculoperitoneal shunt, see Chapter 13). Use systemic antistaphylococcal antibiotic(s) to which the organism is sensitive and that penetrate into CSF. Choice depends on sensitivities – rifampicin or trimethoprim are often used. In addition, vancomycin should be used systemically and through the shunt. The shunt may need to be removed.

Supportive therapy

Ventilation, inotropes, etc. may be needed – see General treatment of severe sepsis, above. Fluid and electrolyte balance need careful attention. Dehydration, if present, must be corrected. Thereafter the essence of management is to support cerebral perfusion pressure while keeping use of crystalloid fluids to a minimum to reduce risk of cerebral oedema. Inappropriate antidiuretic hormone (ADH) syndrome may occur. Anticonvulsants may be needed if fits occur but prophylactic usage is not recommended.

PNEUMONIA

Pneumonia is often a feature of early-onset sepsis. The chest radiograph appearances may mimic those of respiratory distress syndrome due to surfactant deficiency. Management is as described above for early-onset sepsis.

When pneumonia occurs beyond the first 48 hours of life the range of possible causes is very large. In those infants undergoing intensive care, especially when ventilated, the cause is most likely to be bacterial, with the same range of organisms as described under late-onset sepsis. A heavy and relatively pure bacterial growth from endotracheal secretions in the presence of clinical and radiographic deterioration usually provides evidence of the aetiology in ventilated infants. In others, unless the blood cultures are positive, treatment usually has to be empirical. A poor response to antibiotic treatment or an atypical picture should prompt investigation for nonbacterial agents such as viruses and *Chlamydia trachomatis*. Particularly in infants beyond 3 weeks of age, vertically acquired *C. trachomatis* infection should be considered. Infants with this agent may have a history of earlier conjunctivitis (see Chapter 43, p.245).

Viral pneumonia is more common in the winter months and in those neonates already discharged from hospital (see Viral infections, below).

URINARY TRACT INFECTION

This is confirmed by obtaining a positive culture, usually (but not always) with a raised white cell count in the urine. Suprapubic or clean catch urine samples are best. Bag urines are unreliable. Unless the infant is so unwell that antibiotic treatment cannot be deferred (at this age urinary infections may lead to disseminated sepsis), it is best not to treat on the basis of a single bag urine result.

Treatment should be initiated promptly. If the infant is considered to be at least moderately unwell, initial therapy should be parenteral with broad-spectrum agents (e.g. co-amoxiclav if acquired outside hospital or azlocillin and gentamicin if acquired in hospital). Once bacteriological results are available the treatment can be rationalised and often converted to the oral route. Since infection of the renal tissue is common in this age group, antibiotics such as nitrofurantoin that do not achieve bactericidal tissue levels should not be used.

Follow-up

There is a high chance of a UTI in the neonatal period being associated with an underlying abnormality. Therefore all babies with a confirmed UTI in the neonatal period require follow-up and most require further radiological investigation. In the acute phase:

- Examine external genitalia carefully
- Perform ultrasound examination in all cases
- Commence prophylactic trimethoprim when treatment course is completed and continue this until the follow-up appointment
- Arrange follow-up either with a paediatric urologist if history (e.g. poor urinary stream), physical examination or ultrasound suggest underlying abnormality or otherwise in the paediatric clinic so that appropriate investigations can be arranged.

GASTROENTERITIS

This is fortunately uncommon in the neonatal period, particularly in breast-fed infants, but can lead to serious illness. The usual range of bacterial and viral causes can be involved. When severe diarrhoea and vomiting occur, rapid fluid and electrolyte disturbance may occur. Stools should be sent for culture and electron microscopy. Blood cultures (and in sick children a full septic screen) should be performed since *Salmonella* species in particular are liable to cause invasive disease in young infants. Rotavirus infection often causes a very mild or asymptomatic picture at this age. Rarely, any of the recognised infections may precipitate the development of necrotising enterocolitis (see below).

Management is along the usual lines for gastroenteritis in older infants but there should be a lower threshold for intravenous fluid therapy. Systemic antibiotics are required if invasion is suspected in *Salmonella* infection (use trimethoprim, ampicillin or ciprofloxacin depending on sensitivities). Antibiotics may also be required for *Shigella*, *Campylobacter* and *E. coli* diarrhoea. When cases occur in the neonatal nursery, cross-infection is a major risk and the advice of the infection control team should be sought early.

NECROTISING ENTEROCOLITIS

This is a relatively common and potentially devastating disease in which infection of the intestinal wall occurs. The precise pathogenesis remains unclear. The incidence seems to vary quite dramatically from centre to centre and within the same unit from time to time. Two forms can be distinguished epidemiologically, though not clinically. An 'epidemic' form occurring in clusters suggests that there is an infectious process and indeed sometimes intestinal pathogens can be isolated (rotavirus, coronavirus and *Salmonella* are among the organisms that have been implicated). A 'sporadic' form occurs predominantly in low-birth-weight, premature infants, particularly those whose intestines have undergone a period of ischaemia prenatally (placental dysfunction and intrauterine growth retardation), at birth (asphyxia) or postnatally (polycythaemia, abdominal surgery).

The hallmark of the disease is the radiological picture of 'pneumatosis intestinalis' – gas in the wall of the bowel itself – although this is not always present in the early stages of the disease and not necessary for the diagnosis. It is thought that damage to the gut wall allows invasion of bacteria, including gas producers, which then further compromises the blood supply to the mucosa leading to necrosis and preforation. Absorption of endotoxin and bacterial invasion can lead to septicaemia. Enteral feeding seems to be a cofactor, particularly if formula feeds are used.

The diagnosis should be suspected in an infant with any combination of bloody stools, abdominal distension, vomiting – particularly bilious – and nonspecific signs of sepsis.

Investigate with plain abdominal X-ray (and lateral decubitus if perforation suspected) and full septic screen (but defer LP if baby very sick).

Affected infants should be managed in centres with paediatric surgical expertise.

Standard treatment, for 10 days minimum, is:

- nil by mouth with nasogastric drainage and replacement of fluid losses intravenously
- intravenous nutrition
- antibiotics – azlocillin, gentamicin and metronidazole
- surgery may be required for excision of gangrenous bowel, perforation, etc.

Prevention of nectrotising enterocolitis may be achieved by identification of high-risk cases and elective use parenteral nutrition, and avoidance, when possible, of the use of umbilical catheters.

OSTEOMYELITIS

This is rare but it is important not to miss it. The most common causative agents are *Staphylococcus aureus* and group B streptococcus. Other streptococci, Gram-negative enteric bacilli and *Haemophilus influenzae* are other possible causes. Presentation is either with a septicaemic illness or, particularly in group B streptococcal cases, the infant may appear relatively well with swelling or immobility of a limb, the latter sometimes mimicking a nerve palsy – e.g. upper humeral metaphyseal infection presenting as apparent Erb's palsy.

Osteomyelitis should be considered in all cases of *S. aureus* bacteraemia/septicaemia or when sepsis caused by other organisms is slow to respond (especially with persistent positive blood cultures). Clinical signs, e.g. local swelling, tenderness, one limb not moving, may or may not be present. In those with insidious onset, X-ray changes are often present by the time of diagnosis and may show extensive bony destruction, which nevertheless will usually heal well after treatment. In contrast to the situation at other ages, isotope bone scanning is not helpful.

Treatment involves a prolonged course of antibiotics. Initial empirical choice is a broad-spectrum combination such as azlocillin, gentamicin and flucloxacillin for premature neonates in the intensive care nursery, and flucloxacillin and cefotaxime for other neonates. Identification of the causative organism makes ongoing treatment much easier. Surgical intervention may be required in cases that fail to improve on treatment.

SUPERFICIAL INFECTIONS

These should always be taken seriously because of the risk of progression to invasive disease in the immune incompetent host.

Umbilical sepsis

A 'sticky' umbilicus is very common. A swab should be sent (in case infection develops) but antibiotics should not be used routinely. Spirit swabbing by nursing staff should suffice.

True periumbilical infection is indicated by a purulent discharge and/or surrounding erythema. This should be investigated with a swab and blood cultures, and a broad-spectrum antibiotic combination including flucloxacillin should be commenced.

Staphylococcal scalded skin syndrome

This can be a severe and potentially life-threatening infection in newborn infants. It is caused by particular phage types of *S. aureus*, which produce an exotoxin, epidermolysin, that affects the superficial layers of the skin to produce thin-walled bullae that rapidly break down to leave raw areas. The site of the infection itself may be relatively trivial with distant effects produced by the toxin. Circulatory failure may occur. Treatment should be with intravenous flucloxacillin and fluids. Infected infants pose a cross-infection hazard and measures should be taken to control this as large outbreaks have occurred in newborn nurseries.

Paronychia

This is an infection of the nail fold usually caused by *S. aureus* but occasionally by *Candida* species. It is often associated with other superficial staphylococcal infection such as 'septic spots'. A swab and blood cultures should be taken and treatment commenced with oral flucloxacillin if the baby is well and intravenous flucloxacillin and gentamicin if unwell.

Septic spots

These are sometimes difficult to distinguish from erythema toxicum. If in doubt, a 'pustule' should be punctured and a swab sent. Treat as for paronychia.

Candidiasis

Treat topically with nystatin or miconazole. Fluconazole should be considered if candidiasis is a persistent/recurrent problem.

Conjunctivitis

'Sticky' eyes are very common and do not usually indicate an infection. Purulent discharge from an eye needs to be taken seriously. Most commonly it is caused by common bacteria acquired from the environment – *S. aureus* and coliforms. It is best treated with neomycin topically. Possible more serious causes should be considered and the age of onset may be suggestive:

- Under 5 days of age: need to urgently exclude gonococcal infection – ophthalmia neonatorum (see Chapter 55)
- Over 5 days (usually second week of life); need to consider *C. trachomatis* (see Chapter 43).

Never use topical chloramphenicol without first excluding *Chlamydia*. Chloramphenicol partially treats the infection, suppressing symptoms and the true diagnosis. Such babies are at risk of later development of chlamydial pneumonia/myocarditis.

Mothers whose babies are diagnosed as having either gonococcal or chlamydial infection need referral to the department of genitourinary medicine for treatment, contact tracing, etc.

VIRAL INFECTIONS

RESPIRATORY VIRUSES

These may cause serious respiratory compromise in babies with bronchopulmonary dysplasia. Respiratory syncytial virus (RSV), parainfluenza, influenza and adenovirus are the biggest culprits. In Europe, RSV is prevalent in the colder months, November–March each year. It causes common cold symptoms in older children and adults and can be brought into the neonatal nursery by them. Parainfluenza III is prevalent in the late spring.

These viruses can be rapidly diagnosed by immunofluorescence on nasopharyngeal aspirates. A fine catheter is placed in the posterior nasopharynx and a short, sharp suction is applied; the resulting aspirate is flushed through into a trap with sterile saline or viral transport medium. The test requires epithelial cells stripped off by the suction, not mucus itself. Ribavarin treatment should be initiated if compromised babies develop these infections. Cross-infection control procedures are very important, particularly hand-washing and cohorting. High-titre RSV immunoglobulin and an RSV-specific monoclonal antibody have both been shown to reduce the severity of RSV infections in high-risk infants with bronchopulmonary dysplasia when given prophylactically during the winter months. The precise indications for use of these preparations have yet to be established. They are extremely expensive. The use of the former means that measles, mumps and rubella (MMR) immunisation has to be delayed for several months.

HERPES VIRUSES

Herpes simplex

This virus, when contracted in the neonatal period, can cause localised skin or mucous membrane disease, encephalitis or disseminated over-whelming infection. It may be acquired from the maternal genital tract or postnatally from contacts excreting the virus.

Treatment

Exposed babies require close observation and should be isolated with the mother. The use of prophylactic antivirals at this stage is controversial. We prefer not to use them. First signs of disease may be nonspecific (poor feeding, fever, apnoea, jaundice) or specific with a vesicular rash (often one or two spots only initially) or keratoconjunctivitis. When infection is sus-pected the baby needs a full screen, to include virology on the cerebrospinal fluid, aspiration of fluid from vesicles for electron microscopy and culture, and eye and mouth swabs for viral culture. Once specimens have been col-lected, aciclovir treatment is given for a minimum of 10 days. Recurrent dis-ease can occur when aciclovir is stopped. Continuous oral aciclovir given for 6 months should be considered but neutropenia may occur.

Prevention

If the mother is known to have active cervical disease, deliver by cae-sarean section if membranes ruptured less than 4 hours.

Nursing andmedical staff with cold sores should wear masks, employ strict hand-washing and use topical aciclovir to shorten the period of viral excretion.

VARICELLA (SEE ALSO CHAPTER 42)

Most infants are immune to chickenpox by virtue of transplacental anti-bodies from their seropositive mothers. Infants at risk are those born to nonimmune mothers or those who are extremely premature and therefore receive very little maternal antibody. Infants at greatest risk are those whose mothers develop the rash within the period from 5 days before delivery to 2 days after delivery. Untreated, the illness carries a high mortality (30–50%) if contracted in the perinatal period.

Management of babies born to a mother who develops chickenpox in perinatal period

- Babies born to a mother who develops chickenpox between 7 days before delivery and 7 days after birth should be given varicella-zoster immunoglobulin (VZIG; 250 mg intramuscularly regardless of weight)
- Mother and baby should be nursed together in their own side room
- Breastfeeding should be encouraged
- The baby should be carefully followed up with continuing care by the community midwife
- Early antiviral therapy with high-dose intravenous aciclovir 10 mg/kg 8-hourly is indicated in neonatal chickenpox.

Management of varicella-zoster virus contacts and cases on the neonatal unit

It is of paramount important that immediate action is taken in the event of cases/suspected cases. The hospital infection control team should be involved from the start. The measures to be taken are similar to those for prevention of secondary cases of chickenpox at any age (see Chapter 42). It may not be possible to move high-dependency cases to an isolation room/ward. Intravenous aciclovir will reduce the period of virus shedding to 72–96 hours but during this period airborne spread of varicella-zoster virus (VZV) is inevitable. Measures to reduce transmission should be taken and VZV-susceptible babies (see below) should receive VZIG.

The following should be given VZIG:

- Babies exposed to VZV within the first month of life whose mother has no previous history of chickenpox
- Babies receiving systemic steroid therapy or who have received systemic steroid therapy within the last 3 months and whose mother has no previous history of chickenpox
- Babies who are immunocompromised by disease or its treatment, e.g. bronchopulmonary dysplasia, HIV/AIDS, congenital immune deficiency, malignancy/chemotherapy
- Babies born before 30 weeks gestation or whose birth weight was less than 1 kg, regardless of postnatal age and mother's VZV immune status.

Babies who do not fall in these above categories should not be given prophylaxis, regardless of their exposure history, as they are not considered to be at high risk of significant morbidity or mortality following chickenpox.

CYTOMEGALOVIRUS

A newborn infant may be infected:

- transplacentally
- from breast milk
- from blood products.

Congenital infection is discussed in Chapter 3. In most instances, post-natal acquisition of infection is asymptomatic. Occasionally, extremely premature compromised babies may develop pneumonitis and infants with congenital immune deficiency are also at risk.

Treatment

This is only of value for proven cytomegalovirus (CMV) pneumonitis or other organ disease (which is only likely to occur in immune-deficient infants). Ganciclovir is the drug of choice. This is myelosuppressive and blood counts should be monitored.

Prevention

Use CMV-negative blood products and/or white cell filters.

If accidental exposure to CMV-positive products occurs, consider CMV hyperimmune globulin.

ENTEROVIRUSES

This group includes Coxsackie, echo and polio viruses. They can cause a wide spectrum of clinical illness. Coxsackie viruses may be particularly dangerous in the newborn period causing myocarditis, meningoencephalitis and hepatitis. The source of infection is most commonly the mother, with a flu-like viral illness in the week preceding delivery, but she may also have been infected asymptomatically. Postnatal transmission leading to outbreaks has also been described. Specimens for viral culture should be sent – CSF, throat swab and stool are the most useful. Intravenous immunoglobulin has been used therapeutically and for prophylaxis of exposed infants, with some successes reported.

N.B. In very compromised neonates, vaccine-strain polio virus may theoretically cause problems. Therefore live oral polio vaccine should not be used in babies who are going to remain in the neonatal unit.

ENTERIC VIRUSES

See Gastroenteritis, above.

FURTHER READING

Remington J, Klein JO (1995) Infectious diseases of the fetus and new-born infant, 4th edn. WB Saunders, Philadelphia, PA.

Schrag SJ, Zywicki S, Farley MM et al. (2000) Group B streptococcal disease in the era of intrapartum antibiotic prophylaxis. N Engl J Med 342: 15–20.

Just as a fever may not always be caused by an infectious disorder, a rash may not be the result of an infection. The aim of this chapter is to help the clinician decide the likely cause of a rash. Definitive diagnosis and subsequent management are described later in the book. Rashes in the neonate are not covered in this section.

DIAGNOSIS

Diagnosis is based on the history, general examination, features of the rash itself and, in some cases, specific laboratory investigations. In many cases it may not be possible to make an exact diagnosis (in young children, only 1–2% of cases clinically diagnosed as measles are confirmed serologically). This may not matter, as long as important diagnoses have been excluded. However, there are some conditions where the possible consequences are such that an accurate diagnosis is essential. An obvious example is suspected rubella in a pregnant woman or one of her close contacts. Bearing in mind these caveats the following framework is suggested.

History
- **Features of rash**
  - Duration
  - Site
  - Evolution (changes in shape, appearance and possible cropping)
  - Presence of pruritus
- **Accompanying symptoms**
  - Presence of prodromal illness
  - Current symptoms – fever, malaise, headache, etc.
- **Past history**
  - Immunisations
  - Possible contacts
  - Insect bites
  - Foreign travel
  - Known or suspected allergies
  - Previous similar episodes
- **Miscellaneous**
  - Current or recent medication
  - Pets
  - Similar illness in locality of residence, at school or playgroup, etc.

Examination
A complete general examination is necessary. Points to which particular attention should be paid include:

- General appearance, i.e. does the child look well or unwell?
- Fever

- Lymphadenopathy
- Splenomegaly
- Mucous membranes (conjunctivae and mouth)
- General appearance of rash:
  - Vesicular
  - Nodular
  - Maculopapular
  - Punctate
  - Haemorrhagic
- Distribution of rash: look particularly at the soles of the feet, the palms of the hands, behind the ears and at the mucous membranes
- Are all areas and elements at the same stage of evolution or is there evidence of cropping? Has there been scratching?

Investigations

The investigations will depend on the possible differential diagnoses, but may include:

- Full blood count
- A 'saved sample' for serology
- An appropriate specimen for viral culture (throat swab, faeces, vesicular, etc.
- Blood cultures.

Table 5.1 should help in deciding the aetiology of most rashes. Reactions to drugs and other allergic reactions commonly give rise to a maculopapular or punctiform rash and rarely to a vesicular eruption. Scabies often produces a mixed papular and vesicular rash around the fingers, wrists and elbows. Scratching may obscure the characteristic linear burrows.

Table 5.1 Types of rash

	Prodrome	Fever	General malaise	Distribution of rash	Pruritus	Special features
Vesicular rashes						
Chickenpox	None or short coryzal	Mild to moderate	Mild	Mostly truncal	Yes	Contact with sufferers is common; crops
Dermatitis herpetiformis	Nil	Nil	Nil	Trunk	Yes	Sporadic cases; eventually leave depigmentation
Eczema herpeticum	Nil	Moderate to high	Moderate	In areas of eczema	Yes	May be seriously ill
Hand, foot and mouth disease	Nil	Minimal	Minimal	Palms, soles and inside mouth	No	Often occurs as minor epidemics
Herpes simplex gingivostomatitis	Nil	Moderate to high	Moderate (may be dehydrated)	Mouth and lips	Yes (at onset)	Frequent history of contact with cold sores
Impetigo	Nil	Nil	Nil	Face and hands	Yes	Vesicles often replaced by yellow crusting
Insect bites	Nil	Nil	Rare	Variable	Yes	Usually isolated lesions
Molluscum contagiosum	Nil	Nil	Nil	Variable	No	Characteristic pearly vesicles with dimples

Table 5.1 continued

	Prodrome	Fever	General malaise	Distribution of rash	Pruritus	Special features
Maculopapular and punctate rashes						
Enteroviral infections	Short	Mild	Mild	General	No	Rash often pleomorphic
Fifth disease	Uncommon; mild fever and respiratory symptoms	Mild, if any	Minimal	Face ('slapped cheeks'), trunk and limbs	No	Rash may come and go. Heat brings it out. Can have a reticular pattern
Glandular fever	Malaise, mild fever and sore throat	Moderate	Common	General	No	Exudate in throat especially marked. Swollen glands and spleen
Kawasaki disease	Mild fever, malaise and sore throat	Moderate to high and persistent	Mild to moderate	General	No	Palms and soles, lips and conjunctivae affected
Measles	Rising fever, cough and conjunctivitis	Moderate to high	Substantial	Around ears, then face, then trunk. Confluent	No	Koplik's spots in mouth before rash on fourth day of illness
Meningococcal disease	None or short with coryza or fever	Variable	Profound	Variable	No	Petechial rash may be preceded by maculopapular rash. Evolves rapidly
Ptyriasis rosea	Nil	Nil	Nil	Trunk	Initially	Usually in older children; herald patch at onset

Disease					
Roseola infantum (exanthem subitum)	High fever and irritability	Moderate	Moderate	Trunk then face	No	Dramatic improvement in child when rash appears on fourth or fifth day
Rubella	Short; mild fever and malaise	Mild	Mild or absent	Face then trunk and limbs	No	Posterior occipital lymphadenopathy
Scarlet fever	Fever and sore throat	Moderate to high	Moderate	Face, then rapidly generalised	No	Remains blanched for several seconds after pressure; strawberry tongue and perioral pallor
Acute lymphoblastic leukaemia	Mild, nonspecific	Absent or mild/moderate	Moderate	Anywhere, including mucous membranes	No	Pallor, lymphadenopathy and hepatosplenomegaly may be present
Henoch–Schönlein purpura	Mild, sometimes symptoms of upper respiratory tract infection	Mild or moderate	Moderate	Mainly limbs, especially legs and buttocks	No	Rash is urticarial initially. Arthralgia, joint swelling and abdominal pain may be present
Idiopathic thrombocytopenic purpura	Nil to mild	Nil	Nil	Anywhere, including mucous membranes	No	Child is usually well, apart from effects of bleeding
Inherited bleeding disorder	Nil	Nil	Nil	Anywhere, including mucous membranes	No	Spontaneous bruises. Family history may be present

6 The child with a pyrexia of unknown origin

The definition of pyrexia of unknown origin (PUO), also called fever of unknown origin (FUO), varies between different authors. Petersdorf suggested a minimum temperature of 38.3°C for 3 weeks and at least 1 week of intensive hospital investigation, whereas some standard paediatric textbooks set a shorter minimum period of 1 week of fever (see Further Reading).

IMPORTANCE

True PUO is not a common disorder in hospital paediatric practice. Often the patient recovers before a definitive diagnosis has been made, or a viral infection is assumed, but the syndrome is important for a number of reasons. The underlying disorder may have serious implications for the individual, e.g. malaria or neoplasia. A delay in diagnosis may put other individuals at risk from an infectious disease, e.g. tuberculosis. In order to make a diagnosis, a patient may be detained in hospital and extensive investigations carried out. These consume valuable resources in terms of expense and professional time, and may also be hazardous, causing morbidity and rarely death. Therefore it is important that there is some structure to the investigations rather than a 'scatter-gun' approach.

POSSIBLE DIAGNOSES

The list of conditions that may present as a PUO is almost endless, including infectious diseases, autoimmune disorders and neoplasia. The disorders listed in Table 6.1 are those most likely to be encountered in western Europe or North America.

The relative incidence of each will vary depending on the diseases prevalent in a particular area and the extent of initial investigations. A North American study (Table 6.2) considered children who had had a persistent fever for 3 weeks or more and who had previously been immunologically normal.* It included a total of 109 children.

MANAGEMENT

Age is of little help in guiding the diagnosis. All children with a PUO should have:

- A full blood count and film
- A thick blood film for malaria parasites if there is any possibility of this diagnosis
- Repeated blood cultures
- Epstein–Barr virus serology
- Serum saved for other possible serology (e.g. CMV, *Toxoplasma*)

---

* **Steele et al. (1991) – see Reference and further reading (p.39).**

Table 6.1 Likely causes of PUO

Category	Disease
Specific bacterial infection	Brucellosis *Campylobacter* infection Cat-scratch disease Legionellosis Rheumatic fever *Salmonella typhi* infection Tuberculosis
Localised infection	Abscess: abdominal, dental, hepatic, pelvic, perinephric, rectal, subphrenic Cholangitis Endocarditis Mastoiditis Meningitis Osteomyelitis Pneumonia Pyelonephritis Sinusitis
Spirochaete infection	Leptospirosis Lyme disease Syphilis
Viral disease	Cytomegalovirus infection Epstein–Barr virus (infectious mononucleosis) Hepatitis HIV infection Enterovirus infection
Chlamydial disease	Psittacosis
Rickettsial disease	Q fever
Fungal disease	Histoplasmosis
Parasitic disease	Giardiasis Malaria Toxocariasis Toxoplasmosis Trypanosomiasis
Autoimmune disorders	Systemic juvenile idiopathic arthritis Polyarteritis nodosa Systemic lupus erythematosus Undefined vasculitis
Neoplasms	Atrial myxoma Hodgkin's disease Leukaemia Lymphoma Neuroblastoma Wilms' tumour

Table 6.1 continued	
Category	**Disease**
Miscellaneous	Anhidrotic ectodermal dysplasia
	Chronic active hepatitis
	Diabetes insipidus
	Drug fever
	Fabry's disease
	Factitious fever
	Familial dysautonomia
	Familial Mediterranean fever
	Hypothalamic central fever
	Ichthyosis
	Inflammatory bowel disease
	Kawasaki disease
	Pancreatitis
	Periodic fever
	Pulmonary embolism
	Serum sickness
	Thyrotoxicosis

Table 6.2 Final diagnosis in children with a pyrexia of unknown origin (with permission from Steele et al 1991)

Diagnosis		Number (%)
Infectious diseases		24 (22)
EBV infection	8	
Urinary tract infection	4	
Enterovirus infection	2	
Lyme disease	2	
Cat-scratch fever	2	
Osteomyelitis	1	
Psittacosis	1	
Rheumatic fever	1	
Crohn's disease	1	
Bacterial meningitis	2	
Autoimmune diseases		7 (6)
Juvenile rheumatic arthritis	3	
Systemic lupus erythematosus	2	
Periarteritis nodosa	1	
Undifferentiated autoimmune disease	1	
Malignancy		2 (2)
Leukaemia	1	
Lymphoma	1	
Drug-induced fever (paracetamol and methylphenidate)		2 (2)
Factitious (Munchausen's syndrome by proxy)		1 (1)
No aetiological diagnosis		73 (67)

Table 6.3 Pointers to likely diagnoses and helpful investigations in pyrexia of unknown origin

History/examination	Likely diagnoses	Investigations to be considered
Pica	Toxocariasis Toxoplasmosis	Specific serological tests
Exposure to wild or domestic animals	Toxoplasmosis Leptospirosis Lyme disease	Specific serological tests. For leptospirosis, isolation of organism from urine or serology
Possible tick bite	Lyme disease and arbovirus infection	Specific serological tests
Travel abroad	See Chapter 27	
Palpebral conjunctivitis	Measles Coxsackie virus infection Tuberculosis Infectious mononucleosis Cat-scratch disease	Specific serological tests. Tuberculin test for TB and histology for cat-scratch disease. Blood monospot
Bulbar conjunctivitis	Kawasaki disease Leptospirosis	None specific Isolation of organism from urine or serology
Uveitis	Sarcoidosis Juvenile idiopathic arthritis Systemic lupus erythematosus Behçet's syndrome Kawasaki disease	Chest X-ray Angiotensin converting enzyme Antinuclear antibody

Table 6.3 continued

History/examination	Likely diagnoses	Investigations to be considered
Chorioretinitis	Cytomegalovirus (CMV) infection Toxoplasmosis Syphilis	Specific serological tests. Viral culture. Polymerase chain reaction for CMV
Blisters	Infection with *Staphylococcus aureus* *Streptococcus, meningococcus* Malaria Rickettsial infection	Blood cultures. Polymerase chain reaction for meningococcus Blood films Serology
Localised bone tenderness	Osteomyelitis	X-ray and bone scan
Hectic fever with rigors	Septicaemia with renal, liver or biliary disease Malaria Brucellosis Localised pus	Blood cultures Blood film Serology, blood and bone marrow culture Ultrasound scan
Red throat	Infectious mononucleosis Cytomegalovirus infection Toxoplasmosis Typhoid (*Salmonella typhi*) Kawasaki disease Leptospirosis	Serology Serology Serology Isolation of organism (blood culture) Clinical diagnosis Urine culture for *Leptospira*
Abdominal pain and tenderness	Inflammatory bowel disease Collection of pus	Barium meal/enema Abdominal ultrasound scan
Rash	See Chapter 5	

Jaundice	Brucellosis Cholecystitis Hepatitis A–E Infectious mononucleosis Leptospirosis Pancreatitis	Specific serology for most causes of jaundice. Seek *Leptospira* in urine. Cholecystitis is a clinical diagnosis. Pancreatitis is accompanied by raised serum amylase level
Lymphadenopathy (see Chapter 7)	Reactive hyperplasia Cat-scratch disease Cytomegalovirus infection Infectious mononucleosis Mycobacterial infection Toxocariasis Toxoplasmosis Hodgkin's disease Other malignancy	Serology, tuberculin testing if nodes remain enlarged without explanation; biopsy may be needed as well as bone marrow examination
Absence of sweating	Anhidrotic ectodermal dysplasia Familial dysautonomia Atropine poisoning	Careful examination of skin, nails, hair and teeth Tests of autonomic function Toxicology
Erythrocyte sedimentation rate above 100 mm/h	Kawasaki disease Tuberculosis Malignancy Autoimmune disease	Tuberculin test
Pyuria	Urinary tract infection Renal tuberculosis	Renal imaging Early morning urine collections (for TB culture) Tuberculin test

- Urine microscopy (this is important to determine the presence of red and white cells) and culture
- Tuberculin test
- Chest X-ray.

Further investigations should be based on the possible diagnoses suggested by a full history and examination (Table 6.3).

'Blind' imaging is rarely helpful (the exception is abdominal ultrasonography, which is noninvasive), nor is bone marrow biopsy. The value of white cell scans in children has not been proved. When a diagnosis cannot be made, consideration must be given to the possibility of factitious fever (Munchausen's syndrome by proxy). Admission and close observation to ensure that the child is not being given anything to raise the temperature artificially is essential. This can sometimes be difficult to detect.

REFERENCE AND FURTHER READING

Behrman RE, Kliegman RM, Nelson WE, Vaughan VC, eds (1992) Nelson's textbook of pediatrics. WB Saunders, Philadelphia, PA, p 652.

Lorin MI, Feigin RD (1992) Fever without localising signs and fever of unknown origin. In: Feigin RD, Cherry JD (eds) Textbook of pediatric infectious disease. WB Saunders, Philadelphia, PA, p. 1012–1022.

Petersdorf R (1992) Fever of unknown origin: an old friend revisited. Arch Intern Med 152: 21–22.

Steele RW, Jones SM, Lowe B, Glasier CM (1991) Usefulness of scanning procedures for diagnosis of fever of unknown origin in children. J Pediatr 199: 526–530.

7 The child with an enlarged lymph node

This is a common problem in childhood. Most generalised lymphadenopathy in the head and neck is the result of viral upper respiratory tract infection or infectious mononucleosis (Chapter 52). Where a single node is enlarged, other diagnoses have to be considered.

In the child with fever and a warm, tender, enlarged lymph node or group of nodes, bacterial adenitis is most likely. In some cases the gland may be fluctuant. In children with bacterial adenitis there is often a recent history of preceding upper respiratory tract symptoms and the time course of the illness tends to be short.

When the onset of swelling is more gradual and there is less systemic illness, other diagnoses have to be considered. Lymphomas, particularly Hodgkin's lymphoma may present with a firm, single node enlargement. Generalised cervical lymphadenopathy may be a feature of leukaemia; these children tend to look ill and have other signs including anaemia, splenomegaly and petechiae.

Atypical mycobacterial infection is not uncommon in childhood (see Plate 1). This may affect several neighbouring glands. Overlying skin may be dark red/purple in colour and there may be an impression of tethering of firm, cool and painless gland or glands to the skin. Atypical mycobacterial infection is more common than *Mycobacterium tuberculosis*, except in certain high-risk groups.

Other unusual causes of infective lymphadenopathy, discussed in separate chapters, include Kawasaki disease, cat-scratch fever and HIV infection.

DIAGNOSIS AND TREATMENT

Because many cases are the result of viral infection, it is often appropriate, especially in the well child, to watch for a few weeks before embarking on further investigations.

In the child with suspected bacterial adenitis, investigations might include full blood count and blood culture. Although surgical drainage may be necessary if the lymph node becomes fluctuant and forms an abscess, antibiotic treatment alone may be all that is necessary.

The antibiotics selected should be effective against *Haemophilus influenzae*, *Streptococcus pneumoniae* and *Staphylococcus aureus*. Co-amoxiclav or a cephalosporin is recommended.

When antibiotic treatment fails, then surgical drainage may be required and other possible diagnoses should be considered.

Biopsy with possible removal of the lymph node is recommended for suspected cases of mycobacterial infection and lymphoma. Needle aspiration should not be performed in children because it tends to produce insufficient material for both cultures and histology, particularly if a lymphoma is to be excluded. Thus an adequate biopsy or even removal of the complete lymph node (where technically possible) is to be preferred. It is important to ensure that specimens are sent for histology (tumour markers where indicated) and culture for mycobacteria. It is unfair to the child to have to resort to a second unnecessary anaesthetic because of inadequate sampling at the first operation.

Please refer to chapters on Cat-scratch fever (Ch. 41), Nontuberculous mycobacterial disease (Ch. 80) and Tuberculosis (Ch. 105) for more detailed information about treatment.

8 The child with septic shock

EPIDEMIOLOGY AND CAUSES

Organisms responsible for septic shock in infants and children include *Neisseria meningitidis* (most common), *Escherichia coli*, *Haemophilus influenzae* type b, *Klebsiella* spp., salmonellas and other Gram-negative bacteria: *Staphylococcus aureus* and *Streptococcus pneumoniae* are the most frequent Gram-positive pathogens. Below 3 months of age group B *Streptococcus agalactiae* and *Escherichia coli* are more common causes of septic shock among infant admissions.

Surgical patients usually develop septicaemia due to enteric organisms. Immunosuppressed patients may develop septicaemia due to unusual and opportunistic organisms, although Gram-negative bacteria are the major cause of mortality.

TERMINOLOGY AND PATHOPHYSIOLOGY OF SEPSIS

Septicaemia is defined as the presence of organisms in the blood stream accompanied by clinical features of sepsis (tachypnoea, tachycardia, pyrexia/hypothermia and neutrophilia or neutropenia).

Sepsis is the clinical expression of the host's response to bacteria, more specifically to constituents of the cell wall of Gram-negative bacteria – endotoxins – as well as exotoxins produced by Gram-negative organisms. Bacterial infection results in activation of macrophages, which produce the lymphokines gamma-interferon and granulocyte macrophage colony stimulating factor, tumour necrosis factor-alpha (TNF-α) and interleukins 1 and 6 (IL-1, IL-6). These substances are beneficial to the host in mediating the protective inflammatory response but in severe infection an exaggerated, harmful response occurs in which high levels of TNF-α and IL-1 lead to serious damage. Acting with the inflammatory mediators prostaglandin E_2 (PGE$_2$) released by neutrophils, nitric acid released by macrophages and platelet activating factor, a state of shock can develop. Damage to the endothelial cells of blood vessels results in leakage of plasma from the circulation with consequent vascular collapse and breakdown of the normal coagulation mechanisms. The devastating effects of fulminant septicaemia result from the host's response to the bacteria and future strategies for the prevention of septic shock will come not from the development of new antibiotics but from agents antagonistic to endotoxins, the cytokines or inflammatory mediators (see below)

CLINICAL PRESENTATION

Full clinical assessment must include observations of temperature (both peripheral and central), pulse rate, blood pressure, capillary refill, respiration rate and pattern, mental status, conscious level and urine output. Body weight and height should be measured or estimated.

Early features of sepsis typically include fever and tachycardia. Respiration rate may be normal or mildly raised with an irregular breathing pattern. Urine output may be mildly reduced, reflecting mild dehydration, but mental status and conscious level are unaffected.

Later features may include hypothermia, a marked tachycardia, sustained tachypnoea and respiratory irregularity, depressed conscious level and a clinically appreciable reduction in urine output.

Hypotension may also be present but its presence is not essential to the diagnosis of septic shock. Blood pressure may be maintained until a late stage by vasoregulatory mechanisms, especially in a young child. These mechanisms preserve central blood pressure at the expense of impaired perfusion to limbs and organs.

Impaired perfusion may be recognised by cold peripheries, poor capillary refill, tachycardia, tachypnoea and oliguria. Skin core-temperature gradient should be measured with thermistor probes on a toe and in the rectum: a wide skin-core temperature difference (e.g. > 3°C) is a sensitive marker for severe shock.

A capillary refill time prolonged beyond 2 seconds in a room-warm limb is a reliable marker for reduced skin perfusion.

Hypoxaemia or poor cerebral perfusion may result in restlessness, irritability or 'bad behaviour' in a child. Measurement of hypoxaemia with a saturation monitor is an essential adjunct to clinical examination.

INVESTIGATION

Haemoglobin may fall rapidly. The white blood count (showing neutrophilia or, more seriously, neutropenia) and blood lactate (elevated) are helpful measures of response to shock. Blood glucose is often low, and potassium and calcium may be low and need correcting. Evidence of multi-organ failure should be sought with clinical and laboratory evidence of disseminated intravascular coagulation (DIC), adult respiratory distress syndrome, acute renal failure, hepatobiliary dysfunction and central nervous system (CNS) dysfunction.

DIAGNOSIS

The underlying cause can often be inferred from careful history and examination of the patient. Blood cultures should be taken before antibiotics are given: the causative organism usually can be isolated within 24 hours. Bacterial antigen detection in urine or plasma may establish the diagnosis in children who have previously received antibiotics.

MANAGEMENT

See also Chapters 9 and 78.

Immediate treatment

Immediate management is with urgent antibiotic treatment to cover the likely causative organisms, parenteral fluids, vasoactive agents and oxygen. Early drainage of purulent foci should be performed.

Choice of antibiotics for paediatric medical patients should include cefotaxime (initial dose 200 mg/kg/day intravenously 6-hourly). The antibiotic regimen may need variation or supplementation if surgical or immunocompromised patients are being treated. Local or tertiary centre protocols may be available for certain groups (e.g. oncology patients with febrile neutropenia).

Patients with evidence of impaired peripheral perfusion should initially be resuscitated with albumin 4.5% 20–40 mL/kg over 10–30 minutes followed by a further 20–40 mL/kg albumin over the next hour.

Children should be nursed in an area designated for high-dependency care within the paediatric ward where intensive care measures can be commenced if needed. Facilities for intermittent positive pressure ventilation and cardiopulmonary resuscitation should be available.

Admission to the Paediatric Intensive Care Unit

Patients who do not respond to immediate treatment require admission to a Paediatric Intensive Care Unit (PICU) and should be discussed with paediatric intensivists. Requests for admission to a PICU should not be based solely upon a need for ventilatory support, although most patients will be ventilated by the time of transfer. Other factors should be taken into account, including the diagnosis, the natural history thereby implied, the degree of shock, the amount of treatment given and the respiratory pattern. The child should be accompanied on the journey to the PICU by ambulance or within the hospital by paediatric, anaesthetic and nursing staff experienced in the transfer of the critically ill paediatric patient.

Continued resuscitation

Resuscitation should be continued while awaiting the arrival of the transfer team and stability maintained while arrangements are made for transfer. At least one senior member each of medical and nursing staff should remain with the transfer team while preparations are made for departure from the high-dependency area. Most transfer teams spend considerable time achieving optimal stability prior to transfer. The final outcome depends on maintenance of condition during transfer. Albumin and fluid resuscitation should be continued and inotropes commenced. All infusions should be capable of continuing through transfer. The airway should be stabilised – often with endotracheal intubation – and intravenous access secured.

Management of septic shock

Invasive monitoring of blood pressure, pulse, urine output, and differential core–peripheral temperature monitoring should be established. Central venous pressure (CVP) monitoring may allow colloid to be given with confidence until CVP is approximately +12–15 cmH$_2$O. This should be followed by a reduction in the core–peripheral temperature difference and better capillary refill. Children with Gram-negative septic shock may require several times their own circulating volume of colloid because of the capillary leak that is a major feature of the condition. It is important not to be misled by the fluid volumes required into slowing infusion rates or discontinuing volume expansion too early.

Once adequate volume replacement has been completed as shown by CVP and central blood pressure, persistence of signs of impaired peripheral perfusion suggests that either myocardial failure due to endotoxaemia or peripheral vasoconstriction may be present. Myocardial function can be assessed by echocardiography, if available, to measure end-diastolic volume.

The child with established septic shock should be electively intubated and ventilated. This is an urgent requirement if the airway is compromised or there are abnormalities of breathing rate or pattern. Ventilation reduces the work of breathing and myocardial workload. Intermittent positive pressure ventilation can avert the severe deterioration that may occur during a period of unexpected decompensation, and reduces the risk of pulmonary oedema. Midazolam 100 μg/kg/h is given for sedative effect during ventilation: it is also an anticonvulsant. Intravenous opiate infusions such as morphine 20–40 μg/kg/h or alfentanil 30–60 μg/kg/h can be used for sedative and analgesic effect.

Cardiovascular support

Dopamine 2.5–5 μg/kg/min, an inotrope with vasodilator action, should be commenced as first-line supportive treatment when there are signs of impaired perfusion that have not responded to first-line measures. Dobutamine 2.5 μg/kg/min may be added for further inotropic effect and increased to a dose of 20 μg/kg/min while maintaining renal perfusion using dopamine at a maximum of 5 μg/kg/min. If hypotension persists despite adequate CVP dopamine can be increased in 2.5–5 μg/kg/min increments up to a maximum of 20 μg/kg/min. The introduction of a third inotrope such as adrenaline 0.1–1.0 μg/kg/min or isoprenaline 0.1–2.0 μg/kg/min may be considered to keep dopamine at the renal dose of 5 μg/kg/min. Noradrenaline may be used as a fourth inotrope. Other vasodilators that reduce afterload on the heart and improve perfusion include glyceryl trinitrate patch 5 mg/day, and nitroglycerine 1 μg/kg/min. Nitroprusside has also been used. Prostacyclin 1 μg/kg/min acts as a potent vasodilator and an inhibitor of platelet aggregation, which may reduce the risk of disseminated intravascular coagulation. The place of these vasodilators in the management of septic shock has not been established in double-blind placebo-controlled trials in children.

Fluid and electrolyte balance

In septic shock it is important to address fluid balance under the headings of restoration of intravascular volume, maintenance fluid and replacement of ongoing losses. In view of the large amounts of colloid used for the first category (volumes may be 100–200 mL/kg), it is advisable to restrict maintenance crystalloid to half the recommended amount. Ongoing fluid losses (e.g. nasogastric aspirates) should be measured over an hour and replaced with the same volume of intravenous 0.9% saline over the next hour.

Regular electrolyte and blood glucose measurements should be performed. If blood glucose is low, dextrose 10% infusion at 0.5 mL/kg/hour should be commenced. Higher dextrose concentrations may be needed if there is a poor response.

Disseminated intravascular coagulation

Many patients in septic shock show evidence of disseminated intravascular coagulation (DIC), with deranged clotting studies, thrombocytopenia and raised fibrin degradation products. The management of DIC is supportive during correction of the underlying cause. Patients with severely deranged clotting studies should be given fresh frozen plasma or cryoprecipitate. Platelet infusions may be required for patients with severe thrombocytopenia and active bleeding (e.g. from puncture sites), but their effect only lasts 6–8 hours.

Other infusions, such as low-dose heparin (10 units/kg/h), should be considered for individual patients with impending peripheral gangrene and severe coagulation derangement, although this area is controversial and should be discussed with PICU staff before commencement in a high-dependency area. Results of trials of various specific treatments targeted at the disorders of haemostasis that contribute to DIC are awaited.

AREAS OF CONTROVERSY

Administration of corticosteroids is often contemplated as a supplementary treatment in septic shock. While early corticosteroid treatment appears beneficial in animals and adult humans, evidence also suggests that in established septic shock steroid therapy may be detrimental. There are few data available from children, and therefore their use is not currently recommended.

Plasmaphaeresis and blood exchange have both been used to reduce the concentrations of circulating endotoxin and cytokines. There is no convincing evidence of their success.

Modulators of the inflammatory response in sepsis are being extensively studied. These include monoclonal antibodies against endotoxins and cytokines, nitric oxide synthase inhibitors (such as *N*-monomethyl-L-arginine, L-NMMA) and other agents such as polymyxin B and taurolin (anti-endotoxins), and pentoxifylline (a cytokine antagonist). No trial data yet exists on their overall efficacy or safety.

FURTHER READING

Anderson MR, Blumer JL (1997) Advances in the therapy for sepsis in children. Pediatr Clin North Am 44: 179–205.

Astiz ME, Rackow EC (1998) Septic shock. Lancet 351: 1501–1505.

9 The child with toxic shock syndrome

See also Chapters 98 and 99.

The syndrome was first defined in 1978 in a series of children with *Staphylococcus aureus* infection. Since then a similar illness following streptococcal infection has been described. Although it is unusual to isolate *S. aureus* from blood culture in this syndrome, the bacterium is usually isolated from other sites. Several exotoxins are known to mediate the disease, including staphylococcal enterotoxin, also known as toxic shock syndrome toxin-1 (TSST-1), a 22 049 Da protein with a known nucleotide sequence. The group A streptococci identified in toxic shock have been exotoxin-producing M1 and M3 strains.

EPIDEMIOLOGY

This is a rare syndrome in children. Although it was thought initially to be predominantly associated with menstruation and tampon use, this is true in only about half of cases. It has been described following apparently mild staphylococcal skin infection, osteomyelitis and empyema but most consistently in association with bacterial tracheitis. The cases associated with streptococcal infection have been from two main groups – children with varicella infection and those with relatively innocuous streptococcal upper respiratory tract infections.

CLINICAL FEATURES

There is usually a rapid onset of illness with a high fever, vomiting, diarrhoea, headache, pharyngitis, myalgia and hypotension. Multisystem organ failure results from hypotension with poor tissue perfusion and polyclonal activation of T cells with release of cytokines and other inflammatory mediators. Fatal complications include irreversible shock, disseminated intravascular coagulation and arrhythmias. There are very specific dermatological features. These include a diffuse, scarlatiniform rash on the trunk and arms. This tends to be more marked on the flexor surfaces. The palms and soles may become oedematous and the eyes become red. Desquamation may occur in the recovery phase.

DIAGNOSIS

The differential diagnoses include Kawasaki disease and staphylococcal scalded skin syndrome. Most cases of staphylococcal toxic shock have been associated with sterile blood culture but this may be positive in streptococcal toxic shock. Although the portal of entry may not be apparent, investigations should include throat swab with skin wound and vaginal swabs where appropriate. The haematological findings include leukopenia with a high band count, thrombocytopenia and features of disseminated intravascular coagulation with a prolonged coagulation time and fibrin degradation products (FDPs). Other laboratory abnormalities will reflect multi-organ failure if this is present.

MANAGEMENT

This section should be read in conjunction with Chapters 8, 98 and 99.

With the rapid onset of the disease, management has to be prompt and aggressive. Intensive monitoring is very important to assess the degree of intravascular depletion. Large volumes of fluid may be required, supported by inotropic drugs (dopamine). In most patients mechanical ventilation is required. Appropriate antibiotics should be given. Treatment of DIC with fresh frozen plasma may be necessary. Metabolic abnormalities may occur as a result of renal failure and require appropriate treatments.

10 The child with bacterial meningitis

INTRODUCTION

Despite advances in prevention and treatment for this condition it remains the most important bacterial cause of mortality and morbidity in children in developed countries.

EPIDEMIOLOGY

The peak ages of incidence are infancy and early childhood. The incidence fell in the UK following the introduction of the conjugate vaccine against *Haemophilus influenzae* type b (Hib) in 1992. The incidence of meningococcal disease (including septicaemia and meningitis) has risen in recent years. The increase in antibiotic-resistant isolates of *Streptococcus pneumoniae* is a major cause for concern.

The important causative organisms at various ages are shown in Table 10.1. Infection with coagulase-negative staphylococcus is the most common form of meningitis in patients with ventricular shunts (see Chapter 13).

CLINICAL FEATURES

The onset of symptoms may be relatively insidious or there may be rapid progression with coma and prostration. The early features of neonatal meningitis may be completely nonspecific (see Chapter 4). This can also be the case in the young child, particularly with the slower-onset form of the illness in which nonspecific symptoms, including mild upper respiratory symptoms, may be present for several days before the diagnosis becomes evident. Meningitis in young children usually presents with fever, vomiting and lethargy with or without convulsions. Neck stiffness and other signs of meningism may not be present in a child under 18 months of age. Doctors dealing with young children with acute febrile illnesses should have a high index of suspicion and a low threshold for the performing of a lumbar puncture. In the older child headache, photophobia, vomiting and anorexia are common presenting symptoms and neck stiffness is characteristic. Symptoms in older children are usually only pres-

Table 10.1 Important causative organisms of bacterial meningitis

Age	Cause	Empirical antibiotic treatment
0–1 month	Group B streptococcus *Escherichia coli* *Neisseria meningitidis* *Haemophilus influenzae* type b (Hib) *Streptococcus pneumoniae* *Listeria monocytogenes*	Cefotaxime + ampicillin ± gentamicin
1–3 months	*Neisseria meningitidis* *Haemophilus influenzae* type b (Hib) *Streptococcus pneumoniae* Group B streptococcus *Escherichia coli* *Listeria monocytogenes*	Cefotaxime + ampicillin*
3 months –5 years	*Neisseria meningitidis* *Haemophilus influenzae* type b (Hib; rare since 1992) *Streptococcus pneumoniae*	Ceftriaxone or cefotaxime*
6 years or more	*Neisseria meningitidis* *Streptococcus pneumoniae*	Ceftriaxone or cefotaxime*

* If possibility of multiresistant pneumococcal infection add vancomycin.

ent for a maximum of 2–3 days before presentation and often only for a few hours. A longer history should bring to mind the possibility of a subacute cause of meningoencephalitis such as *Mycobacterium tuberculosis* or other agents (see Chapter 11) or, rarely, an intracranial abscess.

The classical purpuric rash of meningococcal sepsis occurs in about half to two-thirds of cases of meningitis caused by this organism. Occasionally, such a rash may be caused by the other meningitic pathogens. A nonspecific maculopapular rash may also occur in meningococcal disease. Arthritis may complicate *H. influenzae* and meningococcal meningitis and in the latter is often multifocal.

NATURAL HISTORY

Outside the neonatal period, the causative organisms are spread by respiratory secretions and droplet transmission. Usually the bacteria first colonise the nasopharynx and from there invade via the blood to the meninges. Factors facilitating invasion into the blood include immaturity of the host defences and possibly, in some cases, intercurrent viral infections such as influenza. Asymptomatic nasopharyngeal carriage of these organisms is not uncommon in the population. Pneumococcal meningitis may be associated with chronic middle-ear sepsis, may follow skull fractures or may complicate congenital defects in the coverings of the central nervous system.

DIAGNOSIS

Lumbar puncture with cerebrospinal fluid examination provides the basis for diagnosis. A Gram stain and cell count should be performed. In cases of bacterial meningitis, more than 50 WBC/mm^3 is usual, although more than 10 is abnormal. Polymorphonuclear leukocytes should predominate: mononuclear cells are seen in tuberculous, viral and partially treated pyogenic bacterial infection. Tuberculous and viral cases can usually be differentiated by history and clinical signs. In tuberculous infection as with bacterial meningitis cerebrospinal fluid (CSF) glucose is low, and protein is elevated. In viral meningitis (Chapter 11) the CSF microscopy usually shows lymphocytes, although occasionally in the early stages a predominance of neutrophils may be seen. Even less commonly in viral meningitis the CSF glucose may be depressed, although it is usually normal.

The causative organism can usually be cultured from the blood, CSF or both and occasionally from other sites such as synovial fluid. In meningococcal sepsis, a throat swab will grow the organism even after the first dose of antibiotics in up to 40% of cases. Gram stain and/or culture of material obtained from skin lesions may also be used to confirm the diagnosis. Antigen detection tests such as latex agglutination may detect bacterial capsular polysaccharide in CSF, blood or urine and enable identification of the causative organism when cultures are negative. Polymerase chain reaction (PCR) tests on blood and/or CSF are highly sensitive and specific for confirming a diagnosis of meningococcal disease when cultures are negative and can also provide information on the group and type of meningococcus. This test has largely replaced serological tests. The PCR and antigen tests are useful if prior antibiotic therapy has been given or if lumbar puncture is contraindicated because of raised intracranial pressure.

MANAGEMENT

The management of neonatal meningitis is dealt with in Chapter 4.

Children with suspected meningococcal sepsis should he given parenteral benzylpenicillin or ampicillin prior to transfer to hospital. In hospital, blood cultures should be performed and a lumbar puncture considered. Intravenous antibiotic therapy should not be delayed; it is acceptable to start this before lumbar puncture, particularly when there are clinical signs of meningococcal infection. Particularly with a prolonged history or focal neurological signs, lumbar puncture may be risky: the fundi should be examined for evidence of papilloedema before this is performed. In the unconscious child, intracranial pressure may be high, even in the absence of papilloedema, and a lumbar puncture may increase the risk of coning. In these cases it should not be performed. Nevertheless treatment of presumed meningitis without a bacteriological diagnosis is unsatisfactory and, because other serious illness may have similar signs, management of this condition without a lumbar puncture should be the exception rather than the rule.

The initial antibiotic therapy is given immediately and before culture results are available. In recent years there has been an increasing problem of penicillin resistance among pneumococcal isolates. While for the moment this remains an infrequent problem in the UK, in some parts of the world such isolates are extremely common. In children older than 3 months, ceftriaxone or cefotaxime is the recommended empirical treatment of choice (Table 10.1 and Appendix III). These agents achieve more than adequate CSF bactericidal levels against all the major bacterial pathogens. Resistance to third-generation cephalosporins can occur in pneumococci as part of a multiresistance pattern but this is still unusual in most countries. If there are concerns about multiple resistance (e.g. if the patient has travelled to an endemic area), vancomycin therapy should be added until culture and sensitivity results are available. In infants of less than 3 months, cefotaxime is preferred (because of poor biliary clearance of ceftriaxone) and ampicillin is added to cover *Listeria monocytogenes*.

The length of treatment varies with the causative organism. For meningococcal disease 5–7 days is adequate. Pneumococcal and Hib disease should be treated for 10 days. Listeria (see Chapters 4 and 74) and Gram-negative bacillary meningitis require a minimum 21 days therapy.

Dexamethasone has been shown to reduce the incidence of neurological sequelae, including deafness, in non-neonatal meningitis caused by Hib. Its effectiveness in pneumococcal disease is unclear, with conflicting reports, and there is a lack of data on its use in meningococcal meningitis. Dexamethasone 0.6 mg/kg/day in four divided doses should be commenced in those (rare) cases where *H. influenzae* is believed to be the cause of meningitis (based on Gram stain findings on CSF). However it is important that antibiotic therapy is not delayed as a result of awaiting the Gram stain results. Similar treatment may be considered in pneumococcal disease but should not be given in meningococcal disease or in any case in which the aetiology is obscure. Proponents of the use of steroids suggest that they are given either with or within 1 hour of the first antibiotic dose; otherwise, they should not be used.

Repeat lumbar puncture is not necessary for the routine management of meningitis due to common organisms but may be useful if treatment failure or relapse is suspected. Since there is a significant risk of relapse in infants after enteric Gram-negative bacillary meningitis, it is useful to document the CSF findings with a lumbar puncture at the end of treatment.

It is important to correct dehydration, which is relatively common in those with a long history or with profuse vomiting. Thereafter, because inappropriate antidiuretic hormone secretion and cerebral oedema may complicate meningitis, crystalloid fluids should be used judiciously. Intracranial pressure is likely to be high and the child may need plasma expanders and inotropic support to maintain cerebral perfusion pressure. Convulsions may occur as a presenting feature or may develop later; these may be difficult to control. Routine use of prophylactic anticonvulsants is not recommended. Intracranial suppuration is a rare complication and specialist advice should be sought in its management.

Long-term complications include sensorineural deafness (approximately 10% of cases) as well as secondary epilepsy and motor and intellectual impairment. All children should be followed up and hearing tests performed as a routine.

PREVENTION

Chemoprophylaxis for close contacts is given when appropriate (see Chapters 57 and 75) in cases of meningococcal and Hib disease: rifampicin to eliminate nasopharyngeal carriage for the latter and rifampicin or intramuscular ceftriaxone or (in adults) oral ciprofloxacin for the former. If a third-generation cephalosporin is used for therapy the index case requires no further treatment to eliminate carriage. Otherwise they too should be treated. Immunisation against meningococci of groups A, C, W137 or Y is used in the control of outbreaks of disease due to one of these organisms. A new conjugate group C vaccine is now routinely in use, and a conjugate group A vaccine may become available soon (see Chapter 78).

Long-term antibiotic prophylaxis (usually penicillin) should be given to children at high risk of disease such as those with hyposplenism or complement disorders.

Routine immunisation against the common causative organisms is discussed in the relevant sections in Part Two, and immunisation in relation to overseas travel in Chapter 26.

11 The child with acute encephalitis or meningoencephalitis

INTRODUCTION

The syndrome of meningoencephalitis covers a range of illnesses from pure encephalitis to an aseptic meningitis with few or no encephalopathic features. Encephalopathy (acute brain dysfunction) can have many causes, some of which are not infection-related – e.g. toxin exposure, metabolic disturbance, tumour, trauma, vascular mishaps, hypoxia, uncontrolled hydrocephalus and status epilepticus. The term encephalitis should be reserved for those conditions in which there is presumed inflammation of brain tissue induced directly or indirectly by microbial infection. Where there is a meningitic component it is more likely that the cause is infection-related, although there are noninfective causes including drug reactions (such as those to nonsteroidal anti-inflammatory agents and to intravenous immunoglobulin), collagen vascular disorders, malignancy and post-neurosurgical. Related disorders that may share the same aetiology include transverse myelitis and polyradiculopathy.

Infection-related meningoencephalitis may vary in severity from mild and self-limiting to a devastating illness with high mortality and morbidity.

ORGANISMS

Table 11.1 lists the important causes. The arthropod-borne viruses, collectively known as arboviruses, include a large number of viruses mainly falling

Table 11.1 Infective causes of acute encephalitis

Viral	Nonviral
Toga(alpha)viruses – includes western and eastern equine encephalitis viruses	*Mycoplasma pneumoniae**
	Mycoplasma hominis
	Leptospira spp.
Flaviviruses – includes dengue viruses, Japanese B encephalitis, yellow fever virus, tick-borne encephalitis viruses	*Borrelia burgdorferi* (Lyme disease)
	Tuberculosis
	Listeriosis
Bunyaviruses – includes sand-fly fever virus	Typhus fever
	Rocky mountain spotted fever
Rabies virus	*Falciparum* malaria
Herpes simplex viruses (I and II)	Toxoplasmosis
Adenovirus	Trypanosomiasis
Enteroviruses	Acute bacterial meningitis
Mumps virus	
Respiratory syncytial virus	
Influenza virus	
Measles virus*	
Rubella virus*	
Reoviruses	
Lymphocytic choriomeningitis virus	
Varicella-zoster virus*	
Epstein–Barr virus	
Cytomegalovirus	
Human herpes virus 6	

* These organisms usually produce the postinfectious form of disease.

into the toga (alpha), bunya and flavivirus families. Many of these only occur in specific geographical locations. Some microbial agents can cause either a pure encephalitis or a meningoencephalitis. Infection with many of the arboviruses and the rabies virus produces a predominantly encephalitic picture. The pathogenesis of meningoencephalitis may involve direct invasion of the central nervous system or an immunologically mediated process leading to inflammation and demyelination in which the organism cannot be demonstrated in nervous tissue (postinfectious encephalomyelitis).

EPIDEMIOLOGY

The incidence of encephalitis induced by any particular organism varies with the prevalence of that organism in the community. For instance, clusters of cases of *Mycoplasma*- or influenza-associated encephalitis are likely to be seen during epidemic years for those particular organisms. Worldwide, the incidence varies considerably in different geographical areas, and sometimes seasonally, depending on the prevalence of arboviruses, rickettsial infections and rabies.

The incidence is relatively low in the UK (where there are few arbovirus vectors) but good epidemiological data are not available. A study in Finland showed an incidence of 8.8 per 100 000 children under 16 years of age.

TRANSMISSION

Arboviruses are insect-borne; rickettsiae, *Borrelia burgdorferi* and typhus are tick-borne. Other causative agents may be spread by droplets (respiratory pathogens) or by the faecal–oral route (enteroviruses).

CLINICAL FEATURES/NATURAL HISTORY

In the directly invasive forms of the illness, meningitic or encephalitic symptoms are normally present from the start (monophasic process) while in the postinfectious forms they usually develop as a second phase after the initial systemic illness (biphasic process). These two forms are not always clinically distinguishable and indeed some agents can induce encephalitis by either or both mechanisms. The early symptoms will usually be non-specific, commonly with fever and vomiting. Symptoms and signs of systemic infection (e.g. rash, lymphadenopathy or pneumonia) may be present. Many agents causing encephalitis, particularly those involving direct invasion, also produce a meningitic process; in which case there is a combined clinical picture of meningism (headache, vomiting, nuchal rigidity and photophobia) and encephalitis. The symptoms and signs of the latter include drowsiness, which may proceed to coma, myalgia, altered behaviour, convulsions, focal or generalised paresis, cranial nerve palsies, ataxia and the signs and symptoms of raised intracranial pressure.

More specific clinical pictures are produced by some agents. The postinfectious encephalitis associated with chickenpox usually produces signs predominantly of cerebellar dysfunction. Focal convulsions and deficits are characteristic of herpes simplex virus encephalitis. An insidious onset of focal neurological abnormalities, particularly if leading to visual loss, with minimal evidence of systemic upset is typical of acute demyelinating encephalomyelitis (ADEM). In such postinfectious forms there may or may not be a history of preceding (usually mild) infectious illness.

Encephalitis is more common in immunocompromised children (acquired or primary states) and in such children is more likely to be severe and to run a more protracted course. Cytomegalovirus and Epstein–Barr virus infections involving the central nervous system are a particular problem among the immunocompromised.

DIAGNOSIS

Not all acute encephalopathy will be infective in nature and noninfective causes should be considered and excluded. The majority of cases are, however, associated with infection and the diagnosis may be evident from the characteristic clinical picture of the infection, e.g. a common childhood exanthematous illness. A careful history covering recent illness/medication, possible exposure to rabid animals and foreign travel is important. In a considerable number of cases the precise microbial diagnosis will not be evident. It is important to initiate specific therapy for treatable causes while pursuing investigations into the aetiology. It should be remembered that acute bacterial or tuberculous meningitis may sometimes produce predominantly encephalitic rather than meningitic symptoms.

Investigations should include radiology – computed tomography, or preferably magnetic resonance, scanning of the brain and a chest radiograph. Such scans may show generalised or focal brain swelling or necrosis, meningeal enhancement or areas of demyelination typical of ADEM. It is important to initiate early a comprehensive battery of investigations to try to establish a microbial diagnosis. This will include appropriate viral and bacterial cultures, Mantoux test, viral (and other) serology and analysis of samples by polymerase chain reaction to look for microbial nucleic acid. Cerebrospinal fluid (CSF) is usually the most useful sample for analysis but care should be taken to assess the risks of lumbar puncture if there is a possibility of raised intracranial pressure. The CSF microscopy and chemistry may be normal in cases of 'pure' encephalitis, particularly in the early phases (e.g. in herpes simplex virus (HSV) encephalitis). However, polymerase chain reaction tests for HSV nucleic acid have a very high diagnostic sensitivity. In aseptic meningoencephalitis, CSF typically shows an excess of mononuclear leukocytes with a raised protein. CSF glucose is typically normal in viral cases and depressed in bacterial (including tuberculous) cases. Occasionally, in the early phase of viral meningoencephalitis the CSF may show neutrophils and/or a low glucose leading to increased diagnostic difficulty.

In cases with a history of foreign travel, specialist advice from tropical medicine experts may be useful both for clinical management and for help in directing samples to specialist reference laboratories.

TREATMENT

This may be divided into supportive and specific therapies.

Supportive care

It is essential, in order to maximise recovery, that careful attention is paid to keeping the brain in optimal condition. More severe cases should be managed in a centre with paediatric intensive care facilities. Correction of biochemical disturbances and maintenance of fluid balance are vital. Haemodynamic and respiratory support may be required. Convulsions will need to be controlled and electroencephalographic monitoring may be helpful in this respect. Raised intracranial pressure (ICP) may need monitoring using invasive techniques in selected cases. Haemodynamic support to maintain cerebral perfusion pressure is vitally important in cases with significantly raised ICP. Ventilatory support may be required because of the consequences of the disease or because of the anticonvulsant therapy and this may be useful in helping to control ICP.

The decision on whether to use steroid therapy depends on the probable causative agent and the type of pathogenic process. It will usually produce clinical improvement in ADEM-type illnesses. It is used in tuberculous meningitis to reduce postinflammatory complications. It may have a role in pyogenic meningitis (see Chapter 10). Anecdotally, it has also produced marked clinical improvement in encephalitis associated with *Mycoplasma pneumoniae* infection. Steroids have been shown to produce no benefit in studies in Japanese B encephalitis. Though there are few data on their use in other forms of viral meningoencephalitis, most authorities would feel that steroids are unlikely to be of benefit and theoretically might produce significant adverse effects in the direct invasion forms of the disease.

Specific therapies

If there is any doubt, empirical antibiotic therapy (see Table 10.1, p. 50) should be initiated to cover the possibility of acute bacterial meningitis and should be continued until this diagnosis has been excluded by the finding of negative cultures and antigen tests. It may sometimes be necessary to commence empirical antituberculous therapy. Many authorities advocate the empirical use of a macrolide antibiotic such as erythromycin or clarithromycin to cover the possibility of *M. pneumoniae* infection, although there is no evidence that such treatment alters the outcome in encephalitis associated with this organism. If there is evidence to suggest the possibility of Lyme disease, ceftriaxone (100 mg/kg/day) should be used until this diagnosis has been excluded on serological testing (see Chapter 75). Many of the other nonviral causes are amenable to specific therapy (see relevant chapters in Part Two).

Of all the viral encephalitides only that due to herpes simplex virus has been shown to respond favourably to specific antiviral therapy. Although the later findings in this condition are fairly characteristic, the early features may be nonspecific. Aciclovir ($500 \text{ mg/m}^2 \times 3$/day) should therefore be commenced in all cases of encephalitis where the aetiology is unclear and will need to be continued until either a firm alternative diagnosis is made or, in the absence of the typical features of HSV encephalitis emerging, there is a negative polymerase chain reaction for HSV on cerebrospinal fluid.

If cytomegalovirus is considered a possible cause (usually in immunocompromised children), ganciclovir can be used as an alternative to cover both HSV and CMV. Pleconaril (pirodavir), a specific antiviral active against enteroviruses, has been shown to be beneficial in chronic echovirus encephalitis in immunocompromised individuals, but its role in acute encephalitis due to these viruses is unproven.

PREVENTION

Acute meningoencephalitis in children in the UK is often caused by common organisms and preventative strategies are dealt with in the individual chapters in Part Two.

For Japanese B encephalitis and tick-borne encephalitis there are good vaccines available, which should be given to travellers at risk. Vaccines are not generally available for the other arbovirus encephalitides – travellers to endemic areas should be given advice on minimising exposure to vector insects (see Chapter 26 and Department of Health booklet *Health Advice for Travellers*).

FURTHER READING

Davies EG, De Souza C (1993) How to investigate and manage the child with suspected acute encephalitis. Curr Paediatr 3: 106–113.

Levin M (1991) Infections of the nervous system. In: EM Brett (ed.) Paediatric neurology, 2nd edn. Churchill Livingstone, Edinburgh: pp. 603–665.

Rantokallio P, Leskinen M, von Wendt L (1986) Incidence and prognosis of central nervous system infections in a birth cohort of 12,000 children. Scand J Infect Dis 18: 287–294.

12 The injured child

INTRODUCTION

Despite improved public awareness of dangers to children both inside and outside the home, accidents and injury remain a major cause of mortality and morbidity in childhood. Advances in immediate retrieval and resuscitation of victims have resulted in higher initial survival rate and in these patients the risk of infective complications is extremely high. In severe multiple trauma and in burn injuries infection is by far the commonest cause of late death.

The mechanisms underlying the increased risk of infection after trauma are complex and poorly understood. In the case of penetrating injuries, open wound trauma and burns there is of course a breach of the first line of the host defences, the skin. Medical care itself, involving indwelling venous and urinary catheters, endotracheal intubation and surgery, leads to further breaching of this innate defence. Furthermore, there is a wealth of evidence suggesting that major trauma in itself has a depressive effect on immune function, particularly cellular function, with evidence for depression of neutrophil chemotaxis, macrophage function and T-cell (especially helper) function. Corticosteroid treatment, used routinely in head-injured patients, further compromises these functions.

This chapter deals with practical aspects in the management of infection in injured children.

MULTIPLE MAJOR TRAUMA

Infective complications are common in multiply traumatised children. These include infections introduced at the time of injury and nosocomial infections associated with treatment: for example, intravenous catheter infections. Table 12.1 lists possible sites of infections.

12 Injured child

Table 12.1 Possible sites of infection in multiple trauma

Infection	Risk factors: direct result of injury	Risk factors: nosocomial infection
Pneumonia	Aspiration	Endotracheal intubation
Empyema	Penetrating chest injury	Insertion of chest drains
Sinusitis	Facial fractures	Nasogastric and nasotracheal intubation
Meningitis	Basal skull fractures with CSF leak	Cerebrospinal fluid drainage procedures (shunt insertion)
Brain abscess	Penetrating brain injuries	Post-neurosurgery
Peritonitis/intra-abdominal abscess	Perforated hollow viscus	Post-surgical
Urinary tract infection	Pelvic trauma	Use of indwelling urinary catheters
Osteomyelitis	Open fractures	Secondary to central line infections
Wound infection	Direct contamination at time of injury	Hospital acquired infection
Bacteraemia	Complicating infection introduced at the time of injury	Indwelling vascular line; manipulation of infected tissues
Septicaemia	Complicating infection introduced at the time of injury	Surgery involving infected tissues

DIAGNOSIS

Diagnosing infection in the severely injured child is made more difficult by the fact that the injuries themselves may lead to signs of infection such as fever, hyperdynamic circulation, leukocytosis and raised inflammatory markers. There should be a low index of suspicion for taking blood cultures and cultures from appropriate sites. The problem with positive cultures from open wounds is that it is often difficult to distinguish between colonisation and infection. It may be necessary to use empirical antibiotics, which should be used in courses that are as short as possible so as minimise the emergence of resistant pathogens.

In infections occurring early after injury the predominating causative organisms include *Staphylococcus aureus*, coliforms and *Pseudomonas aeruginosa*. Later hospital-acquired infection may be with these organisms or with resistant organisms such as methicillin-resistant *Staphylococcus aureus* (MRSA) and vancomycin-resistant *Enterococcus* (VRE). Fungal infections may also occur.

PREVENTION OF INFECTION

Careful wound toilet and early removal of nonviable tissue will reduce the incidence of infection. Abscesses and other infections should be sought and drained in patients with ongoing signs of infection. The role of prophylactic antibiotics is debated; Table 12.2 shows some of the injuries in which there is good evidence that these should be used.

A recent meta-analysis showed that there was no benefit in giving prophylactic antibiotics to patients with basal skull fractures and CSF leakage.

Other prophylactic measures will include checking tetanus immunisation status and immunising if appropriate. Whether lifelong penicillin prophylaxis is required after splenectomy is not fully established. It may be that susceptibility to infection after post-traumatic splenectomy is less than after splenectomy for other reasons. However in the paediatric age group it is sensible at least to initiate prophylaxis in the immediate post-splenectomy period and reassess the patient at a later stage by looking at responsiveness to polysaccharide vaccines and other markers of splenic function such as the presence of circulating Howell–Jolly bodies. Such patients should also be immunised with pneumococcal and meningococcal vaccines.

The use of immune-modulating agents in the traumatised patient may have some role in the future but these are largely untried at present. The use of this treatment in other forms of injury has less theoretical basis and has not been evaluated. Haematopoietic growth factors such as granulocyte colony stimulating factor (GCSF), aimed at correcting the neutrophil dysfunction following trauma and burn injury, and interferon-gamma, which may compensate for the T-cell anergy and macrophage dysfunction that follows major injury, offer promise but are not yet evaluated.

MANAGEMENT OF THE INJURED CHILD WITH ESTABLISHED INFECTION

This should be along general lines used in the treatment of children with infection in intensive care settings. Empirical antibiotic treatment is often necessary and the choice of antibiotics depends on the site of possible infection as well as the time elapsed since the injury. If the child is already on a prophylactic antibiotic regimen a switch of antibiotic may be necessary.

Table 12.2 Injuries in which prophylactic antibiotics are indicated

Injury	Antibiotic prophylaxis
Open fracture	Flucloxacillin
Facial fracture	Co-amoxiclav
Ruptured abdominal hollow viscus	Azlocillin or cefotaxime + aminoglycoside + metronidazole
Burns	Penicillin ± a topical antimicrobial treatment (e.g. sulphadiazine)
Ruptured spleen (requiring splenectomy)	Penicillin

After injury, most early infections are caused by the patient's own endogenous flora and if there is no pre-existing medical condition these are likely to be antibiotic-sensitive. Empirical antibiotic regimens should therefore cover these organisms and a combination such as flucloxacillin, an aminoglycoside and a ureidopenicillin such as azlocillin will cover most of the likely organisms. The choice should be rationalised as early as possible when culture results are available. Later in the hospital course, especially following prophylactic antibiotic regimens, the patient is likely to be colonised with nosocomially acquired organisms. Therefore, suspected infection developing at this stage may require a broader-spectrum range of antimicrobials including an antifungal agent and, if the patient is known to be colonised with MRSA , a glycopeptide antibiotic to cover this infection. Vancomycin-resistant *Enterococcus* is a particular worry in this context. Routine surveillance cultures are useful in guiding therapy by indicating likely colonising organisms but over-reliance on these may be dangerous as sepsis may follow new acquisition of bacteria or fungi.

Failure to respond to antibiotic treatment should prompt a search for occult focal sepsis, which may include sinusitis, cholecystitis or intra-abdominal abscess.

OTHER SPECIFIC INJURIES

Burns

The use of intravenous immunoglobulin therapy in burns patients to replace IgG losses has been shown to be of no benefit. Prophylactic regimens vary widely between units. Topical silver sulphadiazine applied at least daily has been shown to reduce nosocomial infections. There is also fairly general agreement that penicillin prophylaxis is beneficial immediately after the burn and again after skin grafting.

Head injuries

A meta-analysis of the use of antibiotics after basal skull fracture with CSF leak showed no reduction in infections. A watching brief should therefore be adopted.

The use of dexamethasone to reduce brain swelling will enhance susceptibility to infections, especially fungal and especially if other injuries are present.

Closed head injuries can be associated with occult development of cerebral abscess.

Bites

Animal bites in children most frequently involve dogs and cats. There is a wide range of potential organisms that may be inoculated into the bite wound. These include common organisms such as *Staphylococcus aureus* but also less common species, including *Pasteurella multocida* and anaerobes. A prophylactic antibiotic should be given and wound debridement if appropriate. The antibiotic which is most likely to cover the wide range of organisms is co-amoxiclav or, in penicillin-allergic children, a macrolide such as clarithromycin or azithromycin. These antibiotics are also appropriate for human bites. Rabies prophylaxis is indicated if an animal bite occurs in a country in which the disease is endemic (see Chapter 90).

An additional consideration after human bites is the risk of hepatitis B transmission; prophylaxis should be considered.

FURTHER READING

Allgower M, Durig M, Wolff G (1980) Infection and trauma. Surg Clin North Am 60: 133–144.

Monafo WW (1996) Initial management of burns. N Engl J Med 335: 1581–1586.

Rathore H (1991) Do prophylactic antibiotics prevent meningitis after basilar skull fractures? Pediatr Infect Dis J 10: 87–88.

Saffle JR, Davis B, Williams P (1995) Recent outcomes in the treatment of burn injury in the US: a report from the American Burn Association Patients Registry. J Burn Care Rehabil 16:219–232.

Stillwell M, Caplan ES (1989) The septic multiple trauma patient. Infect Dis North Am Clin 3: 155–183.

Talan DA, Citrin DM, Abrahamian FM, Moran GJ, Goldstein EJ (1999) Bacteriological analysis of infected dog and cat bites. Emergency medicine animal bite infection study group. N Engl J Med 340: 85–92.

13 The child with an implant infection

CATHETER-RELATED INFECTIONS

Catheter-related infections are important causes of mortality and morbidity in children. Infection rate varies with the type of catheter and location. The risk of bacteraemia or fungaemia is greater for patients with central lines than with peripheral cannulae. The development of indwelling central venous line access has revolutionised the management of children with cancer, those requiring long-term total parenteral nutrition (TPN), and critically ill patients requiring intensive care support. The downside has been the increasing incidence of bacteraemia/sepsis and superficial catheter-related infections, as well other types of complication such as vascular thrombosis.

CENTRAL VENOUS CATHETERS

Although percutaneously placed central venous catheters are most commonly used for gaining short-term vascular access, they are not suitable for patients requiring long-term access for administration of chemotherapy or TPN. In these cases, either a cuffed, tunnelled catheter (Broviac or

Hickman) or a totally implanted device (Port-A-Cath) is used. In the former system, the catheter is first placed into a central vein (e.g. superior vena cava) and then passed through a subcutaneous tunnel before exiting the skin. A Port-A-Cath consists of a similar system but the catheter is attached distally to a subcutaneous reservoir; access is via needle puncture of intact skin through to the reservoir.

Classification of infections

Infections can occur at the site of insertion, in the subcutaneous tunnel and in the blood stream. Thus they can be divided into:

- superficial infections
  - exit-site infections
  - tunnel infections
- systemic catheter-related infections
  - bacteraemia/sepsis
  - septic thrombosis
  - endocarditis.

Exit-site infections are characterised by the presence of erythema, induration and purulence at the point of catheter exit, while in tunnel infections erythema and induration are present along the whole length of the subcutaneous tract (or subcutaneous port). Bacteraemia and sepsis are the most common manifestations of systemic catheter-related infections. Superficial infections are occasionally associated with a bacteraemia; however, systemic infections are not usually associated with a coexistent exit site or tunnel infection.

Epidemiology/incidence

Infection rates vary depending on the type of catheter used, the age of the patient and underlying disease. Rates are higher in neonates, patients receiving parenteral nutrition and HIV-infected patients, compared to patients with cancer. Accumulated data suggest an overall rate of 2–3 infections per 1000 days of catheter use for Broviac and Hickman lines, with around half being systemic infections. Infection rates for Port-A-Cath are lower at 0.5 per 1000 days. Neonates and patients receiving total parenteral nutrition (TPN) have infection rates of around 4–5/1000 days. The longer the duration of catheter insertion the higher the risk of infection, although most infections tend to occur in the first month after placement of the catheter. Patients with double- and triple-lumen catheters tend to have higher infection rates than those with single-lumen catheters.

Aetiology

See Table 13.1.

Pathogenesis

Organisms tend to be introduced at the time of insertion of the catheter and during periods of manipulation and use. They also gain access by colonising the skin surface and migrating along the catheter tract. Rarely,

Table 13.1 Pathogens responsible for catheter-related sepsis (Adapted from Tapiero and Lebel 1995)

Agent	Percentage of cases
Gram-positive cocci – Coagulase-negative staphylococci (35%) – *Staphylococcus aureus* – Enterococci	71
Gram-negative bacilli – *Klebsiella* spp. – *Escherichia coli* – *Pseudomonas* spp.	20
Fungi – *Candida* spp. – *Malassezia furfur*	6
Multiple organisms	3

the catheter can become infected secondary to a bacteraemia originating at a distant site. The host responds to the presence of a foreign body by coating it with a biofilm (plasma, tissue proteins and fibrin), which is believed to play a role in the adherence of organisms to the catheter surface as well as protecting the microbes from host defences. Some coagulase-negative staphylococci (CNS) produce a 'slime' substance that embeds the bacteria in the biofilm and results in the organisms gaining better adherence to the catheter surface.

Clinical manifestations and diagnosis

Superficial infections are characterised by the presence of erythema, tenderness, induration or purulence at the exit site or along the subcutaneous tract or port. The aetiological agent may be identified by performing a Gram stain, an acid-fast bacilli stain and microbial cultures (bacterial and fungal) from exudate obtained at the site.

The hallmark of systemic catheter-related infections is the onset of fever in the absence of any other obvious source of infection. Rigors that occur after flushing the catheter are particularly suggestive of organisms being released into the blood stream. The presence of embolic phenomena (retina, skin, kidneys) also suggests systemic infection. Malfunctioning catheters should also be assumed to be infected. It is advisable in these latter two circumstances to obtain an ultrasound of the catheter to exclude the presence of a thrombus on the end of the line or the presence of vegetations. It is the practice in some centres to obtain two blood cultures, one from the central line and one from a peripheral vein. The number of colony-forming units (cfu) is then compared from these two sources. Catheter-related sepsis is suggested when the colony count is significantly higher in blood obtained from the catheter. When the catheter specimen is positive and the peripheral sample negative on blood culture, this is suggestive of 'colonisation'. The patient is nevertheless at increased risk of a bacteraemic episode. When there is little difference in colony counts between the two cultures, the scenario is suggestive of a non-catheter-related sepsis/bacteraemia. However in most centres in the UK, and especially in children with cancer, blood cultures are usually only taken from the central line; catheter-related sepsis is assumed when a microorganism (especially a skin commensal) is isolated and there are clinical manifestations of bacteraemia or sepsis, and there is no other apparent focus of infection.

Management

Superficial infections (Table 13.2)

Exit-site infections are generally treated with local therapy, which involves cleaning the site with chlorhexidine and the application of a topical antibiotic (e.g. mupirocin) followed by a sterile dressing. Occasionally, systemic antimicrobials may also be required in the immunocompromised host or in those patients with signs of sepsis. Tunnel infections (or Port-A-Cath infections) generally require removal of the catheter and the administration, intravenously, of empirical antibiotics. Incision and drainage of the tract may be required in some patients.

Systemic catheter-related infections

The infection should initially be treated with an empirical combination of antibiotics administered through the catheter. In double- and triple-lumen catheters, the administration of antibiotics may be rotated around the different ports, on a regular basis, for the first few days. If blood cultures remain positive beyond 3–5 days, the catheter is removed and antibiotics are given via a peripheral line. Catheters should also be removed immediately in those patients with Gram-negative bacteraemia and septic shock. Empirical therapy generally consists of either vancomycin alone or in combination with a third-generation cephalosporin (e.g. ceftazidime) in the non-

Table 13.2 Pathogens responsible for superficial (tunnel/exit-site) infections (Adapted from Tapiero and Lebel 1995)

Agent	Percentage of cases
Gram-positive cocci – S. aureus (16%) – S. epidermidis (14%)	52
Gram-negative bacilli – Pseudomonas spp. (16%)	40
Miscellaneous – Bacillus spp. – Micrococcus spp.	6
Fungi	2

neutropenic patient. Combination therapy would certainly be indicated if there were signs of sepsis. In the neutropenic patient, standard empirical therapy is commenced (e.g. piptazobactam + aminoglycoside) with vancomycin pending the results of the blood cultures. Repeat cultures should be collected and treatment is usually continued for a period of 7–10 days following a negative culture. If fungi are isolated, the catheter should ideally be removed immediately and amphotericin B commenced. A 2-week course of antifungals may be adequate if there is no evidence of any disseminated fungal disease. Atypical mycobacterial infections also call for removal of the line and the administration of a combination of agents with broad antimycobacterial spectrum (e.g. ciprofloxacin, amikacin, clarithromycin).

Associated complications

The presence of an associated thrombus within the central venous line (or on the tip) requires the administration of urokinase as adjunctive therapy, along with the antibiotics. If an atrial thrombus has developed, a longer course of antibiotics is required (as per endocarditis), along with catheter removal and probable surgical excision of the thrombus. Endocarditis, characterised by the presence of valve vegetations and detected by echocardiogram, requires 4–6 weeks of antibiotics and removal of catheter.

Prevention

Education of personnel responsible for catheter care (including parents) is paramount. Local regimens developed for catheter care should be evidence-based and adhered to. Infection rates tend to be lower when catheter care is provided by a specially designated team. Many centres use povidone-iodine applications to the exit site along with dry gauze dressings. The use of heparinised flush solutions containing small quantities of vancomycin has been shown to have no effect on the incidence of Gram-positive catheter-related bacteraemia. The future will see the use of catheters with antibiotics (and heparin) bonded to their surface.

CEREBROSPINAL FLUID SHUNT INFECTIONS

Most shunting procedures involve the use of ventriculo-peritoneal (VP) catheters, and are carried out for the treatment of hydrocephalus. Infections involve the skin flora inoculated at the time of surgical insertion. The aetiology and pathogenesis are similar to catheter-related infections, with *Staphylococcus epidermidis* (> 60%), *S. aureus*, other skin commensals and Gram-negative bacilli being most commonly involved. Infections generally become manifest in the first month after shunt insertion; many are limited to febrile episodes without evident meningitis. Infection rates vary (5–20%) but tend to be higher in younger patients, those undergoing repeat procedures and infants with myelomeningocele.

Clinical manifestations

Symptoms of a shunt infection include fever (variable), nausea, vomiting, lethargy, irritability and drowsiness. Some of these symptoms are a result of shunt malfunction. A shunt series X-ray should be obtained to rule out the possibility of disconnection. Occasionally, shunt malfunctions may lead to an acute shunt blockage and indeed a medical emergency with the development of signs of raised intracranial pressure with or without papilloedema. A computed tomography (CT) scan of the head should be obtained in these circumstances. Some patients may have a shunt wound infection, cellulitis of the shunt tract, a picture of sepsis, or abdominal distension with signs of peritonitis (VP shunts). An ultrasound of the abdomen may be helpful in the assessment of this latter group. It must be remembered that most children with ventriculoperitoneal shunts in situ who develop a fever probably have a coexistent upper respiratory tract infection, although obviously a thorough assessment is required. Patients with infected ventriculo-atrial (VA) shunts may have an associated bacteraemia and may develop an immune-complex glomerulonephritis.

Diagnosis

CSF samples are obtained from the shunt tubing or reservoir using aseptic techniques. The presence of a pleocytosis (with a predominance of neutrophils), elevated protein levels and lowish glucose concentrations are suggestive of a shunt infection. A Gram stain may be positive; however a definitive diagnosis depends on isolation of a microbial agent from CSF cultures. In the absence of a CSF sample, measurement of inflammatory markers such as C-reactive protein may provide evidence to support a bacterial infection. A CT scan of the head may show increased ventricular dilatation associated with shunt malfunction.

Management

Empirical antibiotics (vancomycin plus ceftazidime/cefotaxime) are commenced to cover the likely pathogens pending results of cultures and sensitivities. Ideally, the VP shunt is removed and replaced with an external ventricular drainage system (EVD). CSF fluid samples taken from the EVD system (closed portion) should be sent off daily for cell count, biochemistry, Gram stain and bacterial culture. Once-daily intraventricular antibiotics (vancomycin or gentamicin) are given if there is a poor response to intravenous therapy (persistently positive CSF cultures or little in the way of clinical improvement). Ideally, antibiotic levels in the CSF (ventricular fluid) should be monitored regularly in these patients. Treatment is usually continued for a period of 7–10 days following negative CSF cultures. A new shunt is then reinserted at the end of therapy (re-internalisation). Unfortunately in a small proportion of patients, superinfection of the external ventricular drainage system develops, requiring replacement of the system and further antibiotics.

Complications

Potential complications include brain damage due to the ventriculitis and the development of peritonitis and/or bowel perforation. Nephritis and endocarditis are complications of VA shunts.

Prevention

Good surgical technique at the time of insertion of the shunt, and during any further later manipulation of the VP shunt, is essential. Antibiotic prophylaxis is controversial, but most neurosurgical units tend to give either an antistaphylococcal agent 2 hours preoperatively and repeated postoperatively, or intravenous or intrashunt vancomycin preoperatively only.

FURTHER READING

Salzman MB, Rubin LG (1995) Intravenous catheter-related infections. Adv Pediatr Infect Dis 10: 337–368.

Tapiero B, Lebel MH (1995) Bacteraemia, sepsis and septic shock. In: Jenson HB, Baltimore, RS (eds) Pediatric infectious diseases – principles and practice. Appleton & Lange, Norwalk, CT: pp 347–367.

Yogev R (1993) Central nervous system shunt infections. In: Kaplan SL (ed.) Current therapy in pediatric infectious diseases, 3rd edn. Mosby/Year Book, St Louis, MO: pp 155–158.

14 The child with bone or joint infection

Acute osteomyelitis, an infection of the bone, usually arises by haematogenous spread of bacteria and most commonly arises in the metaphyseal region of one of the larger bones. It may spread to involve the adjacent joint, giving rise to an accompanying pyogenic arthritis. Rarely, it may be multifocal. Up to 10% of cases arise by direct extension from an adjacent infected focus or from a penetrating injury.

Acute pyogenic arthritis may occur as an extension of osteomyelitis or may arise by haematogenous spread without any overt signs of bony involvement. Most cases are monoarticular (usually hip, knee, ankle or elbow) but in about 10% of cases multiple joints are affected.

AETIOLOGY

The majority (around three-quarters) of acute bone and joint infections are caused by *Staphylococcus aureus*. The primary focus of staphylococcal infection leading to bacteraemia is usually not evident. *Haemophilus influenzae* type b (Hib) is now a rare cause of septic arthritis since the introduction of the Hib vaccination programme. Gram-negative bacilli (particularly *Salmonella* spp.), *Neisseria meningitidis*, *Streptococcus pyogenes* and *S. pneumoniae* are other important causes. Gram-negative bacilli are more likely to be the cause in compromised individuals such as neonates, those with immune deficiency or sickle cell diseases. In the neonatal period group B streptococcus is an important cause of osteomyelitis and vertically transmitted *Neisseria gonorrhoeae* can cause pyogenic arthritis (see Chapter 55). Osteomyelitis, often multifocal, caused by nontuberculous mycobacteria is seen in patients with advanced HIV disease and other immunodeficiencies.

CLINICAL FEATURES

In acute cases there is usually a short history (< 24 hours) and the child is ill-looking and feverish. There is a refusal to move the affected limb or to weight-bear on an affected leg. In osteomyelitis there is usually swelling overlying the bone and tenderness. In pyogenic arthritis the affected joint is hot, swollen and tender. In subacute or chronic osteomyelitis the child appears less ill, may not be febrile and the local signs are less acute.

DIAGNOSIS AND MANAGEMENT

In most acute cases the diagnosis can be made clinically. Orthopaedic surgeons should be involved at an early stage and ideally the child's management should be jointly supervised by the paediatric and orthopaedic teams. Particularly in the case of the hip joint, the serious implications of a missed diagnosis make management of suspected arthritis a matter of urgency.

Investigations will show a raised white cell count, sedimentation rate and C-reactive protein. (The last two are also useful in monitoring response to treatment.) Radiographs initially show no bony changes but may show soft tissue swelling and joint effusions (bone changes such as periosteal reaction and areas of rarefaction take at least 10 days to develop). If there is doubt, isotope bone scan will confirm an inflammatory process in joint or bone from a very early stage, except in neonates (see Chapter 4). Blood cultures (multiple if possible) should be taken and are positive in approximately 40% of cases of pyogenic arthritis and 60% of acute osteomyelitis. In septic arthritis, microscopy and culture of aspirated joint fluid and, when appropriate, tests for Hib, *S. pneumoniae* and group B streptococcal antigens in urine or joint fluid may increase the diagnostic rate. Tests for anti-staphylococcal antibody are generally disappointing in children.

The differential diagnosis of osteomyelitis will include trauma (consider nonaccidental injury) and malignancies such as leukaemia, neuroblastoma or osteosarcoma. In acute monoarthritis the differential diagnosis includes: reactive arthritis, which may follow a viral, bacterial or *Mycoplasma* infection; nonpyogenic infections such as tuberculosis; haemarthrosis; vasculitis such as Henoch–Schönlein purpura (arthritis may precede onset of the rash); juvenile idiopathic arthritis; or malignancy. A subacute onset or multiple joint involvement may help distinguish these, but if in doubt a diagnostic tap may be required.

The mainstay of treatment is appropriate antibiotic therapy with or without surgical intervention. In pyogenic arthritis drainage of the joint should always be performed and at the same time the joint space is usually washed out. This is both therapeutically and diagnostically useful. In acute osteomyelitis with a short history, no bony changes on radiographs and no underlying diseases, it is reasonable to treat empirically with antibiotics and reserve surgical exploration for cases that fail to respond clinically or develop complications. If the child has an underlying disorder the infecting organism may be unusual. Therefore in these cases primary surgical exploration is often indicated.

Initial antibiotic treatment should be given intravenously in high dosage. Empirical treatment before culture results are available can be given with flucloxacillin and ampicillin in the child over 6 years or flucloxacillin and cefotaxime (the latter to cover β-lactamase-producing *Haemophilus influenzae*) in the child under 6 years. When culture results are available antibiotics can be modified – the combination of flucloxacillin and sodium fusidate provides good antistaphylococcal treatment while ampicillin is used for streptococcal and non-β-lactamase-producing *H. influenzae* infections. Other antibiotics that may be useful are clindamycin and second-generation cephalosporins. In *Salmonella* osteomyelitis, ampicillin, co-trimoxazole or ciprofloxacin (NB: not licensed for use in children in the UK) may be used depending on the sensitivity of the organism.

Intravenous antibiotic therapy should be continued for a minimum of 3 days or until the fever has been settled for 48 hours, whichever is the longer. Thereafter oral antibiotic therapy is continued for 3–4 weeks for septic arthritis or 4–6 weeks in osteomyelitis. Measurement of serum bactericidal levels may be useful in ensuring adequate oral therapy, especially when there is an unusual causal organism or there is evidence of persisting inflammation (e.g. persisting high erythrocyte sedimentation rate or C-reactive protein). For complicated cases, including those with underlying disorders and particularly if the causative organism has not been isolated, it is prudent to continue giving the antibiotics by the intravenous route for a longer period of time (such as 2–3 weeks) even if there is apparent early clinical response. In chronic osteomyelitis very prolonged antibiotic treatment as well as surgery is required.

FURTHER READING

Davies EG, Monsell F (2000) Managing the child with osteoarticular infection. Curr Pediatr 10: 42–48.

15 The child with an upper respiratory tract infection

The upper respiratory tract consists of the ears, nose, throat, tonsils, pharynx and sinuses. Upper respiratory tract infections (URTI) are common at all ages and especially in young children. Many of these are minor and self-limiting but they may also be associated with considerable morbidity, e.g. the association between febrile convulsions and URTI, or wheezy illness and URTI. Some of these infections are life-threatening because of upper airway obstruction, e.g. epiglottitis or diphtheria.

Most children have several URTIs each year in their first decade. Preschool children attending day care are likely to have more frequent infections than those remaining in the home, particularly in the absence of older siblings. When there is a history of very frequent infections, particularly otitis media and sinusitis, immunoglobulin deficiency should be considered. The most likely is an IgA or IgG subclass deficiency (see Chapter 21).

COMMON COLD (ACUTE CORYZA)

Organisms Rhinovirus, adenovirus, coronavirus, respiratory syncytial virus (RSV).

Incubation period Adenovirus 10–14 days; rhinovirus 2–4 days; coronavirus 2–4 days, RSV 2–8 days.

Transmission Direct droplet spread, faecal–oral transmission.

Clinical features and natural history Fever, rhinorrhoea, sneezing, cough. Poor feeding, especially if nose blocked.

Management Symptomatic, antipyretics. Some small infants with a troublesome blocked nose will benefit from gentle cleaning of nose and saline nose drops. Some infants may benefit from a short course of decongestant drops.

PHARYNGITIS AND TONSILLITIS

Organisms Adenovirus, group A β-haemolytic streptococcus, Epstein–Barr virus, *Corynebacterium diphtheriae*.

Clinical features and natural history Fever, sore throat, cervical lymphadenopathy, tonsillar enlargement. It is impossible to distinguish viral infection from bacterial infection clinically – there may be fever and exudative tonsillitis in both. Adenoviral infection is more likely in children less than 3 years old. In some children with already enlarged tonsils, acute infection may cause severe upper airway obstruction. Diphtheria is rare in the more affluent areas of the world because of routine immunisation but may still occur. There have been recent outbreaks in Russia. Consider this diagnosis in an unimmunised individual who presents with a sore throat and a spreading grey adherent membrane over the tonsils and pharynx.

Management Children with streptococcal infection need treatment with antibiotic because of the consequences of immune complex disease associated with group A β-haemolytic streptococcus (glomerulonephritis, rheumatic fever). Children with streptococcal tonsillitis should be given an antibiotic. The antibiotic of choice is penicillin (erythromycin or other macrolide penicillin-allergic individuals) and must be for 10 days to minimise the risk of relapse. With the difficulty in distinguishing between acute bacterial and viral tonsillitis, children will receive unnecessary antibiotic unless a rapid microbiological diagnosis can be made. There is usually a rapid clinical response in children with bacterial infection – those with viral infection continue to have symptoms and fever. Occasionally, severe tonsillar obstruction will require management with a nasopharyngeal airway.

PERITONSILLAR ABSCESS (QUINSY)
This is more common in adolescents and young adults than young children. It follows severe tonsillitis and will cause a very sore throat, severe dysphagia and asymmetrical tonsillar swelling. The treatment is surgical drainage with intravenous antibiotics and subsequent tonsillectomy.

RETROPHARYNGEAL ABSCESS
This is an unusual condition following bacterial pharyngitis in young infants. There is stridor, fever, drooling, swelling of the neck and lymphadenopathy. This requires surgical drainage and penicillin.

OTITIS MEDIA
Organisms Pneumococcus, *Haemophilus influenzae* (non-type-B), group B streptococci, *Moxarella* (previously *Branhamella*) *catarrhalis*, anaerobes such as *Fusobacterium*, adenovirus, influenza, RSV and parainfluenza viruses.

Clinical features Fever, vomiting, irritability, inconsolable crying. Older children can localise pain to their ears or complain of deafness and dizziness. It is important to carefully examine the ears of all ill children. The ear drum becomes acutely inflamed and may bulge; there is a loss of the normal light reflex. Acute perforation may occur – this often relieves the pain. Recurrent otitis media may lead to glue ear with hearing loss.

Management Relieve pain and fever. Antibiotics are commonly used, although many of these infections are viral. (There is considerable controversy about the role of infection in chronic otitis media with effusion.) In older children penicillin is appropriate because of the incidence of pneumococcal infection, but choose a broad-spectrum antibiotic in children younger than 3 years. Myringotomy is used to treat children with glue ear associated with hearing loss. It is not clear that this is more effective than conservative treatment.

SINUSITIS
The maxillary sinuses increase in size from birth and are usually visible on X-ray between 2 and 4 years, by which time the sphenoidal sinuses have also developed. Frontal sinuses are usually not involved in acute infection until school age.

Organisms Pneumococci, *Haemophilus influenzae* (mainly non-typable), group A streptococci, staphylococci.

Clinical features and natural history Fever, headache, pain and localised tenderness. Complications include orbital cellulitis and very rarely intracranial spread (subdural empyema).

Management Broad-spectrum antibiotics. Consider possibility of intracranial spread if severe headaches develop and always in the presence of neurological abnormality – need CT scan.

ACUTE LARYNGOTRACHEOBRONCHITIS (CROUP)

This is a very common condition of young children, most frequently occurring between the ages of 6 months and 4 years.

Organisms Parainfluenza, influenza, respiratory syncytial virus and rhinovirus.

Clinical features In many instances it is mild. Following coryzal symptoms, a harsh barking characteristic cough develops that is typically worse at night or when the child is upset. The symptoms are intermittent and are improved at rest and the child looks pink, is well perfused and able to drink fluids. In more severe cases there may be increasingly severe respiratory difficulty with chest wall retraction, tachypnoea, tachycardia, agitation and hypoxia.

Management Most children can be managed at home with antipyretics and fluids but parents should be asked to seek help if the child becomes increasingly distressed and agitated. (There is often concern that a child with severe croup may have epiglottitis – it is usually easy to clinically differentiate between the two conditions (Table 15.1) but if the croup is very severe the management will be the same – intubation under controlled anaesthetic conditions.) This is needed in about 5% of cases of croup,

The administration of steroids reduces the severity of symptoms in croup – it does not affect the duration of symptoms. Children with moderate or severe croup (stridor or recession at rest) should be given steroids, which should reduce the need for intubation. Nebulised budesonide has been found to be helpful in croup but it is an expensive drug and the same effect can be achieved with one or more doses of oral dexamethasone, 0.15 mg/kg 12-hourly.

The child with moderate or severe croup needs careful observation. Observe the child's colour, respiratory rate, heart rate and chest wall movement. Keep the parent close to the child. Most children will be able to be discharged quickly. Make sure that the nursing staff have clear guidelines as to when to call for medical help. Review the child frequently if there is deterioration. The child with croup may respond to nebulised adrenaline, 3–5 mL of 1 in 1000 solution, given through oxygen. This effect may last for up to 2 hours. The child needing regular nebulised adrenaline is a child who needs regular observation. Pulse oximetry is helpful and noninvasive. Give oxygen as necessary. Although there are anecdotes about the value of humidity in this condition, frightening a child by placing him/her in a mist tent is counterproductive. If the child is very agitated and thrashing around, it is likely that s/he is hypoxic: give oxygen. If the child is deteriorating, becoming hypoxic or extremely agitated, contact an anaesthetist as the child will need intubation. Each hospital should have guidelines as to which senior medical staff are called to a child with an upper airway obstruction. In some hospitals the ENT surgeon is also called.

75

15 URTI

ACUTE EPIGLOTTITIS

This is a septicaemic illness caused almost always by *Haemophilus influenzae* type b, producing inflammation and swelling of the epiglottis and subsequent respiratory obstruction. (Other organisms are implicated: pneumococcus, *Staphylococcus aureus*.) This is much less common since the introduction of Hib vaccine.

Clinical features   There is acute onset of fever and sore throat. The child may have a muffled voice and drool because of difficulty in swallowing. The child appears unwell, toxic and lethargic. Stridor is quiet. There may be marked tachycardia but the child may be breathing slowly and carefully. Children with epiglottitis adopt a position that is most comfortable for themselves – often leaning forward. Epiglottitis is a medical emergency as the swollen epiglottis may produce severe airway obstruction.

Management   Keep the child calm with the parents while arranging urgent anaesthetic help and intubation. An experienced anaesthetist and ENT surgeon are required in case the child requires an emergency tracheostomy because of failed intubation (fortunately rare.) Do not attempt to examine the throat, take blood or insert a cannula – this should be done once the airway is secured by intubation. There is no place for lateral X-ray of neck in the diagnosis of acute upper airway obstruction. Treat with intravenous antibiotic – cefuroxime or cefotaxime. Recovery is usually rapid and the child may be extubated within 24 hours.

BACTERIAL TRACHEITIS

Organisms   *Staphylococcus aureus*, *Haemophilus influenzae* type b.

Clinical features   It may complicate laryngotracheobronchitis or may occur as primary infection. Children with Down's syndrome are especially at risk. It presents like severe croup but with fever and rapidly progressive airway obstruction. Always consider this diagnosis in a child with upper respiratory tract obstruction who is deteriorating. It requires intubation and intravenous antibiotic.

FURTHER READING

Fahey T, Stocks N, Thomas T (1998) Systematic review of the treatment of upper respiratory tract infection. Arch Dis Child 79: 225–230.

Kilham HA, McEniery JA (1991) Acute upper airways obstruction. Current Paediatrics 1: 17–25.

Macdonald WBG, Geelhoed GC (1997) Management of childhood croup: Thorax 52: 757–759.

Table 15.1 The child with laryngotracheitis versus tracheitis or epiglottitis (see also Table 16.3 for distinguishing these conditions from bronchiolitis and pneumonia)

	Laryngotracheobronchitis	Tracheitis or epiglottitis
Onset	Acute	Acute
Fever	Occasionally	Common
Progression	Tends to be worse at night	Little diurnal variation
General condition	Good	Often shows signs of septicaemia
Episodes of cyanosis	No (unless very severe)	Yes
Treatment	Supportive unless very severe – steroids have a place (dexamethasone)	Usually endotracheal intubation and systemic antibiotics

16 The child with a lower respiratory tract infection

EPIDEMIOLOGY

The respiratory tract is the commonest site of childhood infections and acute respiratory infections make up 50% of all illnesses in children under 5 years. Most involve only the upper respiratory tract but about 5% will involve the larynx and lower respiratory tract and may be more serious. Lower respiratory tract illnesses (LRTIs) are commonest in the first year of life. The incidence of about 20–25 episodes/1000 children/year over the first 2 years decreases with age to around 5/1000 children/year in 9–15-year-olds. During the first decade, LRTIs occur more commonly in boys but thereafter the rates are similar between the sexes. Hospitalisation rates vary considerably but it has been estimated that one in 20 children will be hospitalised because of respiratory infection during the first 4 years of life. LRTIs show marked and unexplained seasonal variations, being commonest in the coldest months. This is particularly striking for the annual winter–spring epidemics of bronchiolitis and pneumonia due to respiratory syncytial virus (RSV) in infants.

PATHOGENESIS

LRTIs develop by two routes. Most agents (respiratory viruses, *Mycoplasma pneumoniae*, *Bordetella pertussis* and *Chlamydia trachomatis*) produce infection by initial involvement of airway epithelium with progression into the parenchyma. The infection typically starts in the upper respiratory tract and then spreads to the lower. In contrast, others (bacteria and certain viruses – Epstein–Barr virus, cytomegalovirus and varicella-zoster virus) spread from the blood stream into the parenchyma and airways. The development and localisation of disease in the LRTIs then depends on a complex interaction between the organism, the host and environmental factors (Table 16.1).

While respiratory viral infections can involve more than one part of the respiratory tract, inflammation usually predominates at a single site. Certain organisms have affinities for particular parts of the respiratory tract, e.g. RSV for peripheral airways, for reasons that are not well understood. In most circumstances, viruses are only isolated from the respiratory tract during an acute infection. Commonly, one virus tends to predominate in a community at any particular time.

ORGANISMS

The spectrum of organisms that cause LRTIs is wide (Table 16.2) and varies with age. In the newborn, pneumonia is usually due to organisms acquired from the mother's genital tract before or during delivery, e.g. group B streptococci, Gram-negative bacteria, *Listeria monocytogenes*, *Chlamydia trachomatis*, *Mycoplasma hominis* and *Ureaplasma urealyticum*, cytomegalovirus (CMV) and herpes simplex virus (HSV). After the first month, over 90% of respiratory infections are due to viruses (RSV, parainfluenza, influenza, adenoviruses, rhinoviruses), *Chlamydia pneumoniae* or *Mycoplasma pneumoniae*. Mycoplasma infection rarely occurs before 3 months and is most common in schoolchildren.

Bacterial infections, particularly *Streptococcus pneumoniae* and *Haemophilus influenzae* (non-typable), causing LRTIs are thought to be uncommon in high-income countries. However, the relative importance of these organisms has been difficult to evaluate because of high carriage rates in the upper respiratory tract in normal children, Other causes of bacterial pneumonia, e.g. *Staphylococcus aureus*, are uncommon in normal children.

Bacterial superinfection during respiratory viral or mycoplasmal infections is uncommon in normal children. There are some well-recognised associations between viruses and bacterial infection, e.g. influenza and staphylococcal pneumonia, which are not understood. Dual viral infections do occur but seem to be uncommon. If they occur, they are often serious,

Table 16.1 Risk factors for lower respiratory tract infections in children

Host factors	Environmental factors
Age	Passive and active smoking
Sex	Exposure to infection via:
Low birth weight	Siblings
Neonatal lung injury	Domestic overcrowding
Congenital malformation	Day care
Bottle-feeding	Low socioeconomic status
Obesity	Atmospheric pollution

Table 16.2 Relative frequency of organisms causing community-acquired pneumonia in otherwise healthy children (Modified from Gilsdorf JR (1987) Community-acquired pneumonia in children. Semin Respir Infect 2: 146–151)

Most frequent	Occasional	Rare
Neonates (< 1 month)		
Group B streptococci	*Haemophilus influenzae*	*Mycobacterium* spp.
Escherichia coli	*Streptococcus pneumoniae*	*Chlamydia* spp.
Respiratory viruses	Group A streptococci	*Listeria monocytogenes*
Enteroviruses	*Staphylococcus aureus*	
		Varicella
		Cytomegalovirus
		Herpes simplex
Young infants (1–3 months)		
Febrile		
Respiratory viruses	Group B streptococci	Varicella
Enteroviruses	*S. pneumoniae*	CMV
	Group A streptococci	Mycobacteria
	H. influenzae	Gram-negative enteric
	Bordetella pertussis	bacilli
	Cytomegalovirus	
	Ureaplasma urealyticum	
	Pneumocystis carinii	
Afebrile		
Chlamydia	Cytomegalovirus	
Mycobacteria	*U. urealyticum*	
	Pneumocystis carinii	
Infants and young children (3 months–5 years)		
S. pneumoniae	*B. pertussis*	
Respiratory viruses	*S. aureus*	
	Group A streptococci	
	H. influenzae	
	Mycoplasma spp.	
	Mycobacteria	
Older children (> 5 years) and adolescents		
Mycoplasma pneumoniae		*S. aureus*
S. pneumoniae	*Chlamydia pneumoniae*	
Respiratory viruses	Mycobacteria	

e.g. measles and adenovirus. While the importance of host factors such as malnutrition or vitamin deficiency in superinfection or dual infections is not known, low body weight has been shown to be associated with impaired cell-mediated immunity.

Often the specific aetiology of LRTI cannot be determined, even in retrospect. Developments in microbial diagnostic technology, particularly techniques based on nucleic acid technology such as the polymerase chain reaction, are increasing the proportion of respiratory infections that can be identified definitively.

CLINICAL PRESENTATIONS AND DIAGNOSIS

The clinical features of LRTIs can include cough with tachypnoea, indrawing, wheeze or stridor. There are well-defined clinical syndromes (Table 16.3) and these clinical patterns are helpful in narrowing the range of likely infectious agents.

In infants, clinical features of pneumonia are often nonspecific and include fever > 38.5°C, refusal to breastfeed and vomiting. Between 1 and 4 years, fever (> 38.5°C) and tachypnoea may occur. The best single finding for ruling out pneumonia is the absence of tachypnoea. The respiratory rate is best measured by observing chest wall movements over 1 minute. Cut-offs that are commonly used to indicate an elevated rate are: > 60/min in infants younger than 2 months; > 50/min between 2 and 12 months; and > 40/min over 12 months. Bronchial breathing and reduced breath sounds are very specific but insensitive indicators of pneumonia. In infants, auscultation is relatively unreliable.

The gold standard for microbial diagnosis of pneumonia is an aspirate obtained from the lower respiratory tract by lung puncture or bronchoalveolar lavage. In clinical practice, chest X-ray films provide a pragmatic alternative. Chest X-rays will be indicated in children with fever and pulmonary findings such as tachypnoea, respiratory distress, decreased breath sounds or bronchial breathing. In the newborn and young infant, respiratory signs may be minimal and only nonspecific features such as apnoea, anorexia, lethargy or vomiting may be present. In infancy, chest X-rays in the absence of signs are rarely positive. In children with immunological deficiency or cardiorespiratory disease, the signs of LRTI may be less obvious and a higher index of suspicion is also needed. Unfortunately, chest X-ray changes in pneumonia are not accurate in distinguishing between bacterial and nonbacterial causes. Lobar or segmental consolidation is characteristic of bacterial pneumonia but bronchopneumonia and interstitial infiltrates can occur in bacterial pneumonia, as can alveolar infiltrates in viral pneumonia. An exception is a large pleural

Table 16.3 LRTI syndromes (infection at or below the larynx) and their clinical features

Syndrome	Presenting symptoms and signs
Croup*	Hoarseness, cough, inspiratory stridor with laryngeal obstruction
Tracheobronchitis*	Cough and ronchi; no laryngeal obstruction or wheezing
Bronchiolitis	Expiratory wheezing with or without tachypnoea, air trapping and indrawing
Pneumonia	Crackles or evidence of pulmonary consolidation on physical examination or chest X-ray

* See also Table 15.1 on page 75.

effusion where a bacterial origin is most likely. Chest X-ray findings may also be negative in early bacterial pneumonia.

For organisms entering via the respiratory tract, airway epithelial cells, sampled usually from the nasopharynx, provide excellent material for microbiological diagnosis. Viral isolation from the upper respiratory tract usually correlates with lower respiratory tract involvement. Rapid, sensitive and specific immunofluorescence tests are available for many viruses, most notably RSV, parainfluenza virus and influenza virus and are increasingly replacing serology and viral culture. Newer molecular diagnostic tests may eventually offer even greater sensitivity.

Unfortunately, it is often difficult to distinguish between viral and bacterial infections on the basis of clinical, haematological or radiological findings. Definite diagnosis of bacterial infections remains difficult. Some nonspecific tests may be useful. There may be a polymorphonuclear leukocytosis. C-reactive protein is more commonly raised in bacterial infections. Cold agglutinins frequently occur in *M. pneumoniae* infections, especially with more severe pulmonary involvement. Young children do not usually produce sputum. Culture of pharyngeal swabs is an unreliable substitute because symptomless nasopharyngeal colonisation with *S. pneumoniae* and *H. influenzae* occurs, particularly in preschool children. While needle aspiration of the lung is the gold standard for defining bacterial lung infection, it is not used frequently in developed countries. Studies using this technique have shown that blood cultures may be positive in as few as 10% of cases. Rapid, bacterial antigen detection tests have not proved particularly helpful in clinical practice. In the severely ill or immune-compromised child, more invasive procedures such as bronchoscopy with bronchoalveolar lavage or lung biopsy may be essential to guide therapy. Where positive, culture of blood or aspirated pleural fluid, if present, may confirm bacterial infection.

SPECIAL PROBLEMS

Immunosuppressed children

The lung is the commonest site of serious infection in immunosuppressed children. They are prone to infection, particularly when the absolute neutrophil count falls below $500/mm^3$. The risk increases with both the severity and duration of neutropenia. Neutropenia for longer than 2 weeks is associated with a high incidence of nosocomial bacterial and/or fungal infections. The array of potential pathogens is wide. Prompt, accurate diagnosis of LRTI is crucial but often very difficult in ill, immunocompromised children because of the lack of specificity of the clinical signs and the wide range of microorganisms encountered. Bronchoalveolar lavage (BAL) provides a safe and accurate method of diagnosis and may provide a specific diagnosis in 50–70% of cases.

Cystic fibrosis (CF)

Respiratory infection is the major source of morbidity and mortality in CF. The lungs are structurally normal at birth but with infection, and the associated chronic inflammation lung, damage develops. The spectrum of pathogens is unusual, with *S. aureus* common in the early years and *Pseudomonas aeruginosa* becoming predominant with increasing age. Prophylactic antistaphylococcal therapy from birth has been shown to improve clinical progress. Because earlier *Pseudomonas* acquisition is associated with worse pulmonary function and earlier mortality, there has been increasing emphasis on strategies, such as intensive antibiotic therapy at first colonisation, to delay chronic colonisation. Once mucoid *P. aeruginosa* becomes established, it is almost impossible to eliminate. Many other microorganisms, including *H. influenzae*, *Burkholderia cepacia*, viruses and more unusual organisms such as *Stenotrophomonas maltophilia*, *Aspergillus fumigatus* and atypical mycobacteria, may all cause LRTI in CF patients. Prevention of infection through good nutrition, regular physiotherapy and appropriate immunisation is the cornerstone of management. In exacerbations, appropriate antibiotic treatment guided by sputum microbiology generally results in clinical improvement. Cross-infection between patients has been increasingly documented, especially with *B. cepacia*. Patients colonised with *B. cepacia* should be kept strictly separate from those uncolonised.

TREATMENT

Treatment is most satisfactory when the causative agent is known and a specific and effective antimicrobial agent can be given.

Respiratory viruses, *C. pneumoniae* and *M. pneumoniae* cause most of the cases of tracheobronchitis, bronchiolitis and croup. Symptomatic mycoplasmal infections are uncommon in children under 5 years. Accordingly, antibiotics will not be indicated in most preschool children, especially if viral infection can be confirmed by rapid diagnostic techniques.

Treatment of RSV infection with nebulised ribavirin has usually been reserved for those at high risk of severe disease. However, there is considerably uncertainty about its efficacy and in many centres it is not now used.

In pneumonia, because of the difficulty of differentiating bacterial from viral infections, antibiotics should be prescribed, particularly for the very young or very sick. The child's age and the likely pathogen will determine the initial choice. Because of the emergence of resistant strains such as penicillin-resistant pneumococci, it is important that this choice is informed by knowledge of local microbial sensitivities. Therapy should be kept under careful review to take account of clinical progress and bacteriological sensitivities. Appropriate antibiotics for less severe cases managed at home would be oral amoxycillin for under-5-year-olds and a macrolide for those over 5 years (when *M. pneumoniae* is more likely). For severe cases requiring hospitalisation, intravenous cefotaxime plus a macrolide is a good empirical choice.

Supportive care and hospitalisation

Most children with LRTIs are managed in the community. Supportive care and antibiotics, where indicated, will be all that is required. Only about 10% will be admitted to hospital. In young children especially, this is usually needed because of respiratory distress, severe systemic features or difficulty feeding. In these more serious cases a number of specific points should be remembered:

Maintain an adequate airway and ensure oxygenation

Hypoxaemia is common. Excessive handling aggravates this and should be avoided. The development of noninvasive monitors has allowed oxygen saturation to be monitored routinely. Low-flow oxygen administered via nasal cannulae will often be sufficient to maintain the oxygen saturation in the normal range (above 95% after the first week of life). About 1–2% of infants with severe bronchiolitis will develop respiratory failure and need mechanical ventilation.

Maintain hydration and nutrition

Children with severe LRTIs often have difficulty feeding. Nasogastric or intravenous fluids may be necessary to avoid dehydration and maintain nutrition. Children with pneumonia and bronchiolitis can develop excessive antidiuretic hormone secretion so mild fluid restriction is usually advisable.

Clear nasal secretions and encourage sputum clearance

Gentle suction clearance of nasal secretions may increase comfort and aid feeding in infants. There is no evidence that physiotherapy is helpful in children with bronchiolitis or pneumonia but it may have an important role in those children where sputum clearance is impaired.

Drain pleural fluid

When present, it may be useful to aspirate fluid for diagnostic purposes. Therapeutic aspiration may only be necessary if breathing is compromised or if the clinical response to antibiotic treatment is poor. Pre-drainage localisation of the fluid and selection of the optimal drainage spot using ultrasound or CT scan is useful. Adequate sedation and analgesia will be necessary for safe and painless drainage, especially in infants and young children. In adults, the installation of intrapleural streptokinase has been shown to lead to greater fluid drainage, smaller effusions at discharge and reduced need for surgical treatment. A multicentre trial is under way evaluating this approach in children.

Hospital cross-infection

Many respiratory infections are highly infectious. Hospital-acquired respiratory infections are common, spread either by droplets (influenza) or by fomites (RSV). Cross-infection rates of up 25% with RSV infection have been noted in children in hospital for more than 7 days during winter epidemics. Such infections can be associated with significant morbidity and mortality in high-risk infants with immune-suppression or cardiorespiratory disease. Effective cross-infection procedures can reduce this rate substantially.

Follow-up

For children with pneumonia, careful clinical follow-up to check that the child is better and that signs have resolved is all that is necessary in uncomplicated cases. Further chest X-rays do not appear necessary if clinical resolution is occurring. In any child with an unusual, persistent or recurrent pneumonia an underlying disorder such as immune-deficiency, cystic fibrosis or a congenital lung disorder should be excluded.

OUTCOME

In developed countries, most LRTIs in children will resolve satisfactorily with appropriate treatment. However, LRTIs remain an important cause of childhood death. A few LRTIs, particularly with specific serotypes of adenovirus (e.g. 7), can cause lasting structural damage to the lung (bronchiolitis obliterans). The longer-term outcome remains controversial. A year after recovery from pneumonia, it has been found that children still have residual lung scan defects. Children with past respiratory illnesses show evidence of airways obstruction in later childhood. Young adults with a history of LRTI in the first 2 years of life have an increased incidence of chronic cough. Cohorts with a high infant mortality from respiratory infection continue to show high death rates from chronic bronchitis decades later. However, recent prospective studies have shown that pre-LRTI lung function is lower in children with wheezing LRTIs. It is not yet clear whether low lung function predisposes to or is a consequence of LRTI.

PREVENTION

Since the immature and rapidly growing lung may be particularly sensitive to permanent injury, the prevention and improved therapy of LRTIs in early childhood may be vital for later pulmonary health. Social and environmental determinants of LRTIs should be avoided. Breastfeeding and the high uptake of childhood immunisations should be encouraged. Influenza vaccination, especially for those with chronic respiratory illness, should be arranged. Vaccine developments such as the introduction of conjugate pneumococcal vaccines may further reduce the incidence of LRTIs.

Where vaccination is not available, immunoprophylaxis such as with high-titre RSV immunoglobulin or monoclonal antibodies may have a role in preventing lower respiratory tract infection in high-risk infants and children.

While more effective therapies particularly for viral infections are needed, one simple measure that would have a substantial impact would be a reduction in parental smoking.

FURTHER READING

Chernick V, Kendig EL (eds) (1990) Disorders of the respiratory tract in children, 5th edn. WB Saunders, Philadelphia, PA.

Loughlin GM, Eigen H (eds) (1994) Respiratory disease in children: diagnosis and management. Williams & Wilkins, Baltimore, MD.

Margolis P, Gadomski A (1998) Does the infant have pneumonia? JAMA 279: 308–313.

World Health Organization (1991). Acute respiratory infections in children: case management in small hospitals in developing countries. Programme Control Acute Respir Infect; ARI: 90.5

Infection of the heart results in endocarditis, myocarditis or pericarditis, with occasional overlap. Connective tissue diseases can cause cardiac inflammation and may mimic infection. Acute rheumatic fever (postinfective) and Kawasaki disease (not a proven infection) have important cardiac sequelae. Cardiac involvement in AIDS leads to ventricular dysfunction, pericardial effusion and arrhythmias. Although these conditions contribute to the differential diagnosis, this chapter will focus on primary cardiac infections.

ENDOCARDITIS

EPIDEMIOLOGY AND CAUSES

Infective endocarditis (IE) is an infection of the endocardium or heart valves. Most affected children have congenital heart disease (CHD). The pathogenesis of endothelial injury and formation of vegetations is related to turbulent and high-velocity blood flow (e.g. aortic stenosis, ventricular septal defect). Therefore IE is very rare in isolated secundum atrial septal defect.

The incidence of IE in neonates without CHD is increasing in association with advances in life support and the use of central venous lines. The presence of prosthetic material within the cardiovascular system predisposes to IE.

Gram-positive cocci are commonly responsible (in 90% of cases when an organism is isolated). Viridans streptococci form the largest group and usually produce a subacute illness. They form part of the normal oral flora and bacteraemia follows mucosal disruption (e.g. dental extraction). Other responsible streptococci are enterococci, pneumococci and β-haemolytic streptococci. The latter two are associated with a high mortality. Pneumococcal IE usually follows an acute course.

Staphylococci (usually *S. aureus*) are responsible for 20–30% of cases of IE. *S. aureus* is the most likely cause of acute disease in patients with previously normal hearts and in intravenous drug abusers. The course is often fulminant. There is a rising incidence of *S. epidermidis* IE following cardiac surgery. This is the main agent responsible for prosthetic valve endocarditis.

Gram-negative bacteria, Gram-positive bacilli and fungi are uncommon causes of IE and associated with a high mortality. Rarely, IE is due to anaerobes or *Coxiella burnetii* (Q fever).

CLINICAL PRESENTATION

Fever, typically low-grade, is usual. It may be absent in 10% of cases. Nonspecific features are common: malaise, anorexia, weight loss and fatigue. Arthralgia or arthritis occurs in a quarter of patients. Chest pain is unusual but may be related to pulmonary embolism.

Murmurs are present in 90% of affected children. However, as most children have pre-existing structural heart disease, a new or changing murmur is found in only 25%. Heart failure occurs in a third and is related to valvular regurgitation. Splenomegaly is found in over 50% of patients.

It is usually nontender but pain and tenderness may indicate splenic infarction or abscess formation. Petechiae of the extremities or mouth are common; splinter haemorrhages, Osler's nodes, Janeway lesions and Roth spots are not. A variety of embolic neurological defects may present in up to 20% of patients.

In infants, IE is acute and presents as overwhelming sepsis with bacteraemia, cardiac failure and a murmur. Among intravenous drug abusers with IE, two-thirds have previously normal hearts, two-thirds have extracardiac sites of infection and in one-third the affected tricuspid valve is regurgitant. Pulmonary complications include infarction, abscess formation and effusions.

DIAGNOSIS

Once IE is suspected, blood cultures are mandatory; ideally three sets in the first 24 hours, followed by a further two sets during the next 24 hours. In 90% of cases, the first two sets will be positive. In fungal endocarditis, blood cultures may be positive only intermittently and the organism is slow to grow.

Blood culture-negative IE occurs in 10% as a result of: prior antibiotic administration; rickettsial, chlamydial or viral infection; slow-growing or nutritionally variant organisms; anaerobes; mural endocarditis; right-sided endocarditis or fungal endocarditis (especially *Candida* and *Aspergillus*). Noninfective endocarditis may be due to nonbacterial thrombotic vegetations or Libman–Sacks endocarditis in systemic lupus erythematosus. Measurement of antibodies against *S. aureus* may be of value.

Elevation of erythrocyte sedimentation rate (ESR) and C-reactive protein (CRP) is usual and recovers with successful therapy. Likewise, serological immune complexes, when present, may follow the course of the disease although, in practice, results may not be forthcoming in time to be clinically useful. Anaemia is present in 40% of cases and, less commonly, haematuria. Transthoracic echocardiography will detect vegetations in two-thirds of patients. However, a 'negative echo' does not exclude IE. The transoesophageal modality is more sensitive than transthoracic and may detect vegetations in up to 95%. Valvular regurgitation may be detected before it is clinically apparent.

MANAGEMENT

Intravenous bactericidal antibiotics are required for 4–6 weeks, except in the case of fully penicillin-sensitive streptococci, when oral amoxycillin may be substituted for benzylpenicillin and gentamicin after 2 weeks. Synergy between agents may produce a rapid bactericidal effect and allow lower doses of each agent. The microbiologist should supervise therapy, which can usually be withheld until initial positive blood culture results are available. In seriously ill patients, antibiotics should be started immediately after initial blood cultures have been taken. Benzylpenicillin and an aminoglycoside are recommended. If *S. aureus* is suspected, flucloxacillin can be used in place of benzylpenicillin. Following recent cardiac surgery, vancomycin is indicated, as hospital-acquired *S. epidermidis* or *S. aureus* infection is likely.

There should be clinical improvement within a few days. Daily physical examination should concentrate on the detection of embolic phenomena and valvular regurgitation, implying progression of local disease. The success of treatment can be monitored by measurement of the peripheral blood white cell count and CRP. Initially, daily ECG will allow detection of arrhythmias and conduction defects. Echocardiography should be performed at least weekly. Surgical intervention is indicated for acute valve destruction, removal of infected prosthetic material, large, mobile left-sided vegetations and persistent or recurrent infection.

PREVENTION OF FURTHER CASES

Good dental hygiene is essential to reduce the risk of IE. Antibacterial prophylaxis is required for any procedure that induces a bacteraemia in patients with a structurally abnormal heart, whether congenital or acquired, native or operated. Patients who have had successful closure of patent arterial duct or secundum atrial septal defect, surgically, or with a device at cardiac catheterisation, no longer require prophylaxis after 6 months have elapsed. Recommendations for prevention of IE in children with structural heart disease are presented in Table 17.1.

MYOCARDITIS

EPIDEMIOLOGY AND CAUSES

Most cases are attributed to viral infection, most commonly Coxsackie B viruses. They are usually sporadic, although epidemics may occur, as happened recently in south-east Asia. Spread is by the faecal–oral route or by droplet infection; intrauterine infection may occur in late pregnancy. Less common causes include Coxsackie A, echo and other enteroviruses, rubella, herpes simplex and varicella zoster viruses.

CLINICAL PRESENTATION

This is variable but can be fulminant in infants. There may be a history suggestive of recent viral illness. There are signs of reduced cardiac output with cool periphery and pallor. Cardiac failure is common with tachypnoea, tachycardia, a third heart sound and hepatomegaly. There may be an apical pansystolic murmur of mitral regurgitation.

DIAGNOSIS

Viruses are infrequently isolated but should be sought in stools, urine, sputum and throat-swab. Paired viral sera may diagnose active infection if there is a fourfold increase in antibody titres. Blood cultures are indicated as it may be difficult to distinguish viral myocarditis from other cardiac infections. CRP is usually elevated.

Electrocardiographic abnormalities are common and include sinus tachycardia, conduction disturbances (notably complete heart block) and,

Table 17.1 Prevention of endocarditis in children with structural heart disease

Dental procedures that require antibiotic prophylaxis are extractions, scaling and surgery involving gingival tissues. Prophylaxis is indicated for tonsillectomy, adenoidectomy and procedures on the middle ear. It should also be given for genitourinary procedures, including bladder catheterisation, and may be indicated for obstetric, gynaecological and gastrointestinal procedures (details to be found in the current issue of the *British National Formulary*).

Dental procedures under local or no anaesthesia

Not more than a single dose of a penicillin in the previous month: oral amoxycillin 1 h before procedure.

< 5 years	750 mg
5–10 years	1500 mg
> 10 years	3 g

If previous endocarditis, add gentamicin.

If more than a single dose of a penicillin given in previous month, or penicillin-allergic: oral clindamycin, 1 h before procedure.

< 5 years	150 mg
5–10 years	300 mg
> 10 years	600 mg

Dental procedures under general anaesthetic

Not more than a single dose of a penicillin in the previous month; no history of endocarditis or prosthetic valve: amoxycillin.

< 5 years	250 mg i.v. at induction; then 125 mg orally at 6 h
5–10 years	500 mg i.v. at induction; then 250 mg orally at 6 h
> 10 years	1 g i.v. at induction; then 500 mg orally at 6 h

Special risk group (prosthetic valve or history of endocarditis)

< 5 years	i.v. amoxycillin 250 mg + i.v. gentamicin 2 mg/kg at induction; then amoxycillin 125 mg orally at 6 h
5–10 years	i.v. amoxycillin 500 mg + i.v. gentamicin 2 mg/kg at induction; then amoxycillin 250 mg orally at 6 h
> 10 years	i.v. amoxycillin 1 g + i.v. gentamicin 2 mg/kg at induction; then amoxycillin 500 mg orally at 6 h

When penicillin-allergic, or more than a single dose of a penicillin given in previous month:
Vancomycin i.v. 20 mg/kg over 100 min, then gentamicin i.v. 2 mg/kg at induction **or**
Teicoplanin i.v. 6 mg/kg and gentamicin i.v. 2 mg/kg at induction **or**
Clindamycin

< 5 years	75 mg i.v. at induction; repeated orally/i.v. 37.5 mg at 6 h
5–10 years	150 mg i.v. at induction; repeated orally/i.v. 75 mg at 6 h
> 10 years	300 mg i.v. at induction; repeated orally/i.v. 150 mg at 6 h

classically, low-voltage QRS complexes with flattened or inverted lateral T waves. Pathological Q waves may indicate severe damage. Echocardiography invariably shows ventricular dilatation with impaired function affecting one or more chambers (commonly the left heart chambers), and, usually, no structural abnormality. Secondary mitral regurgitation may be present. In infants, anomalous origin of the left coronary artery, coarctation of the aorta, incessant tachyarrhythmias and Kawasaki disease must be positively excluded. Endomyocardial biopsy is not recommended routinely, although advocated by some.

MANAGEMENT

Cardiac output must be maintained and heart failure treated. Cautious administration of digoxin, diuretics and captopril is usual. Inotropic agents may be required and dobutamine with or without dopamine is suitable. Arrhythmias demand effective control; patients in complete heart block should be paced. Hypoxaemia and anaemia need correction. The case for using steroids or other immunosuppressive agents is inconclusive. However, if the history is short, intravenous gammaglobulin is typically administered (2 g/kg over 24 hours), particularly if the impression of acute myocarditis is supported by elevated serological acute-phase reactants. Formal anticoagulation may be appropriate in those with particularly poor ventricular function. Cardiac transplantation is reserved for patients with persistent, severe ventricular dysfunction.

PERICARDITIS

EPIDEMIOLOGY AND CAUSES

Causes of pericardial effusion in childhood include viral infection, Kawasaki disease, connective tissue diseases, recent cardiac surgery and renal failure. This section concentrates on the more serious purulent pericarditis, which comprises about 90% of cases of acute pericarditis in children under 2 years. Infection spreads either directly or haematogenously, most commonly from the lungs. The usual organisms are *S. aureus*, *H. influenzae* and pneumococci, but include other streptococci, meningococci and anaerobes. Tuberculous, fungal and hydatid pericarditis are rare in the UK.

CLINICAL PRESENTATION

This diagnosis should be suspected in any septicaemic child who develops cardiomegaly. Patients present with pyrexia, tachycardia and tachypnoea. There may be evidence of pericardial effusion or a friction rub (they may occur together). Older patients may complain of chest pain. Cardiac tamponade can develop with even a moderate-sized effusion if accumulation is rapid.

DIAGNOSIS

Pericardial effusion is suggested radiologically by a rapidly increasing cardiothoracic ratio without increased pulmonary vascular markings. In over

90% of cases, there is ST segment elevation on the ECG. Other typical, although nonspecific, changes include low-voltage QRS complexes with flattened or inverted T waves (see Myocarditis, above). Echocardiography is a sensitive tool for the detection of pericardial effusion and remains the method of choice.

Blood cultures are positive in most cases. Cerebrospinal fluid culture may be indicated. If pericardiocentesis is performed, microbiological examination of the fluid must include Gram stain, microscopy and culture for bacteria (including TB), viruses and fungi.

MANAGEMENT

Children with purulent pericarditis require urgent drainage, about half for tamponade. Should pericardiocentesis fail, immediate surgical drainage is indicated. Free drainage should be maintained as fluid is likely to reaccumulate.

Antibiotic therapy should be tailored to the causative organism. If this is unknown, intravenous flucloxacillin and ampicillin in combination are suitable. If *H. influenzae* is suspected, cefotaxime should replace ampicillin. In some cases, an aminoglycoside may be added. Intravenous therapy should be continued for 3–4 weeks. Tuberculous infection requires steroids in addition to appropriate antibiotics to prevent constrictive pericarditis. As with all of the conditions discussed in this section, general supportive measures are very important in sick children; these include oxygen, appropriate volume expansion and inotropic support. If necessary, these should be provided on an intensive care unit. Follow-up for at least a year will be needed to detect constrictive pericarditis, which can develop rapidly.

FURTHER READING

General

Garson A, Bricker JT, Fisher DJ (1996) The science and practice of pediatric cardiology, 2nd edn. Lippincott, Williams & Wilkins, Philadelphia, PA.

Endocarditis prophylaxis

British Medical Association and Royal Pharmaceutical Society of Great Britain (1999) Summary of antibacterial prophylaxis. In: British National Formulary 38, September 1999. BMJ Books, London, pp 243–244.

Longman LP, Martin MV (1993) The prevention of infective endocarditis – paedodontic considerations. British Society for Antimicrobial Therapy. Int J Paediatr Dent 3: 63–70.

18 The child with diarrhoea and vomiting

INTRODUCTION

Especially in young children, vomiting and, to a lesser extent, diarrhoea may be nonspecific indications that a child is unwell rather than indicating a specific problem with the gastrointestinal tract. Vomiting may be due to an obstruction (particularly in the neonate), infection or metabolic causes.

When assessing a child with diarrhoea and vomiting it is essential to be clear how the terms are being used. 'Diarrhoea' usually means the passage of frequent, loose stools. It is best assessed on the basis of a change from the previous pattern for that child. Vomiting must be distinguished from posseting and the bringing up of small quantities of feed when a baby breaks wind.

The history should include questions about the duration, frequency and magnitude of the problem as well as taking note of the feeding history and any other features of illness that the child may have. General examination, including evidence of weight loss, should allow one to exclude causes other than gastroenteritis. Some of the commoner causes of diarrhoea and vomiting not due to gastrointestinal infection are listed below.

DIARRHOEA
- Systemic infection
- Drugs – especially antibiotics and laxatives
- Lactose or cow's milk protein intolerance (unusual after infancy)
- Toddler diarrhoea – an otherwise well child with often very loose, frequent stools containing undigested food particles
- Malabsorptive syndromes such as cystic fibrosis and coeliac disease
- Crohn's disease and ulcerative colitis
- Urinary tract infection
- Appendicitis
- Others including haemolytic uraemic syndrome (noninfectious variety), Kawasaki disease, malaria, toxic shock syndrome.

VOMITING
- As diarrhoea
- Intestinal obstruction – especially in the newborn or if bile-stained. Usually accompanied by lack of passage of stools/meconium. Pyloric stenosis will present in the first 2 months of life. In the older child volvulus and intussusception are possible causes. Appendicitis and a Meckel's diverticulum should be kept in mind at any age
- CNS infections such as meningitis and encephalitis
- Metabolic disorders, e.g. Reye's syndrome, congenital adrenal hyperplasia and some inborn errors of metabolism
- Miscellaneous – drugs, toxins, periodic syndrome, pregnancy, migraine and cerebral tumours.

GASTROENTERITIS

Gastroenteritis can be defined as the acute onset of watery or very loose stools, with or without vomiting, caused by an infection of the gastrointestinal tract. Infection or other illness outside the gastrointestinal tract must be excluded (see above).

EPIDEMIOLOGY

Gastroenteritis (GE) is still one of the commonest causes of childhood mortality worldwide. WHO estimates that approximately 5 million children die each year of gastroenteritis. For England and Wales there was a dramatic fall in childhood deaths due to GE, from 300–400 per year in the 1970s to 25 per year in 1986. However, the hospital admission rate for GE is unchanged since the 1970s (about 15 000 per year), and the incidence of the disease seen in general practice is also unchanged, with around 10% of children affected in the first 2 years of life. Although the illness now seen appears to be clinically less severe than previously, it is still an important cause of childhood mortality and morbidity. There is clear evidence for the protective effect of breastfeeding.

PATHOGENS

Endemic

The cause of endemic GE varies around the world. In the UK, no pathogen can be isolated from the stools in around 50% of children admitted to hospital with gastroenteritis. The main pathogens in children under 5 years old are shown in Table 18.1.

Food/water-borne

Over 50 000 cases of food poisoning were notified in 1998. The causative organism can usually be predicted by the incubation period and symptoms (Table 18.2). No cause is found in around half of all cases. Early referral of outbreaks and individual cases of important diseases (typhoid, HUS/*E. coli* O157) to the relevant Consultant in Communicable Disease Control (public health specialist) or their equivalent is very important.

Foreign travel

Malaria must be considered in a child recently returned from abroad with a fever and either vomiting or diarrhoea. Other diagnoses to consider include travellers' diarrhoea (enterotoxigenic *Escherichia coli*), *Shigella/Salmonella*, amoebiasis, cholera or helminth infection.

Immunocompromised host

Pathogens include cytomegalovirus, *Cryptosporidium parvum*, *Isospora belli*, microsporidia and atypical mycobacteria. A more interventional approach to diagnosis and treatment may be required, with early referral to a specialist unit.

Table 18.1 Infective agents causing gastroenteritis in children under 5 years old, 1990–94

Infective agent	Age (%)					Total
	0–11 months	12–23 months	24–35 months	36–47 months	48–59 months	
Rotavirus	30 744 (51.8)	23 262 (45)	8042 (28)	2733 (16)	1133 (10)	65 914
Salmonella	8406 (14.3)	6269 (12)	4840 (17)	3661 (22)	2758 (23)	25 934
Campylobacter	5971 (10.1)	7642 (15)	6001 (21)	3736 (22)	2562 (21)	25 912
Adenovirus	5468 (9.2)	2853 (6)	1190 (4)	562 (3)	289 (2)	10 362
Cryptosporidium	1390 (2.3)	3630 (7)	2603 (9)	1557 (9)	1142 (10)	10 322
Giardia	652 (1.1)	2096 (4)	1165 (4)	980 (6)	828 (7)	6221
Shigella	965 (1.6)	1964 (4)	2355 (8)	2412 (15)	2546 (21)	10 242
Escherichia coli	1549 (2.6)	1279 (2)	553 (2)	195 (1)	84 (1)	3660
SRSV*	821 (1.4)	524 (1)	226 (1)	122 (1)	63 (1)	1756
Astrovirus	750 (1.3)	547 (1)	291 (1)	110 (1)	62 (1)	1760
Other	2598 (4.4)	1155 (2)	699 (2)	399 (2)	388 (3)	5239
Total	59 314 (100)	51 221 (100)	28 465 (100)	16 467 (100)	11 855 (100)	167 322

*Small round spherical virus.
Source: PHLS/CDSC.

Table 18.2 Food poisoning causes and features

Incubation period	Fever	Vomiting	Cause	Clinical features, isolation of cause
< 3 hours	–	+	Chemical	Neurotoxic or histamine-like reaction
1–7 hours	–	++	Staphylococcus aureus or Bacillus cereus enterotoxin	Isolate toxin in food, vomit or stool
8–14 hours	–	+/–	Clostridium perfringens enterotoxin	Isolate toxin in food, vomit or stool
16–36 hours	+	+/–	Shigella spp. Salmonella spp. Vibrio parahaemolyticus Enteroinvasive Escherichia coli, Yersinia enterocolitica	Isolate toxin in food, vomit or stool
12–26 hours	–	–	Clostridium botulinum	Botulism, descending flaccid paralysis
1–7 days	–	+	Vibrio cholerae Enterotoxigenic E. coli Norwalk virus Campylobacter spp.	

Other infections may be food-borne but do not typically cause gastroenteritis; examples are brucellosis, toxoplasmosis and some other parasitic infections.
Source: adapted from *Management of Outbreaks of Foodborne Illness*, Department of Health, 1994.

PSEUDOMEMBRANOUS COLITIS (ANTIBIOTIC-ASSOCIATED DIARRHOEA)

Various antibiotics (especially ampicillin, erythromycin and co-trimoxazole) can produce colonic overgrowth of toxin-producing *Clostridium difficile*, with the local production of multiple plaque-like lesions on the mucosal surface. Mild colitis can rapidly lead to toxic megacolon. The diagnosis can be confirmed on finding *C. difficile* toxin in the stool. Treatment is replacing the causative antibiotic with oral metronidazole for 1 week.

VIRULENCE

A number of different mechanisms are involved in the pathogenesis of gastrointestinal infection. Examples include:

- Adherence to mucosal surface by fimbrial adhesins
- Enterotoxin production, e.g. heat-labile (LT) cholera toxin
- Cytotoxin production, e.g. the Shiga toxin of *Shigella dysenteriae*
- Invasion by *Salmonella* spp.

CLINICAL FEATURES

History

Particular note should be made of the presence of bilious vomiting, blood/mucus in diarrhoea, reduced urine output, altered level of consciousness, other affected family members, foreign travel, previous GI problems and medication already received.

Viral infections are relatively short-lived (48–72 h) and are often accompanied by both diarrhoea and vomiting. Upper respiratory tract symptoms are common, especially in rotavirus infection. On the other hand, bacterial infections are predominantly associated with diarrhoea and there may be significant systemic upset. Infection with *Campylobacter jejuni* causes an illness of variable severity. Apart from diarrhoea and vomiting, there is often abdominal pain, fever and general malaise. Bloody diarrhoea is more common in infections with *Salmonella* and *Shigella* spp. and young children may have relatively long-lasting febrile convulsions. *Yersinia enterocolitica* may be associated with an abdominal mesenteric adenitis that can be confused with appendicitis. Invasive salmonellosis is more common in children with sickle cell disease, while children with thalassaemia are particularly at risk from *Yersinia* spp.

Examination – plot on growth chart

The most important points are to assess the state of dehydration of the child, and to identify whether there is any other pathology mimicking gastroenteritis.

Dehydration

This is a clinical diagnosis (Table 18.3). Severe history and infancy are high-risk factors. A recent clinic weight (from the Personal Child Health Record) can be very useful in assessing fluid loss. Hypernatraemic dehydration can be very difficult to assess. The child will usually be drowsy, and other signs of dehydration may be masked.

Table 18.3 Clinical assessment of dehydration

| Sign | Degree of dehydration | | |
	< 5%	5–10%	> 10%
Skin	Normal	Loss of turgor	Mottled, cold with poor capillary return
Fontanelle (if open)	Normal	Depressed	Deeply depressed
Eyes	Normal	Sunken, with reduced intraocular pressure	Sunken, with reduced intraocular pressure
Lips	Moist	Dry	Dry
Peripheral pulses	Normal	Normal	Poor volume and tachycardia
Blood pressure	Normal	Normal	Low
Behaviour	Normal	Lethargic	Prostration, coma
Urine output	Normal	Long periods between micturition	Anuric

MANAGEMENT

Death in children with gastroenteritis is nearly always due to dehydration. The principles of management are therefore as follows.

Important management points

- Check no surgical pathology
- Treat with ORT wherever possible
- Antiemetic and antidiarrhoeal agents are not indicated
- Return to normal diet as soon as possible.

1. Rehydrate

Gastrointestinal infections increase the amount of fluid being secreted into the bowel, either through the action of a toxin or by direct invasion of the mucosa. Rehydration aims to correct those losses. Children that are not clinically dehydrated do not need rehydrating. They should continue on their normal diet and be reassessed if symptoms continue.

Oral rehydration therapy (ORT)

- If the child is breastfed, then the mother should be advised to continue to breastfeed throughout the illness, increasing the length and frequency of breastfeed. Extra fluids as oral rehydration solution (ORS) can be offered if necessary. Any supplemented formula feeds should be stopped.
- If the child has formula feeds, then these should be stopped. ORT should be given alone, for a period of 12 hours, the aim being to completely rehydrate the child in this time (ideally over the first 4 h). The parents should be warned that, although the vomiting and diarrhoea will decrease, they will probably not stop completely. If vomiting is a persistent problem, then very small frequent feeds (e.g. 20 mL every 20 min) is best. A number of commercial ORT solutions are now available (Dioralyte, Rehidrat) and the parents should be instructed how to make them up (the powder is added to a bottle, followed by a measured amount of boiled water and left to cool). The amount given depends on the child. The child's maintenance fluid requirements should be given and the fluid deficit made up. The child should then be given further volumes of ORS with each loose stool. In practice, most parents allow their child to drink as much as they want, and this is safe as long as the ORS has been made up correctly. Ill children may require a nasogastric tube.

Intravenous rehydration therapy (IVRT)

- Children who are shocked (over 10% dehydration) will need IVRT. The principles of fluid management are:
  - Resuscitate
  - Replace deficit
  - Provide daily maintenance
  - Replace ongoing losses.

- Resuscitation should be with 20–40 mL/kg of physiological saline. In a shocked child this can be given over 30–60 min. More may need to be given. Assess progress using pulse, blood pressure and peripheral perfusion. Albumin should not be used.
- Replacing deficit requires an estimate of the deficit from a clinical assessment of the child's percentage dehydration:

  Deficit (mL) = % dehydration × body weight (kg) × 10 mL.

  The deficit should usually be replaced over the first 12 hours. Briefly, if the child has a normal serum sodium, use 4% dextrose/0.18% saline. If the serum sodium is low then use 0.45% saline. In hypernatraemic dehydration, rehydrate more slowly over 48 hours, using 0.45% or 0.9% saline initially. Potassium chloride should be added in standard amounts, once the child has passed urine. Hypernatraemic dehydration should be treated with ORT if at all possible.
- Providing daily maintenance requires a knowledge of basic fluid requirements, which vary with age:

Up to 6 months	150 mL/kg/day
6–12 months	100 mL/kg/day
1–2 years	80 mL/kg/day
2–4 years	70 mL/kg/day
4–8 years	60 mL/kg/day

- Ongoing deficits should be based on the clinical/measured assessment of continuing fluid loss. In severe secretory diarrhoea (e.g. cholera) this can be massive.

2. Return to normal diet

A slow regrade back on to normal feeds is no longer considered necessary. After rehydration with ORT, the child should therefore go back on to normal full-strength milk and solids. Breastfeeding should be continued throughout.

3. Admission/investigation/treatment

Admission

Admit children:

- needing IVRT
- with oliguria (consider haemolytic uraemic syndrome)
- with a severe history
- with adverse social circumstances
- with a doubtful diagnosis.

Investigation

Most episodes of mild GE do not warrant any investigations. Consider:

- stool microscopy – trophozoites, cysts, spores
- stool culture/agglutination – E. coli, Salmonella, Shigella, Campylobacter
- stool virology – electron microscopy/enzyme-linked immunosorbent assay (ELISA)/culture

- blood culture if febrile
- full blood count and electrolytes if child is pale, oliguric or needing IVRT.

Where there is an infectious cause it is important to prevent further cases (see Chapter 33).

18 Diarrhoea & vomiting

Treatment

There is no place for antiemetics, antidiarrhoeal agents, changing to a different cows' milk preparation or starvation.

Antibiotics are needed very rarely. They should be used under the following circumstances:

- Invasive salmonellosis (any species in children under 6 months old or where the organism is *Salmonella typhi* or *S. paratyphi* at any age)
- Shigellosis, if the child is toxic and febrile
- Amoebiasis
- Cholera
- Giardiasis
- Severe *Campylobacter* infection
- Gastroenteritis due to *Clostridium difficile* toxin
- Gastroenteritis due to enterotoxigenic *E. coli* ('travellers' diarrhoea').

4. Chronic persistent diarrhoea

Temporary food intolerance normally occurs in up to 20% of children after GE. The rapid introduction of normal feeds does not appear to increase the incidence of this problem.

All children with GE should be advised to seek further medical advice if the diarrhoea recurs, or persists over 10 days. The stools should then be sent for culture and tested for the presence of reducing sugars (Clinitest, significant if 1% or greater).

- **Lactose intolerance – positive Clinitest (> 1%)**: Return to ORT, then slow regrade back to normal formula feed. If lactose intolerance persists, then change to lactose-free formula.
- **Reinfection or persisting infection**: May indicate immunodeficiency. Consider investigating further.
- **Cows milk protein intolerance (CMPI)**: This is a diagnosis of exclusion without a jejunal biopsy. It produces a clinical picture of continuing diarrhoea and poor weight gain after GE, without either of the above. Treat by changing to alternative milk (casein/whey hydrolysate) for 3 months.

FURTHER READING

Murphy MS (1998) Guidelines for managing acute gastroenteritis based on a systematic review of published research. Arch Dis Child 79: 279–284.

19 The child with urinary tract infection

INCIDENCE

Urinary tract infections (UTI) in children are common. There is a paucity of comprehensive and prospective population-based studies on the annual incidence and prevalence. One exception is a Swedish study, which found that the prevalence of UTIs before the age of 11 years was 3% in girls and 1% in boys. This study also showed that the first UTI occurs most commonly during the first year of life. During the first 3 months, the female to male ratio is 0.4. After this there is an increasing female preponderance.

DEFINITION

The definition of a UTI is the presence in an uncontaminated urine sample of more than 10^8 colony forming units of a bacterium in pure culture per litre in a symptomatic child. The definition of a UTI is confounded by a number of problems. The first is that urinary infections may occur with smaller numbers of organisms. Any growth in a suprapubic or catheter sample indicates infection. Secondly, on the basis of large population studies it is known that between 1% and 2% of school-age girls and approximately 0.03% of schoolboys have asymptomatic bacteriuria. Asymptomatic bacteriuria can be detected during the first year of age in approximately 0.7% of girls and 2.7% of boys. Thirdly, obtaining uncontaminated urine samples from non-toilet-trained children is difficult and significant culture results may be obtained that in fact may represent single-organism contamination. Pyuria, although commonly found in older children with UTIs, may not occur particularly in the infant and its absence does not exclude a UTI. In addition, white cell lysis may occur if there is a long delay before the sample is examined microscopically, particularly if it is left at room temperature or if the urine pH is very high. Pyuria may be present in febrile children in the absence of a UTI.

OBTAINING A URINE SAMPLE

A midstream urine specimen or a clean-catch specimen is ideal. In sick infants a suprapubic bladder aspirate should be considered to avoid delay in initiating treatment. This is a safe procedure that is easily learned and should become available as a service provided by paediatric departments. If the suprapubic aspirate fails and the infant is ill enough to warrant antibiotic therapy then a catheter specimen of urine should be obtained immediately after the first dose of antibiotic.

Hollister urine collection bags are widely used. They are applied after washing the perineum, holding the child upright and taking the bag off as soon as a sample is produced. However, contamination rates are high and although a negative culture result is reliable a positive culture result obtained by this method may not necessarily indicate infection. Repeat urine samples are often needed and results may be confounded if antibiotics have already been started. The use of urine collection bags is best discouraged, certainly within a hospital setting. Urine pads are used in some centres as an alternative to Hollister bags. When used correctly these cause fewer problems with contamination.

Immediate microscopy of a freshly obtained unspun specimen is the gold standard and this can be achieved with basic training. This forms standard practice in a few units and general practices. The advantage is that an immediate diagnosis can be made and only those samples where abnormalities are found on microscopy need be sent to the laboratory. The use of a combined dipstick that contains nitrite to detect bacteriuria and leukocyte esterase for the detection of pyuria in freshly collected urine specimens has been found in recent studies to have very low false-negative rates and high predictive values. However, there are limitations: the rare infection caused by *Pseudomonas* and group B streptococci will not be identified and urine must stay in the bladder for at least an hour for the bacterial conversion of nitrate into nitrite to occur. As yet, this method is not recommended.

There is wide variation in the use of dipslides for urine culture and transport. With this method urine is dropped on to the slide, which is like a mini culture plate. The advantage of this method is that urine culture can start when the urine is still fresh, thereby minimising the proliferation of contaminants. The disadvantage is that urine microscopy is not possible.

If there is going to be a delay in the specimen reaching the laboratory it can be refrigerated for up to 24 hours at between 0°C and 4°C to avoid the proliferation of contaminants.

ORGANISMS

Bacteria giving rise to UTI originate from the bowel flora. In boys there is circumstantial evidence that preputial organisms may be important. There are a number of reports that quote a significantly lower risk of UTI in circumcised boys. This point, however, has not been analysed prospectively.

Escherichia coli is by far the commonest infecting organism, causing 65–85% of infections. Other organisms, such as *Proteus*, *Klebsiella*, other coliforms and *Enterococcus* cause between 1% and 10% of infections. The possibility of urinary calculi should be considered in all children with *Proteus* urinary infection. UTIs may occasionally be caused by *Staphylococcus epidermidis* and *S. aureus*.

CLINICAL PRESENTATION

The modes of presentation of a UTI, especially in young children and infants, are often nonspecific. There may be systemic symptoms such as fever, found to be present in an average of 60% of children over 1 and in over 80% in the under-1-year-old age group. Other symptoms are vomiting, irritability, jaundice, failure to thrive, screaming, abdominal pain, dysuria, frequency and haematuria. UTIs may occur in association with sexual abuse. Hypertension is sometimes found in association with UTIs.

In children presenting with dysuria and frequency it is important to think of other possible diagnoses, such as vulvovaginitis, which may be accompanied by vaginal secretions not seen in a true UTI, threadworms, diabetes and hypercalciuria.

MANAGEMENT

Prompt diagnosis and treatment are essential. However, most children with a UTI are only mildly unwell. For these, treatment with 5–7 days of oral antibiotics is sufficient, although the optimum length of treatment is not known. Most community-acquired infections will respond to trimetho-prim. Nitrofurantoin is also a suitable antibiotic but not for systemically unwell children as significant tissue concentrations are not achieved. In addition, nitrofurantoin is often poorly tolerated, particularly if given in liq-uid form, as it causes nausea and vomiting. Amoxycillin can be used for a therapeutic course but bacterial resistance soon develops as it does with oral cephalosporins such as cephalexin. Children who have had a recent course of antibiotic or are on long-term prophylaxis may be infected with resistant organisms. Lack of clinical improvement within 48 hours can be due to inappropriate antibiotic therapy or to underlying urinary obstruction.

In acutely sick children and infants, intravenous therapy should be used for at least 48 hours or until improvement occurs. Treatment can be continued orally for a total of 10 days. Parenteral cephalosporins such as cefuroxime or cefotaxime are good first-line therapy. Aminoglycosides may be used with careful drug level monitoring but are rarely necessary unless the organism sensitivity pattern dictates. Azlocillin, ceftazidime and ciprofloxacin should be reserved for *Pseudomonas* infections. Some chil-dren, particularly infants and neonates, may be severely unwell with dehy-dration, presenting with signs of shock that may be associated with elec-trolyte imbalance and renal failure. Their early detection and correction is crucial. A transient decrease in the kidneys' urine concentrating ability is common in episodes of pyelonephritis and an increased water intake dur-ing the episode is needed.

RENAL TRACT IMAGING

Abnormalities of the urinary tract may be detected on renal imaging of those children presenting with a UTI. The incidence of these abnormalities varies according to the nature of the studies. Most abnormalities are already present at the time of the first investigation. Obstructive uropathies and neuropathic bladder are specific problems that must be looked for as there is no doubt that surgical intervention and intermittent catherisation in the latter case avert deterioration in renal function.

Vesico-ureteric reflux (VUR) is found in 20–50% and renal scarring in around 10% of all children with a UTI. The natural history of VUR is one of progressive resolution with age, particularly in cases of mild reflux. Renal scarring is associated with problems during pregnancy such as pre-eclampsia and if extensive may lead to hypertension and renal failure.

Investigation aims to exclude obstruction and identify VUR so that antibiotic prophylaxis can be used to reduce the risk of scarring. Although this approach is logical, and recommended, there is no definite evidence from research studies of long-term benefit. Table 19.1 describes the pro-posed investigation. We recommend imaging all children under the age of 5 with their first infection, but accept that there is varying practice. The use of DMSA scanning in all children over 2 years investigated after a first

Table 19.1 Investigation of urinary tract infection in children

All children to be assessed in the paediatric clinic after first UTI
Advice on management of unstable bladder, constipation, high fluid intake to prevent further infections
Advice on the prompt recognition and treatment of further UTI
Parent's information sheet

Under 1 year	1–5 years	Older than 5 years
Ultrasound and DMSA* scan	Ultrasound and DMSA* scan if risk factors†	Ultrasound and DMSA* scan after second infection if no risk factors†
Consider MCUG if abnormalities on ultrasound or DMSA	MAG 3 if hydronephrosis, ureteric dilatation	
+ MAG 3 instead of DMSA if hydronephrosis (> 10 mm AP renal pelvis diameter)		

* 3–6 months after infection.
† Risk factors: febrile/vomiting/loin pain/family history of renal scarring.

UTI remains controversial. Many paediatricians would perform an ultrasound only after an initial episode in a child over 2 with symptoms of a lower urinary tract infection, reserving DMSA scanning for those with any upper tract signs, i.e. systemic illness, fever, loin pain, vomiting. In sick infants an ultrasound should be done during the acute illness to look for obstructive uropathies or evidence of a neuropathic bladder.

ANTIBIOTIC PROPHYLAXIS

Antibiotic prophylaxis is recommended in children with VUR and is often used in infants with normal urinary tracts until 1 year of age and in older children with normal urinary tracts and repeated infections. Many clinicians would follow the initial treatment antibiotic course with prophylactic antibiotics until all investigations are completed and the results are normal. There is no consensus about the length of prophylaxis in children with VUR. It is thought that the risk of renal damage diminishes appreciably after the age of 5–7 years and prophylaxis is often stopped at this point. However, some clinicians would stop earlier in cases of mild VUR and no renal scarring. In the presence of scarring and persistent VUR some clinicians would continue prophylaxis until puberty. There is considerable variation on this practice point. An indirect MAG 3 cystogram may be useful at the age of 5 to identify the persistence of reflux and allow more rational discontinuation in prophylaxis at this age.

Urinary stasis should be avoided by preventing or treating constipation, ensuring regular and complete bladder emptying and encouraging an adequate fluid intake. Some girls with VUR in early childhood develop a recurrence of this problem in pregnancy.

The most commonly used prophylactic antibiotic is trimethoprim, as it is well tolerated. Nitrofurantoin is also used but the liquid form suitable for infants is sometimes difficult to obtain. It is, however, an excellent anti-bacterial although it may cause nausea. Amoxycillin, cephalosporins and nalidixic acid are not suitable as bacterial resistance develops rapidly. In spite of their wide use, the role of antibiotic prophylaxis in preventing renal scarring has not been established in a prospective controlled study.

Urethral catheterisation carries a significant risk of infection. There are a number of reports on the occurrence of a UTI after either an MCUG or cystoscopy. For this reason it is strongly recommended that antibiotic pro-phylaxis should be given for 48 hours in full therapeutic dosage at the time these procedures are carried out.

FURTHER READING

Guidelines for the management of acute urinary tract infection in child-hood (1991) Report of a Working Group of the Research Unit, Royal College of Physicians. J Roy Coll Phys 25: 36–42.

Winberg J, Anderson HJ, Bergstrom T, Jacobson B, Larson H, Lincoln K (1974) Epidemiology of symptomatic urinary tract infection in childhood. Acta Paed Scand (Suppl 252) 63: 1–20.

Verrier Jones K (1990) Antimicrobial treatment for urinary tract infections. Arch Dis Child 65: 327–330.

20 Management of suspected sexually transmitted infections in prepubertal children

There are a number of aspects to be considered when a sexually transmit-ted infection is suspected in a prepubertal child. When should such a dis-ease be suspected? When a potentially sexually transmitted infection (STI) is found in a prepubertal child, what is the likelihood of this actually being due to sexual activity? If a child is suspected to have been sexually abused, what infections should be sought in the absence of any specific clinical indi-cations? There are no simple answers to any of these questions. For man-agement of individual infections, refer to the appropriate chapters.

WHEN TO SUSPECT A SEXUALLY TRANSMITTED INFECTION

Many young girls have a clear or slightly milky vaginal discharge without any symptoms. This is usually of no significance and requires no treat-ment. However, if the discharge is purulent, has an offensive odour or is causing symptoms and/or signs in the genital area, investigations ought to be carried out to exclude infection. Chlamydial, trichomonal and gonorrhoeal infection needs to be specifically looked for and excluded. Although the presence of a foreign body should always be considered, it is uncommon and an examination under anaesthesia need only be carried out to exclude it if all other diagnoses have been ruled out.

SEXUALLY TRANSMITTED INFECTION AND SEXUAL ABUSE

It has become increasingly apparent in children that sexual contact is the most common explanation for these diseases when they have not been acquired perinatally. In some, no other explanation should be entertained, whereas in others alternative modes of transmission occasionally occur. Perinatally acquired anogenital warts and *Chlamydia* may not present in the perinatal period. Some authorities suggest that anogenital warts acquired by this route can first appear up to 2 years after birth. Table 20.1 is compiled from a number of sources and is offered as a guide to the significance of some infections that may be sexually transmitted.

When an STI is found in a child, especially an infant, infection ought to be sought in the mother. If she is found to be positive, it suggests that transmission may have occurred within the family setting. It does not exclude sexual abuse. Most abuse occurs within the extended family and, as the mother is infected, so may her partner be. He is frequently the abuser and should also be examined.

Wherever sexual abuse is considered possible on the basis of one of these infections, others should be sought. The local social services department must be involved at an early stage.

The overwhelming majority of children who have been sexually abused do not develop an STI. A recently published survey of sexually transmitted organisms in sexually abused children (Table 20.2) showed only 3.7% of the girls to be infected with gonorrhoea, *Trichomonas* or *Chlamydia*. All those with trichomoniasis or gonorrhoea and two of the three with chlamydial infection had a vaginal discharge. All those with mycoplasmal infection had either a history or physical signs of penetrative sexual intercourse. However, the significance of mycoplasmas in this situation is unclear and screening for them cannot be recommended.

Although there is variation in results between studies, there are some lessons to be learnt. It is appropriate to look for *Chlamydia trachomatis*, *Neisseria gonorrhoeae* and *Trichomonas vaginalis* in all those where genital-to-genital contact is suspected, as infection may be asymptomatic. Oral and/or anal gonococcal infection must also be considered where the alleged behaviour puts the child at risk. Remember that screening for STIs should ideally take place 10–21 days following the last incident. Accompanying symptoms or signs may suggest further investigations.

It is useful to have a standard kit to test for the main STIs (gonorrhoea, chlamydial infection and trichomoniasis) available wherever a child suspected of being abused is likely to be examined. The exact contents of this kit and handling of specimens will need to be decided in conjunction

Table 20.1 Infections that may be sexually transmitted

Infection	Incubation period of acquired disease	Modes of transmission	Definitive diagnosis	Probability of abuse
Chlamydia	7–14 days	Intrapartum Sexual contact	ELISA/IFAT/PCR Culture*	++ (+++ if child > 3 years)
Gonorrhoea	3–4 days	Intrapartum Sexual contact	Culture	++ (+++ if child > 2 years)
Hepatitis B	Up to 3 months	In utero Intrapartum Child to child (under-5s) in households Sexual contact Blood-borne	Serology	+++[†]
Herpes simplex	2–14 days	Intrapartum Sexual contact Autoinoculation Direct contact	Culture and electron microscopy	++

	Incubation	Transmission	Test	Significance
HIV	Up to 6 months	In utero Intrapartum Sexual contact Blood-borne	Serology/PCR	+++†
Anogenital warts	Up to 2 years	In utero Intrapartum Sexual contact Autoinoculation Direct contact	Clinical/PCR	(++ > 2 years)
Syphilis	Up to 3 months	In utero Intrapartum Sexual contact	Serology	+++†
Trichomonas	1–4 weeks	Intrapartum Sexual contact	Culture and microscopy	+++

++ = abuse likely; +++ = abuse almost certain; ELISA = enzyme-linked immunosorbent assay; IFAT = immunofluorescent antibody test; PCR = polymerase chain reaction.

* Culture is essential in medicolegal cases as there are too many false positives with ELISA. † If in-utero, intrapartum and blood-borne infection can be ruled out by testing the mother and excluding the possibility of blood-borne transmission postnatally.

Table 20.2 Sexually transmitted organisms in sexually abused children – no. of swabs positive/swabs taken

Organisms	< 3	3–10	> 10	Total
Neisseria gonorrhoeae	2/15	0/90	1/54	3/159
Chlamydia trachomatis	0/10	1/67	1/54	2/131
Trichomonas vaginalis	0/15	0/90	4/54	4/159
Mycoplasmas	0/8	6/42	15/46	21/96
Candida albicans	4/15	3/90	12/54	19/159
Bacterial vaginosis	0/15	1/90	2/54	3/159
Anaerobes	0/15	6/90	1/54	7/159

Age (years)

Source: adapted from Robinson AJ, Watkeys JEM, Ridgway GL (1998) Sexually transmitted organisms in sexually abused children. Arch Dis Child 79: 356–358.

with the local microbiology service. A swab and slide for gonococcus, a swab in *Trichomonas* medium and the preferred local option for *Chlamydia* would comprise a reasonable basic kit. The gold standard for *Chlamydia* is polymerase chain reaction (PCR) but culture should also be performed for medicolegal purposes. If the results are to be used in evidence in court, it is important that the 'chain of evidence' is maintained.

When a child has been repeatedly abused by strangers, consideration should be given to testing for other STIs, including human immunodeficiency virus (HIV), syphilis and hepatitis B. If this is to be done, antibody levels should be measured at presentation and again at 3 months and 6 months after exposure. Testing should not be done without counselling the parents, and the child, if s/he is mature enough.

It has been suggested that prophylactic antibiotics might be given to all cases where penetrative sexual abuse is suspected. This course of action is not justified by the low incidence of significant infections. Exceptions to this would be where the child was symptomatic or the abuser was known to have an STI.

HIV INFECTION AND CHILD SEXUAL ABUSE

After consensual sexual intercourse with an HIV-infected partner in adults, the risk of HIV infection for each act of intercourse is of the order of 0.3–1% for receptive penile–anal intercourse and 0.1–0.2% for receptive vaginal intercourse. Although HIV infection has occurred after sexual abuse it is extremely uncommon. While there is strong evidence that treatment of HIV-infected mothers with antiretroviral agents reduces the risk of transmission of infection to the neonate and some evidence that immediate prophylaxis after needlestick injuries also reduces the risk of infection, there is no convincing evidence that treatment after sexual intercourse has a similarly beneficial effect. In view of the rarity of HIV infection after abuse, the potential toxicity of the drugs, the lack of evidence that prophylaxis in this situation is efficacious and the difficulty of initiating timely treatment, HIV prophylaxis is not normally recommended after sexual abuse.

Because the association between HIV and sexual abuse is low in the UK, routine testing of abused children for HIV is not recommended. However the presence of any one of following factors might modify this decision (modified from Moq JYQ (1996) When is HIV an issue after child sexual abuse? Arch Dis Child 75: 85–87):

- Pertaining to the suspected abuser
  - Known to be HIV-positive
  - Is an injecting drug abuser
  - Is bisexual or homosexual, or
  - Comes from a high-prevalence country.
- Pertaining to the child or young person
  - Has had multiple assailants
  - Has another sexually transmitted disease, or
  - Has a history of high-risk behaviour.

If the young person or parent requests testing for HIV infection, it should normally be undertaken

PREGNANCY AND SEXUAL ABUSE

The risk of pregnancy after child sexual abuse is low (c. 1%). It depends on the age of the child, the stage of the menstrual cycle at which the abuse took place, the type of abuse and whether any form of contraception was in use at the time. When genital-to-genital intercourse occurs in a peri- or postmenarcheal girl, and she presents within 72 hours, emergency contraception should be considered.

FURTHER READING

Hobbs CJ, Hanks HGI, Wynne J (1993) Child abuse and neglect: a clinicians' handbook. Churchill Livingstone, Edinburgh.

Management of possible sexual, injecting-drug-use, or other nonoccupational exposure to HIV, including considerations related to antiretroviral therapy (1998) Public Health Statement. MMWR 47: RR-17.

Royal College of Physicians (1997) Physical signs of sexual abuse in children. RCP, London.

21 The child with suspected immunodeficiency

GENERAL PRINCIPLES

While many of the rare major primary immunodeficiencies are now very well defined, more minor degrees of susceptibility to infection in childhood are both common and poorly understood. Indeed, the combination of immunological naivete and immaturity are universal in the first years of life, with consequences familiar to parents and to doctors dealing with children. It is often very difficult to decide, on clinical grounds, whether a child has had more than an average number or severity of infections by chance or because of an underlying problem. A formal strategy for investigation is hard to formulate. However, some guiding principles can be set out.

For practical purposes , recognised immunodeficiencies can be divided into defects of specific immunity – lymphocyte function, including the production of antibodies – and defects of nonspecific immunity, including neutrophils, complement components and other problems such as the breakdown of the protective barriers of the skin and mucosa. There are deficiencies in these barriers around the time of birth as well as defects in other aspects of nonspecific immunity. The main universal deficiency in early childhood is, however, in specific immunity. Most babies encounter no pathogens prior to entering the birth canal and from then onwards face an onslaught of one new potential pathogen after another until, after some years, they achieve a broad repertoire of immunity. Distinguishing between this immunodeficiency of immaturity and that due to a primary (and permanent) immunodeficiency disorder may not always be easy. The major primary immunodeficiency disorders are listed in Table 21.1.

HISTORY

The commonest presentation of a primary immunodeficiency state will be frequent or persistent infection, brought forward by a parent or another physician. Such infections may be bacterial but fungal (candidal) infection is often one of the earliest manifestations of severe combined immunodeficiency (SCID). Alternatively, a single episode of atypical infection such as *Pneumocystis carinii* pneumonia or a family history of a specific disorder may prompt further investigation. Several other less obvious features should also signal the possibility of an immunodeficiency. Unusual erythematous rashes in small infants may suggest graft versus host disease due to maternal lymphocyte engraftment sometimes seen in SCID. Generalised erythroderma, often with lymphadenopathy and hepatosplenomegaly, can be seen in Omenn's syndrome, a variety of SCID. Unexplained poor growth and persistent diarrhoea are also common features of SCID or (less severe) combined immunodeficiency states. Delayed separation of the umbilical cord is seen in leukocyte adhesion defects and sometimes in other congenital

Table 21.1 Important primary immunodeficiency disorders

Disorder	Molecular defect and inheritance	Common presenting features	Important tests*
Humoral deficiencies			
Agammaglobulinaemia (Bruton)	XL Defect of Bruton tyrosine kinase (btk)	Bacterial infections	Serum Igs, B-cell numbers btk analysis
Common variable immunodeficiency	?	Bacterial and opportunistic infections	Serum Igs and antibody responses Lymphocyte numbers and function
Selective IgA deficiency	?	Respiratory/gastrointestinal infections	Serum/salivary IgA
IgG subclass deficiency	?	Respiratory infections	Serum Igs, IgG subclasses and antibody responses
Deficient anticarbohydrate responses	?	Respiratory and other invasive bacterial infections	Response to pneumococcal polysaccharide vaccine
Complement disorders	Factor deficiencies Mostly AR	Bacterial infections, especially meningococcal	Total haemolytic complement If abnormal, individual factor assays
Combined immunodeficiencies (SCID and CID)			
Reticular dysgenesis (T⁻B⁻NK⁻)†	Defect unknown AR	Bacterial infections Candidiasis Pneumonitis Chronic diarrhoea Failure to thrive	Serum Igs Lymphocyte numbers and function
Adenosine deaminase (ADA) deficiency (T⁻B⁻NK⁻)	ADA deficiency AR	As above	As above ADA levels Deoxy ATP levels

Table 21.1 Important primary immunodeficiency disorders continued

Disorder	Molecular defect and inheritance	Common presenting features	Important tests*
X-linked SCID (T⁻B⁺NK⁻)	Defect of common γ-chain of interleukin receptors XL	As above	As above γ-chain expression
Autosomal recessive SCID (T⁻B⁻NK⁺)	Defect of recombination activating genes (RAG) AR	As above	As above T-cell clonality (restricted) RAG mutation analysis
JAK 3 phosphorylase deficiency (T⁻B⁺NK⁻)	Defect of intracellular signalling molecule AR	As above	As above JAK 3 expression
Purine nucleoside phosphorylase (PNP) deficiency	PNP deficiency AR	Infections Developmental delay Autoimmune disorders	As above PNP levels Uric acid
Other forms of SCID	Various defects, known or unknown Mostly AR	As above	As above
CIDs	Known SCID defects with partial expression or unknown defects Mostly AR	Recurrent infections as for classic SCID	Igs, antibody responses, molecular tests to rule out classic SCID disorders
Ommenn's syndrome	Mostly RAG defects AR	Erythroderma, lymphadenopathy, hepatosplenomegaly Infections as for other SCIDs	Igs, including IgE (raised) Lymphocyte numbers and function T-cell clonality

Major histocompatibility antigen (MHA) deficiency	MHC class II deficiency AR	Recurrent infections, especially viral, opportunistic	HLA DR expression
Hyper-IgM syndrome	Defect of CD40 ligand expression XL	Enteropathy, sclerosing cholangitis; Bacterial and opportunistic infections	Serum Igs; Lymphocyte function; CD40L expression
X-linked lymphoproliferative syndrome	Defect of lymphocyte regulatory protein (SAP) XL	Severe outcome after EBV infection (or occasionally other viruses); Severe mononucleosis, aplastic anaemia, hypogammaglobulinaemia, lymphoproliferative disease	EBV serology; EBV PCR; SAP expression

Syndromal disorders

Ataxia-telangiectasia	Defect of cell cycle regulatory protein (ATM) AR	Ataxia; Bacterial and viral infections; Malignancy; Telangiectases	Alpha-fetoprotein; DNA radiosensitivity; Igs, antibody responses; Lymphocyte number and function
Wiskott–Aldrich syndrome	Defect of cytoskeleton associated protein (WASP) XL	Petechiae and bleeding; Eczema; Bacterial infections; Malignancy	Platelet numbers and size; Serum Igs, including IgE; Lymphocyte numbers and function; WASP expression
DiGeorge anomaly	Most have microdeletion at chromosome 22q	Cardiac defect; Hypocalcaemia; Abnormal facies; Bacterial/opportunistic infections	Chest X-ray; Lymphocyte numbers and function; Antibody responses; FISH for 22q deletion
Hyper-IgE syndrome	Unknown defect Probable AD with incomplete penetrance	Skin infections, cold abscesses; Pneumonias and pneumatoceles; Abnormal facies, delayed dentition, osteopenia	IgE, Igs, antibody responses

21 Suspected immunodeficiency

Table 21.1 Important primary immunodeficiency disorders continued

Disorder	Molecular disorder and inheritance	Common presenting features	Important tests*
Neutrophil disorders			
Congenital neutropenia	Defect(s) unknown AR	Bacterial and fungal infections (skin, mouth, deep-seated)	FBC and bone marrow
Cyclical neutropenia	Defect of neutrophil elastase (some) or unknown Mostly AD	Intermittent infections, especially gingivostomatitis	Repeated FBCs (2× per week for 8 weeks)
Chédiak–Higashi syndrome	Defect of secretory organelle protein trafficking AR	Partial oculocutaneous albinism Bacterial infections Development of haemophagocytic lymphohistiocytosis	Neutrophil morphology characteristic NK cell function
Chronic granulomatous disease	Defect of photo-oxidase enzyme system XL (67%), AR (33%)	Pneumonias Deep abscesses Granuloma formation, especially in gastrointestinal and genitourinary tracts	Nitroblue tetrazolium test
Leukocyte adhesion molecule deficiency	Defect of expression of leukocyte function antigen (LFA1) AR	Delayed cord separation Bacterial and fungal infections, especially periodontitis Skin infections	Expression of leukocyte CD11 and CD18

? = often familial but no distinct mendelian pattern; AD = autosomal dominant; AR = autosomal recessive; EBV = Epstein–Barr virus; FBC = full blood count; Igs = immunoglobulins; NK = natural killer; SCID = severe combined immunodeficiency; XL = X-linked.
* In general, where the molecular defect is known, in addition to measuring expression of the defective protein, mutation analysis of the defective gene can be performed. Molecular diagnosis of primary immunodeficiency is centrally funded in the UK and provided at Great Ormond Street Hospital, London. † Lymphocyte phenotype in terms of presence or absence of T, B or NK cells.

neutrophil disorders. Severe or recurrent periodontitis can also be a feature of such conditions.

There are several syndromal associations with immunodeficiency. These include velocardiofacial syndrome (usually associated with a chromosomal microdeletion at 22q), which may result in: the DiGeorge anomaly with immunodeficiency; partial albinism (Chédiak–Higashi and Griscelli syndromes); and short-limbed dwarfism with immunodeficiency. A history of recurrent infections with eczema and thrombocytopenic purpura in a boy should raise the possibility of Wiskott–Aldrich syndrome. Children presenting with ataxia, usually first noticed in the second year of life, may have ataxia telangiectasia (AT). Severe congenital immunodeficiency disorders sometimes may not present until later in childhood. Boys affected with X-linked lymphoproliferative (Duncan) syndrome may not present until they meet Epstein–Barr virus (or occasionally another virus), when they develop one or more of a number of complications, including severe infectious mononucleosis syndrome, aplastic anaemia, hypogammaglobulinaemia or lymphoproliferative disease. In antibody-deficiency states, recurrent ear infections and lower respiratory tract problems, sometimes presenting as asthma, can be present for years before the diagnosis is suspected. Unfortunately some of these children have already developed permanent lung damage by this time.

Recurrent skin sepsis does not usually turn out to be due to underlying problems but rather is due to colonisation with a virulent strain of *S. aureus*, which may also affect other members of the family. However, particularly when there is persistent infection, lymphadenitis, more deep-seated infection or unusual bacterial isolates, an underlying immunodeficiency should be sought. It is worth trying to establish whether there is a predictable temporal pattern to recurrent infection or recurrent mouth ulcers, as neutropenia may be cyclical. Immunodeficiencies are not usually associated with recurrent urinary tract infection. The association of recurrent infection with atypical allergy or unusual autoimmune disorder should merit investigation of immune function. HIV infection will need to be considered in the differential diagnosis of children with recurrent infections, particularly those from high-risk backgrounds. Understanding of the subtleties of immune function is still in its infancy. A considerable proportion of children with a pattern of recurrent infection suggestive of immunodeficiency cannot be given a specific diagnosis. Presumably they have an as yet unrecognised problem. An example is the child with frequent and severe attacks of herpes labialis but normal immune function tests.

EXAMINATION

This should focus on growth parameters, the skin (noting the presence of any rash), the respiratory tract (including the tympanic membranes and, when appropriate, hearing assessment), the presence of absence of lymphoid tissue (tonsillar tissue or palpable lymph nodes) and the presence of an enlarged liver and spleen. Examination for associated features or syndromal conditions (e.g. the presence of cutaneous telangiectasia in AT) may also be appropriate.

INVESTIGATIONS

Investigations for immunodeficiency will often be carried out alongside those for other disorders with overlapping presentation such as cystic fibrosis and recurrent aspiration. Very generally, the following circumstances should prompt investigations for immunodeficiency:

- Single infections with unusual organisms
- Recurrent infections with common organisms – especially bacterial
- Infections associated with failure to thrive
- Infections associated with severe allergy or unusual autoimmune disorder
- Family history of immunodeficiency.

Blood count

The simplest test is the blood count with differential white cell count. Patients will sometimes have had several performed previously and an important abnormality such as lymphopenia may have gone unnoticed. Infants with SCID are often persistently lymphopenic when counts are compared to age-related normal values. Other children may show persistent neutropenia but the degree of associated infectious problems correlates poorly with the neutrophil count. In cyclical neutropenia the neutrophil count falls to abnormally low levels in a regular 3- or 4-weekly cycle, diagnosable only by twice-weekly blood counts over a period. Eosinophilia may be a feature of some T-cell disorders and also certain bone marrow disorders. A low platelet count and small platelets (determined on blood film or by automated measurement of the mean platelet volume) are seen in Wiskott–Aldrich syndrome which may present with infections, bleeding or both. A careful examination of the blood film may reveal abnormal leukocyte granular morphology in Chédiak–Higashi syndrome. Bone marrow examination may be helpful in providing further information if the blood count is abnormal.

Lymphocyte tests

Lymphocyte immunophenotyping ('subsets') provides a more sophisticated count of the different functional types of lymphocytes. Age-related normal value for the main types (CD3 – all T cells; CD4 – helper subset; CD8 – suppressor/cytotoxic subset; CD16/56 – natural killer cells; CD19/20 – B cells) are now widely available. Specialist help with interpretation may be required, particularly if steroid or other immunosuppressive treatment has been given. More sophisticated panels of lymphocyte markers may be required for the diagnosis of certain specific immunodeficiencies (e.g. CD40 ligand deficiency or deficiency of MHC class II expression). Functional tests of the ability of lymphocytes to proliferate and produce cytokines (such as IL-2) or cell-surface-expressed activation molecules in response to different stimuli (mitogens such as phytohaemagglutinin (PHA) or antigens such as *Candida* or tetanus) are important tests to complement the immunophenotyping results.

Antibody tests

Assays for immunoglobulin levels are perhaps the most widely known and used tests of immune function. Measurement of total serum IgG, IgA, IgM and IgE is available in most hospitals and IgG and IgA subclasses can also be measured. Particular caution is needed in the interpretation of these tests in early childhood. Normal newborns have very low levels of IgA, IgM and IgE. Maternal IgG is present and wanes in blood level until the second half of the first year. Some laboratories do not quote well-defined paediatric normal ranges for their own assays, which may be unreliable at the low levels detectable in small children. Furthermore, low values, particularly of one or more IgG subclasses, can be a transient finding of no great significance. It is therefore advisable to investigate any child with suspected humoral immunodeficiency in conjunction with a centre experienced in handling and interpreting paediatric material. Repeat investigations and assays of 'functional' antibody production should be undertaken before gammaglobulin therapy is considered.

Tests of specific antibody responsiveness are a more sensitive index of humoral immune function than are measurements of total immunoglobulin levels. The presence of naturally occurring IgM isohaemagglutinins can be detected in routine cross-matching laboratories. These antibodies are, however, not found in those of blood group AB or, reliably, in infants under 9 months of age. Serum can be sent to reference laboratories for more sensitive analysis by special arrangement and this is particularly useful for measuring antibodies against previously given vaccine antigens (such as diphtheria , tetanus, polio, Hib and MMR) or additional vaccines given during the course of investigation. Hib, pneumococcal, influenza and injectable typhoid (Vi) vaccines can all be used in this way, with the added possible benefit of providing some useful protection as well. Pneumococcal polysaccharide vaccine is potentially the most useful in this respect, since being a pure polysaccharide it is the least immunogenic and therefore potentially the most discriminating test when investigating partial humoral immunodeficiencies. However normal children do not reliably respond to this vaccine before 2 years of age. Furthermore, there is poor standardisation of assays for pneumococcal antibodies, most of which measure antibodies against all the 23 serotypes present in Pneumovax, and these have very variable immunogenicity, particularly in children. Interpretation of 'one-off' levels of pneumococcal antibody is therefore very difficult and pre- and post-vaccine levels should be performed.

Neutrophil disorders

The pathophysiology of neutropenia is often classified for conceptual purposes into either a failure of maturation and release of neutrophils from the marrow or an increased peripheral destruction (often antibody-mediated). Bone marrow examination will usually help distinguish between these two mechanisms. Demonstration of antineutrophil antibodies may also be helpful.

There are two well-defined groups of functional neutrophil disorders. Chronic granulomatous disease, which is a failure of neutrophil production of microbicidal oxidative products, is diagnosed by a simple slide test called the nitroblue tetrazolium (NBT) test. More sophisticated tests can then be performed to confirm the diagnosis. Bactericidal tests can be used to identify other less well characterised neutrophil-killing defects. Deficiency of leukocyte adhesion molecules such as leukocyte function antigen-1 (LFA-1) is due to an absence of the cell surface receptors important for the migration of leukocytes out of the circulation. All leukocytes are affected and there are consequences for specific immunity but the main manifestations relate to failure of normal neutrophil function. These patients have high leukocyte counts and severe cutaneous infections without pus. Diagnosis is by detailed leukocyte immunophenotyping. Defective neutrophil chemotaxis and adherence can also be demonstrated in the laboratory. Individuals with recurrent cutaneous and pulmonary infection, eczematoid rash and very high circulating IgE levels (> 5000 IU/L) – hyper IgE syndrome ('Job's syndrome') – also appear to have a defect in neutrophil chemotaxis, although the reason for this is not clearly understood. Other less well-defined neutrophil disorders are associated with defective chemotaxis but they are difficult to diagnose and characterise because measurement of chemotaxis is fraught with difficulties and can vary considerably from time to time in any one individual.

Complement tests

Deficiencies of many of the individual components of the complement cascade have been described. These are rare. Affected individuals may suffer from autoimmune disorders or recurrent infections or both. Recurrent sepsis occurs in those with C3 deficiency, alternative pathway deficiencies and to a lesser extent in early classical pathway component deficiencies. Recurrent meningococcal infection complicates deficiencies anywhere in the cascade particularly the later (lytic) components, C6–C9. However, very few individuals with single episodes of invasive meningococcal disease have underlying complement disorders. Recurrent meningococcal disease or a family history should prompt investigation. Screening can be performed using a total haemolytic complement (CH50) test, in which antibody-sensitised red cells are lysed in the presence of test serum indicating the integrity of the whole cascade.

Molecular and genetic tests

Where consistent immune function abnormalities are identified it is possible to identify a specific genetic abnormality in some cases. The pattern of immune function observed will help direct appropriate molecular and genetic tests. Such characterisation is helpful not only in the management of the affected child but also in the provision of genetic counselling for the family. However there remain a significant proportion of immunodeficient children in whom the molecular diagnosis has yet to be established. It is important to store material such as DNA and ideally lymphocytes on these children since a retrospective diagnosis may be possible as knowledge of the molecular basis of these conditions advances.

MANAGEMENT

General principles

It is important to minimise exposure to potentially serious pathogens. Chickenpox and measles are particularly dangerous in children with cell-mediated immunodeficiencies. Postexposure prophylaxis should be given using zoster immune globulin or human normal immunoglobulin (see pp. 242 and 348). Children with SCID should ideally be kept in strict isolation until transfer to a designated SCID bone marrow transplant centre. In SCID and some other severe deficiency states blood products should be irradiated because of the risk of transfusion-acquired graft versus host disease.

Antimicrobials

In most cases of immunodeficiency, the mainstay of management is the use of antibiotics, given either in response to infection or on a long-term prophylactic basis. In minor antibody deficiency states a regular prophylactic antibiotic either continuously or through the winter months is the mainstay of management. The choice of antibiotic for prophylaxis against bacterial respiratory infection is not straightforward. In the past, based on largely anecdotal evidence, co-trimoxazole was usually employed. However, concerns over the side-effects of this agent have led to increasing reliance on other agents, except in combined immunodeficiency states where *Pneumocystis carinii* pneumonia (PCP) prophylaxis is also required and co-trimoxazole remains the best option. The issue of emerging antibiotic resistance among pneumococcal isolates is also pertinent. Anecdotally, trimethoprim does not provide adequate prophylaxis for the respiratory tract. The newer macrolides, clarithromycin (given as a single daily dose) or azithromycin (given for 3 days in therapeutic dosage and repeated each fortnight – after an 11-day gap), are suitable alternatives to co-trimoxazole. Once-daily cefixime has also been used. Amoxycillin and co-amoxiclav are not good agents for long-term prophylaxis and the use of ciprofloxacin in this context cannot be justified in children because of its potential for causing arthropathy. Where the bacterial susceptibility is narrow-spectrum (e.g. to meningococcus in late complement component deficiency), simple penicillin V is the appropriate prophylactic agent. Antifungal prophylaxis with fluconazole is used in SCID patients upon diagnosis, switching to itraconazole (to provide cover against *Aspergillus* species) at the time of bone marrow transplantation. Itraconazole prophylaxis is also used in chronic granulomatous disease (where invasive aspergillosis is a significant problem) and in chronic mucocutaneous candidiasis.

Gammaglobulin

Immunoglobulin replacement therapy is used in cases of severe antibody deficiency. It can be administered by intravenous (IVIG) or subcutaneous (SCIG) routes. This treatment should not be embarked upon lightly as it is very costly and administration involves considerable disruption to the patient's life even when arrangements can be made for administration at home. Most children with minor immunoglobulin deficiencies such as IgA or IgG subclass deficiency do not require immunoglobulin and can be managed on prophylactic antibiotics unless breakthrough bacterial infections occur and put the child at risk of chronic lung damage. Immunoglobulin is potentially dangerous in those with minor immunodeficiency associated with complete IgA deficiency, who may develop an anaphylactic reaction to the trace amounts of IgA present in the infusion. Although all commercially available products are made from carefully screened donors and new European regulations require a specific antiviral step in the manufacturing process, they are not totally without risk of transmission of viral infection, particularly hepatitis C.

When appropriately used, immunoglobulin replacement therapy can transform the patient's life from one of chronic invalidity to near normal health. Management involves careful monitoring of the clinical course as well as adjusting dosages to maintain appropriate serum immunoglobulin levels. This should be done in conjunction with a specialist centre.

Cytokines and growth factors

A number of recombinant growth factors and cytokines are available. Treatment with interferon-gamma can replace the stimulus to macrophage function normally provided by T cells. It has been used in combined immunodeficiency states with mycobacterial and other intracellular infections and may be of particular value in those patients with a genetic defects of the interleukin-12/interferon-gamma pathway. It may also be useful as adjunctive therapy in patients with deep-seated fungal infections complicating chronic granulomatous disease. Granulocyte and granulocyte macrophage colony stimulating factors (GCSF and GMCSF) can increase neutrophil counts in neutropenic patients. Experience with these agents in children with primary immunodeficiency remains limited and requires expert supervision.

Bone marrow transplantation

This remains, for the moment, the only curative treatment for immunodeficiency. It is performed in children with major defects such as severe combined immunodeficiency (SCID). Results are best when there is a matched sibling donor and when the diagnosis can be made during the first months of life. Success in SCID transplants particularly depends on early diagnosis and transplantation. For those without a matched sibling donor, matched unrelated donor or parent-to-child haploidentical (mismatched) transplantation can be attempted using fractionation of the donor marrow to remove mature T lymphocytes capable of causing graft versus host disease. This is performed for immunodeficiency disorders in two centres in the UK (Great Ormond Street Hospital, London and Newcastle General Hospital).

Genetic counselling

Since most of the primary immunodeficiencies are inherited, counselling is important and, where appropriate, consideration of antenatal diagnosis.

In an increasing number of disorders the gene has been identified, allow-ing first-trimester diagnosis. In other conditions, such as some SCID cases, this is not yet possible but second-trimester diagnosis can be per-formed on fetal blood. Female carrier detection can be performed for some X-linked conditions such as X-linked SCID and chronic granuloma-tous disease.

FURTHER READING

Chapel HM, Webster ADB (1999) Assessment of the immune system. In: Ochs HD, Smith CIE, Puck JM (eds) Primary immunodeficiency diseases. Oxford University Press, New York, pp 419–431.

Comans-Bitter WM et al (1997) Immunophenotyping of blood lympho-cytes in childhood. Reference values for lymphocyte subpopulations. J Pediatr 130: 388–393.

22 Management of the immunocompromised child with infection

INTRODUCTION

Those working in paediatrics increasingly have to deal with children whose immunity to infection is compromised. This may be by virtue of immaturi-ty of immune responses (very low birth weight infants, particularly those who are sick), a primary defect of immune function – congenital immuno-deficiency – or, more commonly, through acquired defects of immunity secondary to human immunodeficiency virus (HIV) infection, chemothera-py or other immunosuppressive treatment (including corticosteroids). Other children who behave in an immunocompromised way include those who have been splenectomised and those with sickle cell anaemia, cystic fibrosis, primary ciliary dyskinesia syndrome and those with chronic debil-itating diseases.

Infections in immunocompromised children are liable to be more fre-quent and more severe. They may show atypical features and may be caused by atypical (opportunistic) organisms.

Since immunocompromised children are susceptible to a wide variety of organisms it is not always easy to predict the class of organism caus-ing infection, let alone the species. However, there are some broad gen-eral rules depending on whether the predominant defect lies within phago-cytic cells (usually the neutrophils), antibodies or the cell-mediated immune system (Table 22.1). In view of the broad range of possible infect-ing organisms and the varying clinical presentation there should be a low threshold for thorough investigation to identify the cause of any illness (Table 22.2).

Table 22.1 Important pathogens in the immunocompromised child

Neutrophil disorders

Bacteria	Staphylococci, enteric Gram-negative bacilli
Fungi	*Candida* spp., *Aspergillus* spp., *Nocardia* spp.

Antibody disorders

Bacteria	Encapsulated organisms (*Streptococcus pneumoniae*, *Haemophilus influenzae*)
	Enteric Gram-negative bacilli
	Staphylococcus aureus
Viruses	Enteroviruses
Protozoa	*Giardia lamblia*

Cell-mediated immune disorders

Bacteria	Intracellular pathogens (*Salmonella, Listeria, Mycobacterium, Legionella*)
Viral	Herpes group (herpes simplex virus, varicella-zoster virus, cytomegalovirus, Epstein–Barr virus)
	Respiratory (adenovirus, influenza virus, respiratory syncytial virus)
	Enteric (rotavirus, adenovirus)
	Papovavirus
Fungal	*Candida, Aspergillus, Nocardia, Cryptococcus, Pneumocystis*
Protozoa	*Toxoplasma, Cryptosporidium*
Helminths	*Strongyloides*

NEUTROPHIL DISORDERS

Neutropenia

Neutropenia is one of the commonest forms of immunocompromise encountered. It may be congenital or autoimmune in origin but most commonly it will be secondary to myelosuppressive treatments. Affected children tend to suffer infection with bacteria, particularly staphylococci and Gram-negative enteric bacilli, including *Pseudomonas aeruginosa*. They may also develop fungal infections with *Candida* and *Aspergillus* species and this is most likely to occur if the neutropenia is profound ($< 0.1 \times 10^9$/L) and prolonged (> 1 week). Other risk factors for fungal sepsis are the prior use of broad-spectrum antibiotics or systemic corticosteroids.

A significant fever (> 38°C) in a neutropenic child ($< 0.5 \times 10^9$/L) should be treated very seriously. A careful examination is required, looking for focal signs of infection – skin, mouth, chest, abdomen and perineum being particularly important. Blood cultures from each lumen of any indwelling central line and by direct venepuncture should be collected, swabs taken from any focal infective lesions and a chest radiograph performed. Empirical broad-spectrum antibiotic therapy should then be commenced immediately. Suitable therapy includes an antipseudomonal β-lactam (such as piperacillin, piptazobactam or ceftazidime) plus an aminogly-

Table 22.2 Diagnostic techniques in the diagnosis of infection in the immunocompromised

Pulmonary
- Nasopharyngeal aspirate
  - Immunofluorescence and culture
- Bronchoalveolar lavage
  - Microscopy and culture
  - Immunofluorescence
  - Special stains (silver stain, Ziehl–Neelsen) in histology
  - PCR
- Lung biopsy
  - As above

Gastrointestinal
- Stool
  - Microscopy and culture
  - Ziehl–Neelsen stain
  - Electron microscopy
  - ELISA
  - PCR
- Biopsy
  - As above

Liver
- Biopsy
  - Bacterial, viral, fungal cultures and histological stains
  - PCR
- ERCP
  - Bile sampling

Central nervous system
- Computed tomography/magnetic resonance imaging scans
- Cerebrospinal fluid
  - Bacterial, viral, fungal microscopy and culture
  - Antigen detection tests
  - PCR

ELISA = enzyme-linked immunosorbent assay; ERCP = endoscopic retrograde cholangio-pancreatography; PCR = polymerase chain reaction.

coside. Some centres use single broad-spectrum agents such as ceftazidime or meropenem but most still use combination therapy. The most common organism isolated from blood cultures in this situation is a coagulase-negative staphylococcus and this is usually associated with an indwelling central venous catheter. Gram-negative bacillary sepsis is less common but is more feared because of the possibility of a fulminant illness with endotoxic shock. *Staphylococcus aureus* and streptococcal sepsis are also found.

If blood cultures are positive, antibiotic therapy can be tailored appropriately. However, quite commonly they are negative and if the fever doesn't settle this presents a problem. Empirical changes in antibiotics become necessary and these should be performed by the third day of unremitting fever. The choice at this stage is either a new combination of antibacterials such as a glycopeptide (vancomycin or teicoplanin) and an agent active against Gram-negative bacilli (ceftazidime, ciprofloxacin) or the addition of intravenous amphotericin to cover fungal infection. The latter should be introduced early in patients at high risk of fungal infection (prolonged and profound neutropenia).

The process of empirical change is repeated again after 48 hours if the fever persists and cultures remain negative. By this stage it should be obligatory to add amphotericin.

When focal signs develop during episodes of febrile neutropenia new problems are faced. Soft tissue infections can occur anywhere but particularly around the head and neck and the perineal region. These often produce relatively mild signs of inflammation (until neutrophils return) but usually do cause some local swelling and often disproportionately severe pain. Donor white cell infusions, ideally obtained from donors primed with granulocyte colony stimulating factor, may have a role in containing these local infections. Problems with leukocyte infusions include the need for a pool of available donors, the risk of cytomegalovirus (CMV) transmission and the need for the use of CMV-negative donors in seronegative children, particularly those who might require a bone marrow transplant at a later date.

'Embolic' skin lesions may occur from circulatory dissemination of infection. Necrotic skin lesions (ecthyma gangrenosum) are characteristic of pseudomonal sepsis.

Intra-abdominal focal sepsis is relatively common in neutropenic patients, particularly after chemotherapy, which induces a mucositis. Characteristic features of typhlitis (necrotising colitis) are diarrhoea with/without bleeding, abdominal pain, distension and later an ileus. Management should be conservative with intravenous fluid therapy, nasogastric drainage and antibiotics – metronidazole should be added to the regimen, although there is a lack of evidence of its efficacy in this situation.

Pneumonia in neutropenic children will present with the usual symptoms, although chest pain is relatively more common in this group than in immunocompetent children. Chest signs are notoriously unreliable and radiography, while confirming the presence of a likely infective process, rarely gives specific clues as to the microbial diagnosis. It is reasonable to start empirical treatment with a standard neutropenic broad-spectrum antibiotic combination but if there is failure of response after 24–48 hours then bronchoalveolar lavage (BAL) should be undertaken to try to obtain a microbial diagnosis. It should be borne in mind that children who are neutropenic because of chemotherapy will also have depressed cell-mediated immunity and will therefore be susceptible to the whole gamut of opportunistic pneumonias. Specimens obtained at BAL should therefore be tested accordingly (see below).

Neutrophil function disorders

Children suffering from neutrophil function disorders are liable to the same spectrum of infections as neutropenic children, although generally with a less fulminant and more focal nature. Unless the patients have indwelling venous lines, staphylococcal infections are usually of the coagulase-positive (*S. aureus*) variety. Skin and lymph node sepsis and pneumonia are common. while more deep-seated focal infection in liver, brain or bone may also occur. Depending on the defect, there may be a tendency to less intense inflammation than might be expected. Fungal infection, particularly with *Candida* and *Aspergillus* species, also occurs. Treatment is with antibiotics and judicious surgical intervention. In chronic granulomatous disease where there is a failure to kill phagocytosed organisms it is important to use agents that penetrate well into the cells, such as co-trimoxazole (although this is less useful therapeutically in these patients as it is usually used prophylactically), ciprofloxacin and rifampicin. Adjuvant treatments with recombinant cytokines such as granulocyte colony stimulating factor (GCSF), granulocyte macrophage colony stimulating factor (GMCSF) or interferon-gamma have been shown to be useful in some situations. Donor leukocyte infusions using GCSF-primed donors can be used in severe non-responding cases.

ANTIBODY DEFICIENCY

In addition to those with primary immunodeficiencies, antibody disorders are found among children with HIV infection, on prolonged immunosuppressive treatment, after bone marrow transplantation and in protein-losing states such as enteropathies and nephrotic syndrome. Splenectomised and otherwise hyposplenic patients such as those with sickle cell anaemia produce poor antibody responses to capsulated organisms. Bacterial infections are the hallmark of antibody deficiency states, whether partial, as in IgA or IgG subclass deficiencies, or profound as in X-linked agammaglobulinaemia. The predominant bacterial types are different from those causing problems in neutrophil disorders. Capsulated organisms such as *Streptococcus pneumoniae* and *Haemophilus influenzae* are the most common pathogens found, although enteric Gram-negative bacillary and staphylococcal infections also occur.

Infections are most common in and around the respiratory tract (otitis, sinusitis, pneumonia) but more disseminated infections may occur – bacteraemia, cellulitis, meningitis, septic arthritis. Febrile episodes with or without focal signs should be treated early with a broad-spectrum antibiotic such as co-amoxiclav or ceftriaxone. Care should be taken if immunoglobulin infusions are to be given during a febrile episode since reactions are more common at this stage.

If there is failure of response to first-line antibiotics, other infections to consider include those due to *Mycoplasma* and *Ureaplasma* species, which can cause arthritis as well as respiratory and genital infections in these patients.

While 'pure' antibody deficiencies rarely result in opportunistic infections, some syndromes such as common variable hypogammaglobulinaemia may include subtle defects of cell-mediated immunity. Therefore, opportunistic infection (see below) may need to be considered when treating these patients.

Nonbacterial infections can occur in pure humoral deficiency states. *Giardia lamblia* can cause acute or chronic diarrhoea and may require repeated courses of treatment. Some viruses, particularly enteroviruses, are poorly handled in profoundly hypogammaglobulininaemic patients. Thus vaccine strain poliomyelitis may occur and echoviruses may produce a chronic infection of the nervous system and/or of muscle tissue.

These viral infections are rare in those already on immunoglobulin replacement therapy. When they occur they are very difficult to treat, although they may respond to very-high-dose intravenous immunoglobulin or intraventricular immunoglobulin for established central nervous system infection. A newly developed antiviral agent, pleconaril, with activity against enteroviruses, is currently under trial and offers the potential for treating these problems.

CELL-MEDIATED IMMUNE DEFICIT

Children with primary congenital disorders of the T lymphocytes, those undergoing chemotherapy, immunosuppressive therapy (including steroids) or bone marrow transplantation and those suffering from moderately advanced HIV disease will be vulnerable to a wide variety of different pathogens, including opportunistic infections. Since disordered cell-mediated immunity usually results in defective antibody production, these disorders therefore produce a combined immunodeficiency and the spectrum of microbial susceptibility includes bacterial pathogens.

The wide range of potential pathogens in these children is shown in Table 22.1. A history of antimicrobial prophylaxis is helpful since its use will alter the balance of possibilities. For instance, *Pneumocystis carinii* pneumonia (PCP) is much less likely to occur if the child has been given prophylactic co-trimoxazole. If the child is also neutropenic this alters the spectrum of possibilities. Febrile episodes without localising signs should be treated initially with broad-spectrum antibiotics (as for the neutropenic child if neutropenic, otherwise as for the antibody-deficient child – see above). Many episodes settle on this regimen but if not a wide diagnostic trawl needs to be initiated. Pneumonitis has the widest spectrum of causes and early intervention with bronchoalveolar lavage to look for bacteria, fungi (including *P. carinii*), mycobacteria and viruses is indicated. For viral diagnosis, immunofluorescence looking for a panel of respiratory viruses (respiratory syncytial virus, influenza A and B, parainfluenza, adenovirus and measles) and herpesviruses (cytomegalovirus, herpes simplex virus) should be performed as well as polymerase chain reaction tests on blood and respiratory secretions to include testing for cytomegalovirus (CMV), Epstein–Barr virus (EBV) and adenovirus. If BAL fails to provide a diagnosis and the patient fails to improve, more aggressive diagnostic intervention such as lung biopsy may prove necessary. While awaiting the results of tests a broad range of antimicrobial cover may be needed and then the treatment can be rationalised in the light of the results (Table 22.3).

Gastrointestinal infections may occur with common or opportunistic pathogens. Acute episodes of diarrhoea may fail to resolve completely

Table 22.3 Initial therapies to be considered for 'atypical' pneumonia

Therapy	Organism
Piperacillin (or piptazobactam) + aminoglycoside	Bacteria
Clarithromycin	*Mycoplasma, Chlamydia, Legionella*
High-dose co-trimoxazole	*Pneumocystis, Nocardia*
Liposomal amphotericin	*Candida, Aspergillus, Cryptococcus*
Ganciclovir	Cytomegalovirus, herpes simplex virus, varicella-zoster virus, Epstein–Barr virus
Ribavirin	Respiratory syncytial virus, influenza virus, parainfluenza virus, adenovirus

and the resulting chronic symptoms may lead to nutritional problems and failure to thrive. Cytomegalovirus may cause a colitis with clinical and radiological features mimicking pseudomembranous colitis. Stools need to be examined for the usual bacterial and viral pathogens and particular care taken to look for *Giardia lamblia*, *Cryptosporidium*, *Microsporidium* spp. and *Isospora*. These are notorious for causing chronic diarrhoea in patients with AIDS. *Cryptosporidium* in particular is a cause of chronic severe diarrhoea. Treatment with paramomycin may reduce the stool output but is not curative in these patients. Albendazole may be useful in microsporidial disease.

In patients with HIV infection and certain immune deficiencies affecting the handling of intracellular pathogens (particularly CD40 ligand deficiency), *Cryptosporidium* and to a lesser extent *Microsporidium* may affect the biliary system, leading to a cholangiopathy, which may present acutely or lead to chronic subclinical infection resulting in the development of sclerosing cholangitis. Once established this is very difficult to treat. The combination of paramomycin and azithromycin may suppress the process in some patients.

Central nervous system infection may present as acute meningitis. In addition to the usual pathogens, *Cryptococcus neoformans*, *Salmonella* species and *Listeria monocytogenes* all need to be considered. A generalised encephalitic illness may be generalised and acute or subacute and due to a wide variety of pathogens but especially cytomegalovirus, Epstein–Barr virus and enteroviruses. Focal encephalitis presenting as focal neurological deficit or focal convulsions may occur as a result of rekindled *Toxoplasma* infection (usually in older children who have had previous exposure to *Toxoplasma*), herpes simplex or focal fungal infections in disseminated *Aspergillus*, *Candida* or *Nocardia* infections. Computed tomography or magnetic resonance imaging will help define some of these infections.

Retinitis is a problem increasingly recognised in children affected with HIV and congenital immunodeficiencies. Cytomegalovirus is the most likely viral cause and the diagnosis is made by the clinical appearance combined with a positive viral test (polymerase chain reaction, antigen test or culture) in the blood. Sampling of material from the eye is not normally undertaken. *Toxoplasma* should also be considered – the ophthalmological appearances are characteristic and identification of *Toxoplasma* nucleic acid in blood or cerebrospinal fluid confirms the diagnosis. CMV retinitis is treated with foscarnet, ganciclovir or a combination of both. Long-term maintenance therapy may be required. In difficult cases where tolerance of the drugs was poor vitreous implants of ganciclovir have been successfully employed. *Toxoplasma* eye disease is treated along the usual lines (see p.429), although the role of steroids is less clear than in immunocompetent patients.

Skin and lymph node infections can be caused by bacteria, including salmonellas and mycobacteria (mainly atypical), and by fungal infection. To facilitate diagnosis and institution of appropriate treatment, biopsy material should be obtained early.

PREVENTION OF INFECTION IN THE IMMUNOCOMPROMISED CHILD

This should start with education of the family and their health professionals about the risks of infection and the need to seek prompt medical advice after contact with infections such as chickenpox or measles. Avoidance of mixing with large numbers of people in crowded spaces will reduce the likelihood of viral respiratory infections, which, even if not considered dangerous in themselves, may lead to the need for hospitalisation and antibiotic therapy because of the possibility of other more serious infections. Avoidance of individuals with symptomatic infections is sensible, although not always possible. In children considered at risk for severe cryptosporidiosis, continuous special precautions may be appropriate (Table 22.4).

In children beginning chemotherapy, antibody status against measles and herpesviruses (varicella-zoster virus, herpes simplex virus and CMV) should be measured on samples taken before blood products (and thus passive antibody) are given. This will help determine subsequent susceptibilities.

Table 22.4 Reducing the risks of cryptosporidiosis in immunocompromised children

- Drinking water to be boiled or filtered* and avoid bottled water
- Avoid 'toddler' swimming pools (high risk of inadvertent defecation)
- In over-5-year-olds allow swimming in pools but discourage excessive swallowing of water
- Avoid contact with farm animals (especially lambs and calves) and with surface water on farmland
- Minimise contact with kittens and puppies – wash hands after any contact
- Treat confirmed infection with paramomycin
- Consider prophylaxis with paramomycin in very-high-risk cases, although there is no evidence for its effectiveness

* The use of filters fitted to the domestic water supply has not been fully evaluated. They need to be of high specification with a pore size of less than 1 μm. Changing the filters poses a high risk to the operator and the manufacturer's instructions should be followed.

Postexposure prophylaxis is given for measles and chickenpox using zoster immune globulin or human normal immunoglobulin. In children of CMV seronegative or indeterminate status with conditions that may require bone marrow transplantation, CMV-negative blood products should be used.

During periods of neutropenia, precautions against nosocomial infection are required. Avoidance of high-risk foods such as salad or fruit without skin is sensible but completely sterile food is unnecessary unless gut decontamination is being attempted. Broad-spectrum nonabsorbable antibiotic combinations are rarely used in children as they are poorly tolerated and of doubtful benefit. Either nonabsorbable or systemic antifungals should, however, be used prophylactically in all neutropenic patients. Prophylactic absorbable antibiotics are used in some centres – quinolones such as ciprofloxacin have replaced co-trimoxazole in this situation. There are, however, concerns about using these powerful therapeutic tools on a prophylactic basis, particularly when they are not yet licensed for use in children.

In other situations such as the partial immunoglobulin deficiencies prophylactic antibiotics have an important role. The choice of antibiotic for prophylaxis depends on the range of pathogens that need to be covered and patient acceptability. As a general rule the narrowest-spectrum drug to cover the relevant pathogens is used (Table 22.5).

In some situations judicious use of vaccination may be helpful (see Chapter 25).

Table 22.5 Prophylaxis in the immunocompromised

Drug	Condition
Penicillin	Sickle cell anaemia, nephrotic syndrome, complement disorders
Flucloxacillin	Some neutrophil disorders
Azithromycin/clarithromycin	Antibody deficiency
Co-trimoxazole (daily)	Antibody deficiency; some neutrophil disorders
Co-trimoxazole (3 ×/week)	Cell-mediated disorders, including HIV; leukaemia
Nystatin/fluconazole	Intensive chemotherapy; neutrophil and cell-mediated disorders
Itraconazole	When high risk of *Aspergillus* infection – intensive chemotherapy; bone marrow transplantation; chronic granulomatous disease
Aciclovir	Cell-mediated disorders; standard dose – HSV prophylaxis; high dose – CMV prophylaxis after solid organ or bone marrow transplantation

CMV = cytomegalovirus; HIV = human immunodeficiency virus; HSV = herpes simplex virus.

FURTHER READING

Patrick CC (ed.) (1992) Infections in immunocompromised infants and children. Churchill Livingstone, Edinburgh.

23 The child with HIV infection

ORGANISM

Human immunodeficiency virus (HIV) in an enveloped RNA virus of the family Retroviridiae. There are two major types – type 1 (HIV-1) and type 2 (HIV-2). HIV-1 is far more numerous and predominates outside West Africa.

EPIDEMIOLOGY

By the year 2000 it was estimated that about 40 million people would have been infected with HIV infection worldwide, including 10 million children. By the end of 1999 UNAIDS estimated that 33 million people were living with HIV/AIDS, of whom two-thirds were in Africa and one-fifth in south/south-east Asia. In 1997 alone there were 5.8 million new infections, including 600 000 new infections in children; and 2.3 million people died of AIDS, more than the total number of deaths from malaria globally. The large majority of new infections in children occurred in Africa (about 530 000) and south/south-east Asia (47 000) through mother-to-child (vertical) transmission of the virus, with fewer than 500 children becoming newly infected in Europe and a similar number in the USA. There has been a marked decrease in the incidence of vertically acquired HIV infection and of paediatric AIDS in both the USA and most countries in western Europe since 1994, with the advent of interventions that can reduce the risk of vertical transmission to under 2%. Outbreaks of nosocomial transmission have taken place through poor infection control, e.g. in Romania and Russia, where a number of children were infected via blood products. Also, numbers of children continue to be infected through blood transfusions in low-income countries where it is not possible to always screen all blood donations.

Because of the importance of vertical transmission, the epidemiology of paediatric HIV-1 infection reflects patterns of infection in women. In industrialised countries, injecting drug use has been a major risk factor for infection in women in southern Europe and the USA, but this is being overtaken in some areas by acquisition via heterosexual sex, which is the major route of acquisition of maternal infection in low-income countries and worldwide. In the UK and Ireland, risk factors vary by area. In Edinburgh and Dublin, the major risk factor has been injecting drug use while in the other high-prevalence area, London, the majority of vertically infected children are born to women who acquired their infection in association with time spent in sub-Saharan Africa.

By September 2000, 1900 babies born to HIV-1-infected women had been reported in the UK and Ireland, of whom 681 are known to be infected. Over 70% were reported from London, where data from unlinked anonymous serosurveys also show a high prevalence of HIV in pregnant women (approximately 1 in 500, compared with about 1 in 6000 in the rest of England and Wales). In the UK in 1998, only about 30% of infected women knew their HIV diagnosis by the time of the birth of their baby. This situation appears to be have been worse in the UK than in other countries in Europe or the USA. With recent official guidance (Department of Health, England) to routinely offer and recommend HIV screening as part of standard antenatal care in all areas, this situation has begun to improve, with the percentage of HIV-infected women diagnosed in Inner London being 70% in 1999. Economic analyses indicate that under almost all scenarios, screening is cost-effective in industrialised countries from the health-care perspective if testing costs can be kept to the minimum. However, there are also real issues of the societal costs of caring for increased numbers of orphaned children (both infected and uninfected) born to infected women who subsequently die. This is a major issue in parts of the world where antiretroviral therapy is not affordable and there is no state support for the care of such mothers and children.

Transmission

The most important routes of transmission are vertical (mother to child) and through blood and blood products. Vertical infections can take place in utero, intrapartum or postnatally via breastfeeding. The relative contribution of each of these is becoming increasingly clear, with increasing evidence to suggest that at least two-thirds of transmission occurs at the time of delivery or in very late pregnancy. It has been established that breastfeeding increases the risk of mother-to-child HIV transmission about twofold.

Vertical transmission rates of HIV-1 infection have been found to vary in different parts of the world; typical values found in prospective studies of nonbreastfeeding populations are 15–25% in Europe and the USA and 25–35% in Africa. Known risk factors that explain some of this variation are shown in Table 23.1. The transmission efficiency of HIV-2 is considerably

Table 23.1 Risk factors for vertical transmission of HIV infection

Maternal
- HIV disease status (related to virus burden)
  - Primary infection*
  - Advanced clinical disease*
  - Low CD4 count or low CD4/CD8 ratio*
  - High viral load*
- Presence of sexually transmitted disease/chorioamnionitis*

Delivery
- Mode of delivery (elective caesarean delivery reduces risk)
- Prolonged labour/rupture of membranes increases risk*
- Premature delivery*

Breastfeeding*

Other
- Viral phenotype
- Genetic factors

* Associated with increased risk of transmission.

less. The risk of vertical transmission of HIV-1 may be higher (because of increased viral load) during the primary 'seroconversion illness'.

Cases of 'casual' transmission from an infected child without the possibility of blood-to-blood contact have not been reported. There have been a very few reported cases of transmission between children within households and in all of these cases there were possibilities for blood-to-blood contact such as sharing of toothbrushes or injection equipment, biting and spillage of blood or other body fluids.

Transmission from sexual intercourse to children occurs. Heterosexually and homosexually acquired HIV-1 infection is seen among teenagers in the USA. There are also reports of HIV-infected children who have been infected by being sexually abused by HIV-1-infected perpetrators.

NATURAL HISTORY

The virus predominantly infects and affects the T4 lymphocyte (CD4, T helper cells) but also other cells, including macrophages and neuronal and glial cells in the central nervous system. HIV-1 does not cause any congenital syndrome and infected babies appear normal and have normal weights at birth. In untreated cohorts of infected children, about 20% develop acquired immunodeficiency syndrome (AIDS), of whom half will die, during the first year (called 'rapid progressers'). The major cause of death in these children is from *Pneumocystis carinii* pneumonia (PCP) acquired in the first 6 months of life, and there are indications from US and UK data that preventing this by use of prophylactic co-trimoxazole may reduce progression to AIDS in infancy. Children not progressing early in life progress to AIDS at a rate of about 5–7% per year (slow progressers) and a few vertically infected children are now well even in their teenage years. The reasons for differences in progression are unclear but may be related to timing of HIV-1 acquisition, the infecting dose and virulence of the virus.

Monitoring T-cell subsets and HIV-1 RNA

Even in the completely well child, it is now standard practice to monitor the CD4 cell count and HIV viral load (measured by HIV-1 RNA using the Roche Amplicor, Nasba or Chiron test kits) every 3–4 months in the well child not on antiretroviral therapy and more frequently at the start of therapy. This is particularly important with the increase in options for treatment with antiretroviral drugs that has occurred recently.

CD4 counts in uninfected children under 5 years of age differ from those in adults in that they are high at birth and reduce gradually to about 5–6 years of age, by which time they are near adult values. Only after this age can absolute numbers of CD4 cells be usefully used to guide commencement and response to treatment in a similar way to adults. Prior to this, age must be taken into account and it is preferable either to follow the CD4% (percentage of total lymphocyte count) or to follow the fall in CD4 count using reference centiles (available in AVERT (1998) *Guidelines for Management of Children with HIV Infection*, 3rd edn).

HIV-1 RNA is measured in RNA copy numbers per millilitre and varies between less than 20 and over 1 million/mL. Values are very high (several thousand to over a million) in infancy, following acquisition of infection at or around the time of birth. There is a gradual fall up to 5–6 years of age by 1–1.5 $\log^{10}$ copies/mL (e.g. from 500 000 to 20 000–50 000/mL) in the absence of antiretroviral therapy. Although high values are predictive of progression of disease in children as in adults, there is considerable overlap between values in children with rapid and slow progresser disease.

CLINICAL MANIFESTATIONS

The main manifestations of HIV-1 are shown in Table 23.3, which, with Table 23.2, outline the Centers for Disease Control and Prevention 1994 classification of HIV/AIDS in children. Many signs are nonspecific in young infants and an index of suspicion is required. Paediatric AIDS is defined by the appearance of a number of AIDS indicator diseases: opportunistic infections; recurrent severe bacterial infections; severe failure to thrive; encephalopathy and malignancy (most commonly non-Hodgkin's lymphoma). Lymphocytic interstitial pneumonitis (LIP) is now recognised to be associated with a better prognosis and is not be included as an indicator of severe disease (category C). The type of AIDS indicator disease to an extent predicts survival. Children with opportunistic infections (especially PCP and cytomegalovirus disease), encephalopathy and lymphoma have a worse survival than those with LIP and recurrent bacterial infections.

AIDS indicator diseases

Opportunistic infections

These are less likely to be due to reactivation of prior infection than to primary disease in children with vertical HIV-1 infection. In the UK PCP is the most commonly reported opportunistic infection (Table 23.4), diagnosed most frequently in infants where the mother was not known to have HIV infection in pregnancy. It occurs most frequently at 3–6 months of age, often when the CD4 cell count is relatively high, and has a high mortality. Cytomegalovirus (CMV) may cause disseminated dis-

Table 23.2 Revised human immunodeficiency virus paediatric classification system 1994 – immune categories based on age-specific CD4+ t lymphocytes and percentage (modified from Centers for Disease Control (1994) Revised classification system for human immunodeficiency virus infection in children less than 13 years of age. MMWR 43(No. RR-12): 1–10)

Immune category	< 12 months No./μL (%)	1–5 years No./μL (%)	6–12 years No./μL (%)
Category 1: no suppression	≥ 1500 (≥ 25)	≥ 1000 (≥ 25)	≥ 500 (≥ 25)
Category 2: moderate suppression	750–1499 (15–24)	500–999 (15–24)	200–499 (15–24)
Category 3: severe suppression	< 750 (< 15)	< 500 (< 15)	< 200 (< 15)

Table 23.3 Revised human immunodeficiency virus paediatric classification system 1994 – clinical categories (modified from Centers for Disease Control (1994) Revised classification system for human immunodeficiency virus infection in children less than 13 years of age. MMWR 43(No. RR-12): 1–10)

Category N: Not symptomatic

Children who have no signs or symptoms considered to be the result of HIV infection or who have only **one** of the conditions listed in category A.

Category A: Mildly symptomatic

Children with **two** or more of the following conditions but none of the conditions listed in categories B and C:
• Lymphadenopathy (≥ 0.5 cm at more than two sites; bilateral = one site)
• Hepatomegaly
• Splenomegaly
• Dermatitis
• Parotitis
• Recurrent or persistent upper respiratory infection, sinusitis or otitis media.

Category B: Moderately symptomatic

Children who have symptomatic conditions other than those listed for category A or category C that are attributed to HIV infection. Examples of conditions in clinical category B include but are not limited to the following:
• Anaemia (< 8 g/dL), neutropenia (< 1000/mm³) or thrombocytopenia (< 100 000/mm³) persisting ≥ 30 days
• Bacterial meningitis, pneumonia or sepsis (single episode)
• Candidiasis, oropharyngeal (i.e. thrush) persisting for > 2 months in children aged > 6 months
• Cardiomyopathy
• Cytomegalovirus infection with onset before age 1 month
• Diarrhoea, recurrent or chronic
• Hepatitis
• Herpes simplex virus (HSV) stomatitis, recurrent (i.e. more than two episodes within 1 year)
• HSV bronchitis, pneumonitis or oesophagitis with onset before age 1 month
• Herpes zoster (i.e. shingles) involving at least two distinct episodes or more than one dermatome
• Leiomyosarcoma
• Lymphocytic interstitial pneumonitis (LIP) or pulmonary lymphoid hyperplasia complex
• Nephropathy
• Nocardiosis
• Fever lasting > 1 month
• Toxoplasmosis with onset before age 1 month
• Varicella, disseminated (i.e. complicated chickenpox).

Category C: Severely symptomatic

Children who have any condition listed in the 1987 surveillance case definition for acquired immunodeficiency syndrome with the exception of LIP (which is a category B condition).

Table 23.4 Most frequent manifestations of vertically acquired HIV infection in children

AIDS (severe HIV disease)	Approximate percentage of reported first AIDS indicator diseases*
Opportunistic infections	
Pneumocystis carinii pneumonia	30–40
Candida oesophagitis	5–10
Cytomegalovirus infection	5–10
Atypical mycobacteria	5
Cryptosporidiosis	< 5?
Toxoplasmosis	< 2
Cryptococcus	< 1
Other manifestations	
Recurrent bacterial infections	20–30
HIV encephalopathy	10–15
Neoplasms (mainly lymphomas)	< 5
Wasting	10–15

ease, especially early in life, but retinitis alone (which occurs in adults) appears to be less common in children than in adults. As in adults, CMV is often cultured from asymptomatic children with or without HIV-1 infection, and difficulty may arise in defining its role in the pathogenesis of symptoms. As in adults, cryptosporidiosis and atypical mycobacterial infections are observed in children with profound immune deficiency. However, since the advent of highly active antiretroviral therapy (HAART), including treatment with protease inhibitor (PI) drugs, there has been a decrease in the observed rate of severe opportunistic infections in adults. Except where children were previously undiagnosed, the same is occurring in children.

Invasive bacterial infections

The organisms most frequently responsible are polysaccharide encapsulated bacteria such as streptococci and *Haemophilus influenzae* and *Salmonella* species. Pneumonia is the commonest infection, causing significant morbidity, and children with lymphocytic interstitial pneumonitis (see below) are particularly prone to recurrent bacterial lung infections often resulting in bronchiectasis.

Failure to thrive

HIV wasting disease is multifactorial. It may occur secondary to infections, poor oral intake or from HIV-1 enteropathy. In older children, poor growth and pubertal development are observed. Again this is decreasing in industrialised countries with the advent of HAART for children and more focus on prevention of malnutrition.

Malnutrition, diarrhoea and bacterial infections remain the major problems for HIV-infected children in Africa where the estimated median survival without effective antiretroviral therapy is in the order of only 4–5 years.

HIV encephalopathy

Early encephalopathy presents in the first 2 years of life with motor developmental delay and progressive motor signs, particularly spastic diplegia. A CT or MRI scan may show generalised atrophy and/or basal ganglia calcification. There is an association with early development of opportunistic infections such as PCP and CMV. Expressive language delay, behavioural abnormalities and memory loss may occur in older children.

Lymphocytic interstitial pneumonitis

LIP is observed in about 40% of vertically infected children although it is rare in adults and children acquiring HIV-1 infection later in childhood. It is often initially asymptomatic and without chest signs and can be diagnosed in the second year of life on the basis of a persistently abnormal chest X-ray only. Children may have associated parotitis and very high immunoglobulin levels (IgG > 50 U/L). The pathogenesis is unclear but LIP may be due to HIV-1 itself or to early acquisition of another virus such as Epstein–Barr virus. The differential diagnosis includes other causes of interstitial pneumonia, including tuberculosis. A presumptive diagnosis can usually be made on clinical and radiological grounds without resorting to lung biopsy.

Diagnosis of HIV infection

Children born to HIV-infected mothers all have maternal HIV antibody (anti-HIV) detectable at birth. Therefore testing for anti-HIV is not useful for diagnosis of an infected infant until loss of maternal antibody from the infant. The median time to loss of maternal antibody is 10 months and all have lost it by 18 months, so that a child over 18 months of age who has HIV antibody is HIV-infected. Early HIV diagnosis in the first weeks of life can now be routinely made by detection of the HIV genome by polymerase chain reaction (PCR). Undertaking HIV culture or the p24 antigen tests can also be done but are expensive and time-consuming and, in the case of culture, it takes time to get results. The sensitivity of PCR, however, is only 40–50% in the first week of life, rising rapidly to over 90% by 2 weeks. Therefore a negative result during this time does not exclude infection. Two positive results on separate specimens are required to confirm infection and two or more negative results, one at over 3 months of age, will confirm that a baby is uninfected, so long as the mother is not breastfeeding. A negative HIV antibody test between 12 and 18 months will absolutely exclude infection. High immunoglobulin levels (especially IgG), reversed CD4/CD8 T-lymphocyte ratio or low CD4 for age, and clinical signs (e.g. persistent candidiasis beyond the neonatal period, axillary lymphadenopathy, splenomegaly, poor feeding and weight gain) are other pointers to an infected child.

MANAGEMENT

Therapy for specific infections is discussed under individual diseases in other chapters. The following discussion focuses on prophylaxis and anti-retroviral therapy.

PCP prophylaxis

PCP in infancy is a preventable disease. Provided mothers are identified in pregnancy, infants can be commenced on PCP prophylaxis with co-tri-moxazole from 4–6 weeks of age (after stopping zidovudine if given to prevent mother-to-child transmission) and before a definitive diagnosis of HIV status has been made. Prophylaxis can then be stopped in infants established to be uninfected. Infected children should all continue pro-phylaxis throughout the first year of life. Thereafter, it can be stopped in children with CD4 counts consistently above 20%, provided they are being regularly monitored, but many clinicians prefer to continue as it may also help to prevent bacterial ear and chest infections. Alternatives to co-trimoxazole in the unusual event of an allergic reaction include dapsone 2 mg/kg daily or inhaled pentamidine (300 mg by Respigard II inhaler monthly), but PCP breakthrough has been documented with both.

Prevention of bacterial infections and LIP treatment

Immunisation against *H. influenzae* and *S. pneumoniae* is recommended for all children with HIV infection. Monthly intravenous immunoglobulin (IVIG) therapy may help to reduce bacterial infections in some children with recurrent bacterial infections and not responding to co-trimoxazole, although this has no effect on other aspects of HIV disease progression or mortality. Other prophylactic antibiotics may be helpful in children with LIP and recurrent chest infections. In children with severe LIP, a short course of steroids followed by low-dose maintenance oral or inhaled steroid (with or without a bronchodilator if evidence of bronchospasm exists) may improve lung function.

Immunisations

Children infected with HIV should receive all immunisations with the exception of BCG, which should be withheld from those with symptomatic disease and where tuberculosis is uncommon because there have been some reports of severely immunocompromised children developing dis-seminated BCG-osis. As tuberculosis incidence is low in the UK and most children born to HIV-infected mothers are followed closely, BCG is not usually given to these children at birth. If, when the child's infection status is resolved, s/he turns out to be uninfected then BCG may be given.*

Adverse reactions to other live vaccines have not posed a problem. Inactivated polio vaccine (IPV) is recommended because of a possible risk

---

* **If, however, the child is shortly returning to a country with a high tuberculosis prevalence and will not be closely followed, s/he should receive BCG at birth; this is WHO policy for low-income countries.**

of transmission of live polio virus to an infected child and other immuno-compromised family members. Immunisation should not be delayed as the immunogenicity of vaccines in children with severe immune suppression is reduced. Normal human immunoglobulin and zoster-immune globulin (VZIG) are recommended after exposure to measles and chickenpox respectively. Booster immunisation against measles may be helpful and this approach is under evaluation. Pneumococcal vaccine is recommend-ed for children over 2 years of age; the new conjugate vaccines may be of value for younger children and require further evaluation. HIV-infected children with reasonable immunological function (including those on ther-apy) show good immunological response to MMR vaccine.

Antiretroviral therapy

In the last 2 years many new antiretroviral drugs have been introduced, including a new class of more potent drugs, the protease inhibitors, and there have also been advances in knowledge about how to use existing drugs. Of the 10 antiretroviral drugs licensed for use in adults in the UK, five have so far been licensed for children and others are available on compas-sionate programmes from the drug companies. Clinical trials of antiretrovi-ral therapy combinations continue to be set up through the Paediatric European Network for Treatment of AIDS (PENTA) and are open to all cen-tres in the UK (contact MRC HIV Clinical Trials Centre, 020 7380 9991).

When to start?

Opinions differ as to when to start therapy in adults, as reflected by dif-ferences in national guidelines. Recent guidelines for adults produced by two UK groups (BHIVA and PACT) can be summarised as suggesting starting when one or more of the following occur:

- The CD4 count is less than about 300–350 cells/mm^3
- Viral load is greater than 10 000 or somewhere between 10 000 and 50 000 copies/mL
- CD4 count is falling rapidly even if viral load is less than 10 000 copies/mL
- Clinical symptoms are developing.

Paediatricians in countries and centres in Europe also vary as to when they commence therapy in children but tend to be more conservative than in the USA. US guidelines suggest starting therapy in all infants under 12 months of age and in any child under 3 years with a viral load over 100 000 copies/mL. However, issues of adherence, the wishes of the family and telling the child his/her diagnosis are further important issues when con-sidering when to start. Ongoing studies in the US and commencing in Europe (PENTA 7 trial) are investigating the impact on disease progres-sion of commencing aggressive therapy with three or four drugs very early in life (< 12 weeks of age – i.e. as soon as the diagnosis is made).

What to start with?

Increasingly the gold standard, as in adults, is to start children on triple therapy with either two nucleoside analogue reverse transcriptase inhibitors (NRTIs) and a protease inhibitor (PI) or two NRTIs and a non-nucleoside analogue reverse transcriptase inhibitor (NNRTI). Choice of a PI is limited in children, with only nelfinavir or ritonavir available for young children in appropriate formulations. The latter has a very bitter taste, which may hinder compliance; nelfinavir is available as a powder or tablet that can be crushed and given with food. The PI drugs are metabolised at a faster rate than in adults, requiring comparatively high doses to be given.

When to switch?

In adults one aim of therapy is to achieve undetectable HIV-1 RNA viral load. In children, probably because of higher viral loads, this has been less achievable to date. Therefore there is a risk, if this goal is pursued, that children's therapies would be switched frequently and they would rapidly run out of and become resistant to available therapies. Falling CD4 count (taking account of age), deteriorating clinical status, in particular poor weight gain and/or growth, and rising viral load all help determine the time to change therapy. As a general rule, if a protease inhibitor is being started, at least one and preferably two NRTIs should be changed at the same time. At the time of writing (2000), tests of HIV resistance to antiretroviral therapies are not routinely available in many centres in Europe, but are likely to become so soon, and this may help clinicians to decide about what therapies to switch to. A trial randomising children to resistance testing or not and comparing HIV RNA 12 months later is planned in Europe and will run alongside a similar trial in adults.

Care in the community

Children with HIV infection may attend school normally and the need to know within the school setting should be influenced by needs of the HIV-infected child and not those of teachers and other children. Universal precaution guidelines for dealing with blood in schools should be carried out, also for prevention of transmission of other blood-borne infections such as hepatitis B and C (see Chapter 33, pp. 219–220).

Social/psychological aspects of management

The social and psychological aspects of management are among the most difficult. Issues include testing of children and mothers, telling children their diagnosis, and confidentiality. HIV infection usually remains associated with stigma in every country and two (mother and child) or more family members may be sick or dying at the same time. The association with sex and injecting drug use add to the stigma and families are often overwhelmed at the time of diagnosis, especially if the family members only learn of the diagnosis through illness in the child. Social and cultural isolation and fear of disclosure of the diagnosis are common.

Management of the wide range of medical, psychological and social issues requires coordination between disciplines, between hospital and community services and voluntary and statutory sectors, while at the same time allowing the family to maintain control over who knows. Family clinics have been set up in higher prevalence areas so that parents and children benefit from coordinated care from a multidisciplinary team. As the numbers of infected children are still small and the issues are often complex, some centralisation of expertise is required. This will also allow opportunity for children to participate in multicentre treatment protocols. Development of shared care protocols similar to those set up for shared management of children with cancer and leukaemia provide models of care. Coordination between adult genitourinary medicine physicians, obstetricians and paediatricians is essential if pregnant women with HIV infection are to benefit from therapy and future developments to prevent vertical HIV transmission.

PREVENTION OF FURTHER CASES

Approaches to reduction of vertical transmission

Breastfeeding increases the risk of vertical transmission by about 15%, thereby doubling the risk of transmission in Europe. The most significant reduction in transmission is from the use of zidovudine in pregnancy, at delivery and to the newborn, which has been shown to reduce the risk by two-thirds in a randomised placebo-controlled trial in 1994 (ACTG 076 trial). Elective caesarean section has now also been shown to significantly reduce transmission risk by about half. In clinical practice use of these interventions has translated into reductions of vertical transmission to under 2% where HIV infected women do not breastfeed. In 1998, it was shown in a study on nonbreastfeeding women in Thailand that transmission can be reduced by half if zidovudine is only given for the last month of pregnancy, given orally during delivery (it was given by the intravenous route in the 076 trial) and not given to the baby at all. There are short-term safety data on the use of lamivudine (an NRTI) and nevirapine (an NNRTI), which are at present being used in clinical trials designed to evaluate the effect of combination therapy in further reducing mother-to-child transmission rates. Increasingly, mothers are already taking or are being prescribed triple therapy (including a PI) for their own disease during pregnancy. The effects of this on the fetus are unknown and long-term follow-up to observe any adverse effects on exposed children is essential.

Further research in this area continues, including most importantly the long-term effects of antiretroviral therapies on transmission among women from parts of the world where breastfeeding is important for child health. The logistic and economic issues that need to be overcome in order to make therapies available to prevent mother-to-child transmission in the many countries in the world where antiretroviral therapies are not currently affordable are being actively discussed by WHO, UNICEF and UNAIDS.

Another possible intervention to reduce mother-to-child transmission that may be of particular relevance for low-income countries include cleansing of the birth canal (vaginal lavage). Trials in this area are in the progress or being planned with collaboration between the USA, European countries and countries in the developing world.

Antenatal HIV testing

In the UK and other developed countries it is now clearly advantageous for an HIV-infected pregnant woman to know her HIV status. The health-care needs of the mother herself can be met and she can make informed plans for the future. Information can be given about the risks of mother-to-child transmission, in particular breastfeeding, and the options of taking zidovudine and other therapies to further reduce transmission, or termination of pregnancy, can be considered. The subsequent follow-up of the infant and advantages of early diagnosis can also be discussed. It is now important that detection of previously undiagnosed HIV infection in pregnant women increases in the UK. The 1998 guidelines from an intercollegiate working party (see Further reading) and government policy should be followed. Antenatal testing should be routinely offered and recommended and integrated with other tests performed during pregnancy. It is incumbent on health professionals to ensure that this takes place.

FURTHER READING

AVERT (1998) Management guidelines for HIV-1 infected children, 3rd edn. AVERT, Horsham, West Sussex, tel. 01403 210202; http://www.avert.org.

Department of Health (1999) Reducing mother to baby transmission of HIV (HSC 1999/183). NHS Executive, London.

Intercollegiate Working Party for Enhancing Voluntary Confidential HIV Testing (1998) Reducing mother to child transmission of HIV infection in the UK. Royal College of Paediatrics and Child Health, London.

Sharland M, Gibb D, Tudor-Williams G, Walters S, Novelli V (1997) Paediatric HIV infections. Arch Dis Child 76: 293–296.

Recommendations for the use of antiretroviral agents in paediatric HIV infection, at http://www.hivatis.org/guidelines/pediatrics.

Consideration for antiretroviral therapy in HIV-infected pregnant women and interventions to reduce perinatal HIV-1 transmission (November 2000), at http://www.hivatis.org/guidelines/adult.

24 Management of the child with systemic fungal infection

INTRODUCTION

The great majority of systemic fungal infections that are seen in paediatric practice in this country are opportunistic in that they afflict children who are susceptible by virtue of some severe debilitating disease, such as acute leukaemia, or as a consequence of the treatment of that disease. The principal fungal groups are *Candida* spp., *Aspergillus* spp. and *Cryptococcus neoformans*.

Recent large surveys in the USA have highlighted *Candida* as a leading cause of hospital-acquired blood-stream infections in patients suffering from a broad range of medical and surgical conditions that might increasingly be seen in paediatric intensive care units (PICUs). *Candida albicans* is the principal pathogenic species although the proportion of systemic *Candida* infections due to non-albicans species has also noticeably increased.

Cryptococcosis is the leading systemic mycosis in AIDS patients although it can also occur in lymphoma and in the chronically immunosuppressed, classically presenting in these groups as meningitis.

There are also fungi that hitherto have been quite rare as human pathogens but are believed to be generally increasing in incidence in the immunocompromised. These include *Fusarium*, *Pseudoallescheria boydii* and phaeohyphomycetes such as *Phialophora*.

Histoplasmosis, blastomycosis and coccidioidomycosis arise rarely in the UK, typically following acquisition of the causative agent (a dimorphic fungus) from endemic areas abroad.

ANTIFUNGAL DRUGS

The antifungal armamentarium (Table 24.1) is still relatively limited in terms of the number of drugs that have proven efficacy and are relatively safe for treating systemic mycoses. The polyene amphotericin B is still widely regarded as the gold standard therapeutic agent even though efficacy data from controlled trials are relatively limited, despite its use over three decades.

The advantages of amphotericin B are its broad antifungal spectrum of activity and the fact that fungal resistance to the drug has rarely been documented. The disadvantages are that the normal mode of administration, by slow intravenous infusion, is often accompanied by unpleasant febrile reactions and that nephrotoxicity is an almost invariable complication of prolonged treatment. A liposomal preparation of amphotericin B (AmBisome) is available and is now licensed for use in the UK for the same indications as 'conventional' amphotericin B. Its principal advantage is that the incidence of nephrotoxicity is greatly reduced even when much higher daily doses are given. Whether at the same time this is associated with greater efficacy has yet to be fully established in paediatrics, where experience with the drug is limited. There are two other lipid formulations

Table 24.1 Drugs used to treat systemic fungal infection in children

	Amphotericin B (Fungizone AMB)	Liposomal AMB (AmBisome)	AMB colloidal dispersion (Amphocil)	Fluconazole (Diflucan)	Itraconazole (Sporanox)	5-flucytosine (Alcobon)
Preparation	Micellar suspension made with sodium desoxycholate	AMB in liposomal vesicles	Complex of AMB and sodium cholesteryl sulphate → disc-shaped particles	Bis-triazole	Dioxolane triazole	Fluorinated pyrimidine
Route of administration	Intravenous	Intravenous	Intravenous	Oral, intravenous	Oral (variable bioavailability)	Oral, intravenous
Kinetics	High protein binding; poor concentrations in CSF, eye, urine	High concentrations in liver and spleen; high serum concentrations; low concentrations in kidney	Same as AmBisome but lower serum concentrations	Low protein binding; excellent penetration of most body sites; > 50% serum concentrations in CSF; excreted unchanged in high concentrations in urine	High protein binding; low levels in CSF and urine; no adjustment of dose in renal failure	Low protein binding; excellent penetration of body sites including CSF and urine
Toxicity	*Immediate: fever, chills; kidney toxicity; hepatic toxicity	Immediate: less frequent; reduced kidney toxicity	Immediate: less frequent; reduced kidney toxicity	Low rate of mild side-effects	Low rate of mild side-effects	Myelosuppression, hepatotoxicity

Table 24.1 Drugs used to treat systemic fungal infection in children

	Amphotericin B (Fungizone AMB)	Liposomal AMB (AmBisome)	AMB colloidal dispersion (Amphocil)	Fluconazole (Diflucan)	Itraconazole (Sporanox)	5-flucytosine (Alcobon)
Interactions	Occur with other drugs if mixed in infusion	As for AMB	As for AMB	Serum levels reduced by rifampicin	Serum levels reduced by rifampicin	
Dose	0.5–1 mg/kg/day	3–5 mg/kg/day	3–5 mg/kg/day	3–6 mg/kg/day	3–5 mg/kg/day	100–150 mg/kg/day
Antifungal spectrum	*Candida* spp.; *Aspergillus* spp.; *Cryptococcus neoformans*; dimorphic fungi; wide range of other fungi	Same as AMB + better activity against *Mucor* or *Fusarium*	Same as AMB + better activity against *Mucor* or *Fusarium*	*Candida albicans*; *Cryptococcus neoformans*	*Candida albicans*; non-albicans species; *Cryptococcus neoformans*; *Aspergillus* spp.; dimorphic fungi; *Sporothrix*	*Candida* spp.; *Cryptococcus neoformans*

* Rare 'anaphylactoid' reactions have been reported. AMB = amphotericin B; CSF = cerebrospinal fluid.

recently licensed (Amphocil and Abelcet). Again, data in children are very limited but, as for AmBisome, kidney-sparing would be an expected property such that either could replace conventional amphotericin B in the event of nephrotoxicity. The place of these new formulations and how precisely they should be used is yet to be established, especially bearing in mind that they are considerably more expensive than conventional amphotericin B. In view of the lack of clear evidence of greater efficacy, the present recommendation is to consider their use in place of amphotericin B when renal function is already impaired or is rapidly deteriorating. There have been a few reports of use of amphotericin B with intralipid, also with the aim of preventing nephrotoxicity; however this preparation has yet to be properly evaluated and so its use cannot be recommended.

5-flucytosine has a narrower spectrum of activity, principally restricted to *Candida* and *Cryptococcus*. However, it needs to be given in combination with amphotericin B, since the emergence of drug resistance is very likely when it is used alone. Good concentrations are achieved in the central nervous system and urinary tract, so that infections at these sites are the main indication for use of 5-flucytosine. In view of its myelosuppressive effects, serum drug concentrations should be monitored on a twice-weekly basis and dosing needs to be reduced in the event of renal impairment.

Of the azole antifungal drugs, the triazoles fluconazole and itraconazole are licensed for use in children in the UK. Fluconazole has good activity in vitro against both *Candida albicans* and *Cryptococcus neoformans* and proven efficacy against these pathogens when they cause systemic infections. Side-effects are infrequent and generally not serious, although when high doses of the drug are given it would be wise to regularly monitor liver function. Pharmacokinetic data are interesting in that in neonates there is prolongation of the half-life, and consequently the dosing interval should be increased, whereas in infants more than 4 weeks old, and in children, the half-life is reduced so that higher doses than those used in adults are recommended. Oral administration of the drug achieves comparable serum concentrations to the intravenous route. It should be noted that some of the non-*albicans Candida* species are resistant to fluconazole, including *C. krusei* and *C. glabrata*. For this reason it is important that *Candida* isolates are fully identified to species level and that their antifungal susceptibility is determined when they cause a significant clinical infection.

The use of itraconazole for treatment of systemic fungal infections has been hampered by the fact that there is no licensed preparation of the drug for parenteral administration, although one is undergoing clinical trial. When given by the oral route its bioavailability is variable and is dependent on low gastric pH. However, preliminary results with a new solution formulation suggest that this achieves much improved absorption, although patient compliance may not be so good because of the large volumes of suspension that require to be swallowed. Potentially, this drug has a number of important advantages over fluconazole with respect to its antifungal activity. Firstly, it is effective in treatment of aspergillosis, which fluconazole is not, and secondly it may be active against strains of *Candida* spp. that are fluconazole-resistant.

Although cerebrospinal fluid concentrations of itraconazole are poor it appears that it does achieve therapeutic concentrations in the brain and anecdotal case reports of successful treatment of fungal brain abscesses appear to support this.

While there is no evidence to warrant combining one of these azoles with amphotericin B to achieve greater therapeutic effect, at the same time there is no clear evidence that they would be antagonistic in vivo.

There is considerable interest at present in the therapeutic role of colony stimulating factors (e.g. G-CSF, GM-CSF) in opportunistic fungal infections, especially in what is probably the most susceptible group, the neutropenic patient. Even though CSFs have been shown to reduce the duration of neutropenia after immunosuppressive therapy, there is as yet less conclusive evidence that fungal infections have been reduced in frequency.

SPECIFIC FUNGAL INFECTIONS

Systemic candidiasis

Intrauterine *Candida* infection is rarely encountered but can result in fetal death. Premature rupture of membranes leading to ascending infection of maternal origin may be the mechanism involved. No particular maternal risk factors have been identified apart from vaginal candidiasis and antibiotic therapy.

Candida spp. are acquired by the newborn from mother's vaginal flora to form part of their normal intestinal flora. The prolonged administration of broad-spectrum antibiotics, especially cephalosporins, is likely to lead to fungal overgrowth as a prelude to invasion of the intestinal mucosa, resulting in candidaemia. Very – or extreme – low birth-weight babies are most at risk of systemic infection in this situation and may develop disseminated disease with deep organ involvement. A factor in this may be immature phagocytic cell responses. Other well-recognised risk factors for candidaemia are the presence of indwelling vascular catheters and parenteral nutrition therapy. The use and need for any or all of these support therapies should be continually reviewed to try and reduce the risk of fungal infection. Studies on neonatal PICUs have shown that the colonising yeast flora progressively change from *C. albicans* to non-*albicans* species; this may be the result of cross-infection due to transmission between patients of these strains on staff hands.

Systemic candidiasis often has an insidious onset without any specific signs, although once the infection becomes established the infant will be clinically septic. A perineal rash or peroral septic spots may be observed, as may oral thrush. In order to establish the diagnosis it is essential to take repeated blood cultures, as the documentation rate with single or few cultures is poor. A single isolation of a yeast from blood or other sterile site should be regarded as evidence of systemic infection. Overall, documentation rates run at only 50–70% with currently available mycological tests. New molecular tests based on amplification and detection of fungal DNA in blood or other samples should improve these figures once they have been properly validated. What is important is to have a high level of awareness of which infants are most at risk and to consider early empirical antifungal therapy when the presentation requires it. There is a high incidence of meningitis complicating candidal sepsis in neonates such that there should be a readiness to obtain spinal fluid for laboratory examination: features consistent with this diagnosis would be pleocytosis, elevated protein and lowered sugar. Culture of the spinal fluid can be positive for *Candida* while blood cultures are sterile. There may be involvement of the brain with abscesses as another feature of this infection, which has a worse prognosis. Also, there is a high incidence of endophthalmitis complicating candidaemia, which can be diagnosed by careful examination of the fundi.

A suprapubic urine culture can also help in diagnosis as involvement of the urinary tract occurs in as many as 50% of cases. This may be complicated by renal parenchymal infection and more rarely the development of fungus balls obstructing the renal pelvis, a complication that may require urgent surgical intervention. Endocarditis is a rare but well-recognised complication of candidaemia believed to arise most often from seeding off an infected indwelling vascular catheter.

The most important therapeutic considerations in cases of neonatal candidaemia are as follows. When arising as a complication of vascular line sepsis, in the absence of obvious organ involvement, will removal of the implicated catheter be sufficient? The answer is no and the recommendation is to give antifungal therapy. Amphotericin B is first choice with a total dose for the course of 15–25 mg/kg. 5-flucytosine 100mg/kg/day should be added in all cases of CNS infection in view of its excellent penetration across the blood–brain barrier. Serum levels of this drug must be measured at least twice weekly (and not exceed 80 mg/L) to prevent marrow toxicity. At least 3 weeks' therapy will be required. Systemic candidiasis in older children may be complicated by pneumonia, meningitis or endocarditis. Endophthalmitis and skin rash are particularly associated with this infection.

Aspergillosis

Disseminated aspergillosis, with involvement of vital organs, typically occurs as a complication of prolonged profound neutropenia after leukaemia chemotherapy or bone marrow transplantation. The initial focus of the infection is pulmonary, characterised by single or multiple pulmonary infiltrates; the presence of fungus balls (mycetoma) within cavitary lesions is best detected by CT scan. At least 25% of case will have extrapulmonary dissemination to other sites, especially skin, brain, kidneys and heart. Amphotericin B or itraconazole are agents of first choice for treatment. Mortality is characteristically more than 90%.

In the febrile neutropenic child, the possibility of a systemic fungal infection due to either *Candida*, *Aspergillus* or, less commonly, *Mucor* arises when there is a failure to respond to 5–7 days of broad-spectrum antibiotics.

The need for empirical antifungal therapy at this point is well accepted. Amphotericin B has traditionally been used here (0.5 mg/kg/day) with adjustment according to how the patient's illness progresses. AmBisome is now licensed for this indication. If the fever abates and the patient improves, then amphotericin B can be stopped after 7 days. However, when a fungal infection has been documented, treatment should be continued for at least 4–6 weeks, according to the causative agent. As yet, there is no established fungal chemoprophylaxis regimen for neutropenic patients, although itraconazole would be the most appropriate choice in view of its spectrum of activity and oral administration.

CRYPTOCOCCOSIS

For treatment of cryptococcosis the choice of regimen is either amphotericin B (+ 5-flucytosine) or fluconazole for at least 6 weeks. In AIDS cases life-long suppression with fluconazole is necessary to prevent relapse.

25 Immunisation of the child with a potentially impaired immune response

INTRODUCTION

When vaccines are considered in the child with impaired immune responses, the reflex is often to avoid them altogether. This takes its origin in the very real fear of potential damage that live vaccines can do to children with some severe immunodeficiencies, e.g. live polio virus vaccine in X-linked agammaglobulinaemia. There is an additional common perception that killed vaccines, which pose no such risk, are 'not worth using' because the child's immune response will be inadequate.

Such children are at particularly high risk of serious infections and therefore among those most in need of protection by immunisation, where it can be done safely. Thus there is a great need for specific vaccines to be tested in different groups of 'high-risk' children to assess their safety, immunogenicity and efficacy. There is a renewed consciousness of these issues in the context of the improving survival of children with malignant diseases, including leukaemia, the increased intensity of treatments used, including haematopoietic stem cell transplantation and the small but growing population of children with HIV infection. Although there is good evidence regarding the use of some vaccines in some of these groups, there are also large gaps in our knowledge, so that in many instances recommendations have to be made on the basis of extrapolation from what may be known about other vaccines and conditions, rather than direct evidence.

The vaccines

The live vaccines currently licensed in the UK are bacillus Calmette–Guérin (BCG), trivalent oral polio vaccine (OPV), measles, mumps and rubella

(MMR), yellow fever and oral typhoid. A live varicella vaccine is available but is rarely used. All other licensed vaccines are not live. The enhanced inactivated polio vaccine (eIPV) given by injection is highly immunogenic.

CHILDREN WITH MALIGNANCY, INCLUDING LEUKAEMIA

Children diagnosed as having malignant disease and treated with cytotoxic drugs should avoid all live vaccinations during and for 6 months after cessation of chemotherapy. Live oral polio vaccine (OPV) should not be given to household contacts during this time. Children who have completed a primary course of immunisation before the development of their malignancy are generally considered to be adequately protected against diphtheria, tetanus, pertussis and polio, although measles antibody titres decline in some children. It is not yet known whether Hib antibody titres are maintained for this group. If the normal immunisation schedule was interrupted by the onset of disease then the schedule for the killed components (and eIPV) should be completed while on treatment provided the child's condition is stable. In acute lymphoblastic leukaemia (ALL) this will be while on the maintenance phase of chemotherapy. Influenza vaccine should be considered in the autumn months. Currently, in the UK, malignancy alone is not an indication for pneumococcal or hepatitis B immunisation.

Six months after cessation of therapy, booster doses of diphtheria, tetanus, OPV, Hib, meningococcus C, MMR and, if under 7 years of age, acellular pertussis vaccines should be given. If the child is considered to be in a high-risk group for tuberculosis, a tuberculin test followed if appropriate by BCG vaccine should be undertaken.

Chickenpox (varicella)

This infection is usually mild and self-limiting in normal children but can be devastating in children with malignancies, especially leukaemia. It is essential that all children diagnosed with malignancy have varicella-zoster virus (VZV) antibodies measured at diagnosis and prior to blood product administration. Susceptible patients with a recent history of exposure to varicella should be passively immunised with zoster immune globulin (VZIG), ideally within 72 hours of exposure, although there is some evidence that VZIG given up to 10 days after exposure may attenuate subsequent infection. Those who develop the disease are treated with high-dose intravenous aciclovir and supportive measures.

Although there are no published data to support this practice, there is increasing use of aciclovir prophylaxis in these patients instead of, or as well as, VZIG. If employed it should be used orally in full therapeutic dosage for 14 days commencing 7 days after exposure.

Attenuated varicella vaccine is available in the UK on a 'named patient' basis and has been used in several trials in children with malignancies in the USA and Japan. It now has a licence in both countries. In a large North American study a mild rash occurred in 50% of leukaemics given the vaccine but severe illness did not occur. When there was clinical concern, aciclovir, to which the vaccine virus is very sensitive, was given. The efficacy of the vaccine was assessed by the rate of development of disease

25 Immunisation & impaired immunity

after household exposure to varicella. The vaccine produced 100% protection against severe disease and 86% protection against all forms of disease. It has been suggested that the vaccine could be given to children with ALL under the following circumstances:

- The child must have been in remission for at least 1 year
- The total peripheral lymphocyte count should be at least 700 cells/mm^3 or more on the day of vaccination
- Immunosuppressive chemotherapy should be withheld for 1 week before vaccination and 1 week afterwards. Steroids should not be given for 2 weeks after vaccination. It is not necessary to withhold chemotherapy at the time of the second dose of vaccine where this is required.

Even if it is felt inappropriate to immunise the index case the vaccine could be given to siblings lacking a clinical history of chickenpox since household contacts constitute a significant source of infection.

Measles

Measles can cause encephalitis, pneumonitis and death in children with malignancy even if passive protection is attempted with gammaglobulin. The incidence of measles has declined in the UK with universal immunisation but vaccinated children may lose their immunity while on cytotoxic therapy so that seropositivity at the time of diagnosis does not necessarily mean that the child will remain immune. At present we rely on herd immunity to protect the at-risk population. It is particularly important to ensure that the patient's siblings and other frequent contacts have been immunised. Human normal immunoglobulin should be given to those at risk with a history of exposure but it does not provide complete protection.

The cautious approach to measles vaccination stems from a study carried out in 1962 in the USA. Of 12 children with ALL immunised with measles vaccine, one died of atypical measles. However, more recent studies have demonstrated that the current live vaccine induces seroconversion without severe adverse effects in children with leukaemia who are in remission but still on treatment. Nevertheless, the current guidelines state that children with malignancies should only receive MMR 6 months after cessation of chemotherapy.

CHILDREN WHO HAVE HAD INTENSIVE CHEMOTHERAPY AND/OR HAEMATOPOIETIC STEM CELL TRANSPLANTATION

These patients are at much higher and more prolonged risk of serious infection than those receiving cytotoxic therapy alone. The degree and length of immune suppression depends on a number of factors including the original disease, the conditioning chemo/radiotherapy regimen, the type of donor and, most importantly, whether or not T-cell depletion of the marrow (or blood) was undertaken. In addition, graft versus host disease (GVHD) and its treatment may further impair immune reconstitution.

In theory, the recipient of an allogeneic transplant should be immunologically naïve. However, this is not always the case and the ability to make specific antibody may persist, although in many cases it tends to decline slowly over 12–24 months.

All children who have had a haematopoietic stem cell transplantation should be re-immunised provided they have been off immunosuppression for at least 6 months and do not have chronic GVHD at the following times after transplant:

- 12 months for matched sibling donor and autologous transplants
- 18 months for unrelated donor or related mismatched transplants.

They should receive three doses each of diphtheria, tetanus, pertussis (omit if over 7 years), Hib and eIPV. They should also receive single doses of pneumococcal and meningococcal vaccines. Finally, they require two doses of MMR vaccine, the first of which should be given 6 months after the commencement of the vaccination schedule (18–24 months after transplant). Measurement of antibody responses is not necessary as a routine but may be checked if there is doubt about the patient's ability to respond. Partly because it is poorly immunogenic and partly because it does not cover all the disease-causing serotypes, the use of pneumococcal vaccine does not allow penicillin prophylaxis to be discontinued early and this is continued for at least 2 years and in some cases for life. Influenza vaccination should be given yearly each autumn. Postexposure measles and VZV prophylaxis should be given to post bone marrow transplant cases regardless of pre-transplant antibody status.

Patients with GVHD need individual assessment. Some will have markedly impaired immunity and passive protection using replacement doses of intravenous immunoglobulin may be required. In others it may be appropriate to use killed vaccines.

CHILDREN UNDERGOING SOLID ORGAN TRANSPLANTATION

Before elective organ transplantation it is important to ensure that routine immunisations are up to date. Hepatitis B vaccine should be given and a strong case can be made for use of varicella vaccine for those who are nonimmune.

After transplantation these children require long-term immunosuppression and live vaccines are contraindicated. Pneumococcal vaccine should be given and repeated after 5 years if antibody levels are found to be low. Influenza vaccine should be offered each autumn.

CHILDREN WITH HIV INFECTION

These children have mostly acquired their infection by vertical transmission. Initially, it may not be clear whether or not the child is infected (see Chapter 23). Extensive infection with BCG has followed immunisation of infected individuals. As tuberculosis incidence is low in the UK and most children born to HIV infected mothers are followed closely, BCG is not usually given. If the child's infection status proves to be noninfected then

BCG should be given as the child is at high risk of exposure to tuberculosis in a household with at least one other HIV-positive individual. If, however, the family is returning shortly to a country with a high prevalence of tuberculosis and will not be closely followed, s/he should receive BCG at birth, This is WHO policy for low-income countries. Routine infant immunisations are given as normal with the exception that eIPV should be substituted for OPV since, although paralytic disease with OPV is extremely rare, it has been described and the risk is not only to the child but also other immunocompromised household members.

MMR seems to be safe and efficacious in HIV-infected children regardless of disease status.

CHILDREN WITH PRIMARY IMMUNODEFICIENCIES

The seroresponse to specific vaccine antigens is being used increasingly in the investigation of children with suspected immunodeficiency (see Chapter 21). However, immunisation is also an important part of their management and, as with children with malignancies, efforts should be made to provide these children with as much protection as possible, bearing in mind that in some cases they may be unable to respond to vaccines. The same broad principles apply – care being needed in the use of live vaccines while nonlive vaccines are safe and should be used freely. Unfortunately, the routine use of BCG and polio vaccine occasionally reveals the unsuspected underlying diagnosis of severe immunodeficiency.

The deficiencies can be classified into:

* Severe disorders of antibody- and/or cell-mediated immunity. These children should not be given live vaccines. The use of killed vaccines is debatable, particularly in those on intravenous immunoglobulin therapy.
* Less severe disorders such as IgA, IgG subclass or specific antibody production deficiency. Many of these children will have been immunised with live and killed vaccines before diagnosis. The response to these vaccines is used as an indicator of disease severity. Occasionally, there may be progression of the immune defect, in which case further use of live vaccines may need to be ruled out. However, in general these children can continue to receive the full range of vaccines.
* Defects of innate immune mechanisms including neutrophil and complement disorders. With the one exception that BCG should not be given to patients with chronic granulomatous disease, these children are at no increased risk from live vaccines and should be immunised in the normal way. Those with complement disorders seem particularly vulnerable to meningococcal infection of rare serogroups. They should be given meningococcal C conjugate vaccine and also the polysaccharide meningococcal vaccine containing antigens of groups A, C, W135 and Y.

CHILDREN WITH SICKLE CELL DISEASE AND OTHER CAUSES OF HYPOSPLENIS

Individuals with absent spleens or reduced splenic function, including those with sickle cell disorders and coeliac disease, are not at any increased risk from viral infections nor from live vaccines. These can be given according to the standard programme. Annual influenza vaccine is advised as it reduces the possibility of serious bacterial respiratory superinfection.

Overwhelming pneumococcal infection is a significant hazard. The current vaccine (23 valent unconjugated polysaccharide) has a lower efficacy in children under 2 years of age but should be given to older children. When splenectomy is a planned procedure, the vaccine should be given as far in advance as possible. Reimmunisation may be required. Invasive Hib infection sometimes occurs in hyposplenic individuals well beyond the age of 5 years and meningococcal infection can also be a problem. The vaccines against these agents should be given. Clear recommendations regarding reimmunisation cannot be made, although monitoring of antibody titres may be helpful.

CHILDREN WITH MALNUTRITION AND CHRONIC DISEASE

The important questions of how chronic malnutrition may influence the immune responses to both infections and vaccines are not of major importance in the UK, although they are elsewhere. Children with chronic diseases in whom adequate nutrition can be a problem – such as those with cystic fibrosis – should receive all the routine immunisations and be offered additional protection with pneumococcal and influenza vaccine.

CHILDREN WITH THE NEPHROTIC SYNDROME

These children are at increased risk of pneumococcal infection and should be immunised with pneumococcal vaccine. Except when in remission, they also require passive immunisation after exposure to measles and varicella.

CHILDREN BORN PREMATURELY

While such children respond appropriately to most immunisations, there is some evidence that, after Hib and hepatitis B vaccination, a small number of premature babies may not be adequately protected. Nevertheless, it is recommended that all immunisations should be scheduled on the basis of the child's actual date of delivery and no allowance should be made for prematurity. Antibody tests to Hib and hepatitis B can be used to detect the minority of infants that do not make an adequate response and it is recommended that they are performed in those infants born at less than 28 weeks gestation.

CHILDREN WITH INFLAMMATORY CONDITIONS BEING TREATED WITH SYSTEMIC CORTICOSTEROIDS AND/OR IMMUNOSUPPRESSIVE DRUGS

Children being treated with replacement doses of steroids should receive all the usual immunisations. A number of conditions require pharmacological doses of steroids. The dose and period of systemic steroid treatment that results in significant immunosuppression is usually given as prednisolone 2 mg/kg/day for more than a week or 1 mg/kg/day for more than a month (see Contraindications to Immunisation in the current Department of Health Guide).

Further immunosuppression may occur in those on additional or alternative immunosuppressive agents such as azathioprine, methotrexate or cyclosporin. From the safety point of view, the general rules concerning the use of immunisation apply: avoid live vaccines, but give non-live vaccines normally. There are theoretical concerns in children with certain inflammatory diseases such as juvenile idiopathic arthritis that immunisation may exacerbate the underlying disease. There is no good evidence to support this and decisions over vaccination therefore need to be made in this context. It is recommended that the routine vaccination schedule is followed (with the exception of giving live vaccines to those on significant immunosuppressive therapy). Any child with significant immunosuppression should receive VZIG if exposed to chickenpox, unless s/he is known to have had chickenpox previously. The situation becomes increasingly unclear with lower doses or alternate-day steroid regimens for longer periods and individual discretion is called for. With regard to measles, the current recommendation is that children on 2 mg/kg/day or more of prednisolone should receive normal immunoglobulin if in contact with the disease, unless they are known to be immune. Live vaccines can be given once the child has been off immunosuppression for at least 3 months.

FUTURE DEVELOPMENTS

Conjugate vaccine against the common pneumococcal disease-causing serotypes is likely to become available soon. This will be of particular importance to children potentially at risk of such infections because of immunodeficiency or other chronic disease. In the meantime there is an urgent need for further specific studies of the safety and efficacy of existing vaccines in well-defined high-risk groups so that clearer, evidence-based recommendations can be made.

FURTHER READING

Department of Health (1995) Immunisation against infectious disease. HMSO, London.

Plotkin SA, Orenstein W (eds) (1999) Vaccines. WB Saunders, Philadelphia, PA.

Royal College of Paediatrics and Child Health Working Party (2001) Report on Immunisation in the Immunocompromised Child. RCPCH, London, in press.

26 Preparation for travel abroad

International travel is increasing. European families are increasingly likely to travel abroad for business or pleasure. For example, in 1999 UK residents made over 54 million trips abroad compared with 31 million in 1990. Over 7 million visits were to countries outside western Europe and North America. Increasing numbers of trips were to exotic locations and around 2 million visits in 1999 from the UK were to countries with endemic malaria.

Children travelling abroad generally fall into one of three major groups:

- those taking a holiday in Europe, the Mediterranean or further afield
- those going to spend an extended period abroad with their parents
- those returning with their parents to their countries of origin, of which the Indian subcontinent is the most common, followed by West Africa.

This third group is the group of children who are most at risk as they are more likely to be going to home villages where risk of exposure is highest; also, their parents frequently do not appreciate that the children are at risk, not having developed immunity from lifelong exposure to pathogens such as malaria, hepatitis A, etc.

The infections to which a child may be exposed include those commoner in less developed countries, many of which are amenable to immunisation or chemoprophylaxis (e.g. polio, diphtheria, yellow fever and especially malaria) and also those that remain prevalent in the UK (gastroenteritis, whooping cough, hepatitis A, measles, tuberculosis). With air travel, almost all diseases contracted abroad may be incubating on return. Hence, a history of recent travel must be sought in any child with fever, gastrointestinal or other symptoms suggestive of infection (see Chapter 27).

Health advice for travel is a complex subject and a text can never be up to date. Also, the protection recommended for a holiday may be very different from that for an extended stay. This section simply outlines the advice most commonly sought and lists the sources that the health-care worker or traveller can consult for more detailed and current information.

GENERAL ADVICE

Travel abroad has many potential hazards, not all associated with infection. These include different safety standards, exposure to extremes of climate, and language difficulties, all compounding ignorance of the local medical system. To a certain extent, parents must exercise their own common sense regarding their child's visit. A family checklist is: appropriate clothing, entertainment for the journey, adequate protection against sunburn, protection against insect bites, medical insurance, immunisation, prophylaxis and simple medications.

These topics are well covered in many popular and professional publications, examples of which are listed in Further reading. Specific guidelines suitable for the public visiting individual countries are also provided in the Department of Health leaflet *Health Advice for Overseas Travel* (see Further reading), which is updated annually and is available on Prestel.

SIMPLE PRECAUTIONS

Water- and food-borne infections

Most holiday-acquired infections (particularly the various forms of gastroenteritis) are water- and/or food-borne and, although they are not preventable by immunisation, simple precautions will help to protect all family members. Some guidelines are given below. The extent to which they are followed will depend on local conditions and family preference. However, it is wise to emphasise to parents that diarrhoea is a common cause of a spoilt holiday and may be a serious risk.

1. Scrupulous attention to hand hygiene, especially after using the toilet, nappy-changing, and before meals. Soap and/or toilet paper may be unavailable locally.

2. Where the water supply is of uncertain quality (i.e. most countries outside northern Europe, North America, New Zealand, Australia and urban South Africa), the traveller should not drink water from taps or other sources unless it is known to be purified. Hot, bottled or canned drinks with well-known brand names are likely to be safest. Alternatively, water can be treated. If visible matter is present, the water should first be strained through a closely woven cloth. Sterilisation is achieved by boiling for 5 minutes or disinfecting. Where bioled or safe bottled water is not available, appropriate disinfectants are chlorine and iodine (either liquid bleach, tincture of iodine or 'sterilising' tablets). Iodine is preferable as chlorine is less effective. All tablets have makers' instructions. Tincture of iodine (2%) should be used at a concentration of 4 drops to 1 L of water; the water is then allowed to stand for 30 minutes before use. The above ingredients are available from some chemists, travel clinics and by mail order from MASTA (see Advice services).

3. In the same countries as those where water precautions are advised, the following should be avoided: uncooked vegetables, salads, unpeeled fruit, uncooked shellfish, cream, ice-cream, underdone meat or fish, uncooked or cold precooked food and ice cubes. Similarly, unpasteurised milk (unless boiled) and cheese apart from that known to be made from pasteurised milk may also carry infection.

4. Families preparing their own food should cook meat well. Fruit and vegetables should be washed thoroughly in clean, soapy water. If they are not then being cooked, they should be soaked for half an hour in treated water at three times the concentration of disinfectant used for purifying drinking water (see point 2, above).

5. In case a child develops gastroenteritis, the family need to pack some oral rehydration mixture (e.g. Dioralyte), although care must be taken over reconstitution so as not to provide too concentrated a solution. One cupful for each loose stool is a memorable dosage, but parents must seek medical help if excessive vomiting, severe diarrhoea, drowsiness or other signs of dehydration occur, especially in a young baby (see Ch. 18).

6. Children (and adults) should not play on beaches or swim in water visibly polluted with sewage. This also applies in European countries, including the UK.

Insect bites

Another important source of ill health is insect bites, which can result in a spectrum of problems from mild irritation to death from malaria. Hence, protection against insect bites is highly advisable. Insect repellents can be highly effective against flying and crawling insects, although their effectiveness varies according to constituents. For children, conservative use of low concentrations of diethyl toluamide (known as 'deet'), ethylhexanediol or dimethylphalate are effective. These are nontoxic to children if used according to the manufacturer's instructions (which require avoiding excessive applications in babies and small children) and should be put on the skin before going out, especially in the evening when biting is most common. Insect bites can also be reduced by keeping arms and legs covered when out after sunset. Where night-biting flying insects present a hazard and bedrooms are not air-conditioned, use of a 'knock-down' insect spray is advisable. A mosquito net will give additional protection but must be well-tucked in around the end of the bed and without holes. Nets can be made much more effective if impregnated with permethrin (which must be repeated 6-monthly) and families spending extended periods in malarious countries will often invest in their own. (Special nets are available to fit cots.)

Animal bites

Rabies is endemic in most low-income countries and the Mediterranean (see Chapter 90). Even though the risks from a single bite or scratch of a dog, cat or wild animal are small, they are a considerable source of anxiety: parents need to educate their children against approaching animals on holiday and families going to rabies-endemic areas should know how to treat a bite (see Chapter 90).

SPECIFIC ADVICE FOR PARTICULAR COUNTRIES AND DISEASES

Because the specific advice can change so frequently, it is best for the traveller or the professional either to consult regularly updated publications or to contact designated information centres. The former are: the pamphlet *Health Advice for Overseas Travel* (updated regularly), the Department of Health/PHLS publication *Information for Overseas Travel*, HMSO 2000 (intended for professionals), the yearly booklet *International Travel and Health – Vaccination Requirements and WHO Health Advice*; the medical newspaper *Pulse* (table and chart updated monthly). These list the advice and requirements by country. However, the advice is not always consistent or complete. Requirements tend to lag behind the times, local officials at times operate their own rules and protection in addition to the formal requirements is very often advisable. Also, what is necessary for a trip to a country's main city may be radically different from the protection appropriate for an extended stay up-country. The main information centres are listed below. Risks will also be dependent on the season, duration of stay and type of accommodation.

Parents taking children abroad would normally consult their GP or practice nurse for advice in the first instance, who would use one of the sources above. When a complicated tour or extended trip is planned the commercial Medical Advisory Services for Travellers Abroad (MASTA) company is useful (see below for details). It does charge a fee. Family application forms are available directly from MASTA and some chemists.

ROUTINE IMMUNISATIONS FOR TRAVEL

Polio

There have recently been cases of poliomyelitis in the children of African and Asian immigrant parents. Although born in the UK, these children had either not started or not completed their immunisation before being taken on visits to the home country where they acquired their infection. Some parents do not realise the need for continuing the course. Such high-risk babies must be fully protected before they leave, by starting in the neonatal period if necessary. It is equally important to advise that children of any age visiting an endemic area (for practical purposes all less developed countries) should be fully immunised against polio. Adults accompanying them should have boosters if they have had none in the preceding 10 years. Recommendations on polio vaccination for people travelling abroad should appreciate that polio has been eliminated in the Americas so that vaccination with polio is no longer necessary for tourists to South, Central or North America.

Diphtheria, measles

Both are common in the Indian subcontinent, Africa and part of the Middle East, including Turkey. An epidemic of toxigenic pharyngeal diphtheria has been under way in the newly independent states of the former Soviet Union since 1991. All British children should be protected by ensuring immunisation is up to date while those travelling to an endemic area should consider a booster if they have not had an immunisation in the prior 10 years, especially if they are going to mix closely with the local population, such as on school exchanges. Children going to the USA (and some other countries) and entering school or registered day-care will be required by law to produce documentary proof of immunisation.

Tuberculosis

Children at risk are those making extended visits to low-income countries. If the child has not had BCG as a neonate, it must be given before visiting an endemic area for a month or more. Forward planning is needed as a tuberculin (Heaf or Mantoux) test must be used first (if the child is over 3 months) and 6 weeks should elapse between BCG and departure.

Tetanus

Whatever and wherever the holiday, the consultation for advice should include ensuring up-to-date tetanus vaccination (NB. Not more frequently than 10-yearly after the primary course) and once the primary 5 doses have been given no booster is necessary.

ADDITIONAL IMMUNISATIONS AND CHEMO-PROPHYLAXIS COMMONLY RECOMMENDED FOR TRAVEL

Hepatitis A

The vaccine is now used in preference to immunoglobulin, which has become difficult to obtain for use in travellers. The vaccine should be given at least 2–4 weeks prior to travel if time allows, although there is some preliminary evidence to suggest it may at least modify the disease when given close to departure. A paediatric vaccine is licensed for use in children who are 1 year and over, but the age at which the adult preparation is recommended varies with each manufacturer. Immunisation is thought to give protection for at least a year and probably longer; its exact duration is unknown but a booster produces some years' protection. It needs to be remembered that hepatitis A is best prevented by good hygiene and food/water precautions (see above) and that the greatest risk is to older members of the family as the disease is most severe beyond childhood.

Typhoid

There are between 100 and 200 notifications of typhoid in the UK each year, the majority having been acquired overseas, chiefly in the Indian sub-continent. Prevention is most effectively achieved by good standards of personal hygiene and avoidance of contaminated food and water. The risk of infection in children under 1 year is low. A range of typhoid vaccines are available but these are considered moderately protective only (see Chapter 106) and not all specialists recommend their routine use in short-term travellers to countries where risk is low.

Cholera

The disease is endemic in most low-income countries (see Chapter 44), and occasionally infections are also acquired in the Mediterranean. A handful of cases occur annually in the UK, all acquired abroad. As for typhoid, good hygiene is the best prevention and the vaccine is of very limited effectiveness. It is not recommended and is not available in the UK at the present time (see Chapter 44).

Yellow fever

The disease occurs in two endemic zones, central Africa and the northern zone of South America, with cases occurring in both urban and rural settings. Cases are almost unheard of in the UK but travellers to these countries are certainly at risk and must be protected. Yellow fever immunisation is mandatory for entry to some countries with the endemic zone for all travellers. For other countries travellers direct from the UK do not have to show a yellow fever certificate but those travelling from infected areas must do so. Listing for these two types of countries are published in the sources of further reading. Immunisation is always advised (whether mandatory or not) for travel to rural areas within the endemic zones. Many general practices are now registered as yellow fever centres offering immunisation and the Department of Health booklet *Health Advice for Overseas Travel* contains a current list. For a description of the disease, see Chapter 58.

Malaria

Around 2000 cases of malaria are imported annually into the UK. In 1995 there were 2055 cases reported, 261 in children under age 15 years including one death. Malarious countries include almost all of Africa, most of the Middle East, south and south-east Asia, Oceania and Latin America. Examination of the ethnic group of children affected in the UK suggests that children from ethnic minority groups are most at risk, partially because they are most likely to travel to places where malaria is hyperendemic and partially because parents do not always appreciate the importance of protection. Children and adults brought up in Europe will possess far less exposure-derived immunity than their peers who have grown up in malarious surroundings. Protection against malaria infection and severe disease is based on three strategies: prevention of bites (see Insect bites, above), chemoprophylaxis and prompt diagnosis.

Chemoprophylaxis

This is highly effective when the recommended regimens are taken properly; even when breakthrough infections occur the use of chemoprophylaxis will almost always prevent the most severe sequelae. Essential points to make to families are that medication must be taken throughout the trip and continued for 4 weeks after return and that if a febrile illness develops it may be malaria, hence should this happen medical assistance must be sought immediately and the doctor informed about the travel abroad (see Chapter 27). The choice of chemoprophylaxis is a complex subject and recommendations differ according to the part of the world in question, patterns of malaria resistance to antimalarials and experience of new medications. A general guide is contained in Chapter 76 and the most authoritative source of guidance for the UK at the time of this publication is the article by Bradley and Warhurst listed in Further reading, below. Current guidance can be sought from the latest published material or expert sources of advice (see below). Because of the increasing rise in resistance to more traditional prophylaxis, mefloquine is recommended for Africa and Oceania, although currently (2000) this drug is not recommended for children under 2 years, pregnant women in the first trimester or during breastfeeding, while the more traditional daily proguanil (Paludrine) and weekly chloroquine remains reasonably effective.

Meningococcal disease

Vaccination is recommended for travellers to high-incidence areas such as the countries of west, central and east Africa and much of the Middle East (see Chapter 78). Vaccination is essential for travellers going to large gatherings such as the Hajj pilgrimage to Mecca in Saudi Arabia. However advice on specific countries changes with time and it is advisable to check with one of the sources below.

FURTHER READING AND SOURCES OF ADVICE

Bradley DJ, Warhurst DC on behalf of an expert group of doctors, nurses and pharmacists (1997) Guidelines for the prevention of malaria in travellers from the United Kingdom. CDR Review 10: R138–151.

*†Dawood R (1992) Travellers health: how to stay healthy abroad. Oxford Paperbacks, Oxford.

Department of Health (2000) Health advice for overseas travel. Stationery Office, London. Updated annually and available on Prestel.

Fisher PR (1998) Travels with infants and children. Inf Dis Clin North Am 12: 355–368.

Samuel BU, Barry M (1998) The pregnant traveller. Inf Dis Clin North Am 12: 325–354.

*World Health Organization (2000) International travel and health – vaccination requirements and health advice – updated annually

Advice services

NB. This information is correct for August 2000 but changes are frequent.

Birmingham	*Department of Infection and Tropical Medicine, tel. 0121 766 6611 (x 4403/4382/4535)
Liverpool	*School of Tropical Medicine, tel. 0151 708 9393
Manchester	†Department of Infectious Diseases and Tropical Medicine, Monsall Hospital, tel. 0161 720 2267
London	†Hospital for Tropical Disease, London has a payline for the public, tel. 09061 337755
	†MASTA, Keppel Street, London WC1E 7HT, tel. 020 7631 4408 (mail order service and provides individual health briefs, tel. (payline) 0891 224100) – charges a fee
Oxford	*John Warin Ward Churchill Hospital, tel. 01865 225214
National	†British Airways Travel Clinics – these are in many cities and prescribe medicine and vaccines; details of the nearest clinic can be obtained by telephoning 020 7831 5333 but no advice can be given over the phone
	*Communicable Disease Surveillance Centre, tel. 020 8200 6868 (open to enquiries by health professionals, does not give advice on individual cases but is happy to advise on policy that is applicable to particular circumstances)
	Malaria Reference Laboratory:
	*doctors 020 7636 3924
	†public 0891 600 350 (payline) or 020 7636 3924 (9.30–10.30am and 2–3pm)
	*Scottish Centre for Infection and Environmental Health, tel. 0141 300 1111 (policy on individual cases as for CDSC). SCIEH also provides a subscription website for professionals

* Services for doctors, nurses and pharmacists giving advice. † Suitable for enquiries by members of the public

27 Management of the child with an infection contracted abroad

THE SIZE AND NATURE OF THE PROBLEM

Until recently, there have been no studies looking specifically at the incidence of infectious diseases in children who have returned from travelling abroad. Surveys had included children but it was often difficult to separate them, and their problems, from the greater number of adults. This is important because the risks and consequences of travel-related illnesses are very different in children from those in adults. Children are at little risk of acquiring hepatitis B and human immunodeficiency virus (HIV) infections while on holiday, as these are predominantly spread by sexual intercourse. On the other hand, they are more likely to contract hepatitis A, as immunity in young children from developed countries is low. However, the consequences of the disease are rarely serious in children, whereas it can be fatal in adults.

An extensive survey of travellers from Scotland showed that 33.5% of children aged 0–9 years experienced an episode of illness compared with 41% of those aged 10–19 years, 48% aged 20–29 years, 38% aged 30–39 years and only 20% of those aged over 60 years. One imagines that the main explanation for this pattern is the behaviour of the travellers.

A recent report* looked at admissions to one hospital of children with a fever within 4 weeks of returning to the UK from the tropics. Of 31 children, 14 had a nonspecific self-limiting illness, four had malaria, three bacillary dysentery, two dengue fever, two typhoid and one each hepatitis A, bacterial lymphadenitis, pneumonia, *Pneumocystis carinii* pneumonia (this child had newly diagnosed HIV infection), acute myeloid leukaemia and streptococcal sore throat. A study in Birmingham showed that notifications were not an accurate reflection of the true situation. Of 19 cases of malaria seen in hospital, none had been officially notified. Other diseases seen were diarrhoea from various causes, typhoid, paratyphoid, hepatitis (mainly hepatitis A) and amoebiasis. The most common place of travel was the Indian subcontinent but a large number had been to Europe and a few to Africa.

Table 27.1 shows the risk of illness and use of medical resources in relation to travel. Most of the illnesses are trivial and many are no different from those acquired at home. However, in 1993 there were 253 cases of imported malaria in children in the UK and in 1994 a child died of diphtheria acquired on a visit to Pakistan. As a generalisation, the risk of developing a travel-related illness increases the further south and east the destination; however, there are illnesses found in parts of Europe that are exceedingly rare in the UK. Examples include tick-borne encephalitis in some parts of Austria, Germany and Scandinavia; diphtheria in the countries of the former USSR; and rabies in many parts of Europe. Remember

---

* Kelin JL, Milman GC (1998) Prospective, hospital based study of fever in children in the United Kingdom who had recently spent time in the tropics. Br Med J 316: 1425–1426.

Table 27.1 Estimated monthly incidence of health problems per 100 000 travellers (all ages) to tropical areas (redrawn from Steffen R, Lobel HO (1996) Traveller's diseases. In: Cook GC (ed.) Manson's tropical diseases, 20th edn. WB Saunders, London.)

Infections		All problems
	100% ⊤ 100 000	Any health problem (used medication or felt ill)
Traveller's diarrhoea		
		Felt ill
		Consulted physician during
	10% ⊥ 10 000	travel or on return home
Malaria (no chemoprophylaxis, west Africa)		Stayed in bed
Acute febrile respiratory tract infection		Incapacity for work after return
	1% ⊥ 1000	
		Hospitalised abroad
Hepatitis A		
Gonorrhoea		
Animal bite with rabies risk		
Hepatitis B (expatriates)	0.1% ⊥ 100	Air evacuation
Typhoid (India, north and north-west Africa)		
HIV infection	0.01% ⊥ 10	
Typhoid (other areas)		
Poliomyelitis, asymptomatic		
Legionella infection (Mediterranean)	0.001% ⊥ 1	Died abroad
Cholera		
Paralytic poliomyelitis		

that some illnesses, e.g. malaria and schistosomiasis, may not become apparent until months or even years after exposure. Some travellers return from sojourns abroad with more than one acquired infection. It is therefore important not to assume that all of a patient's symptoms may be explained by the first infection diagnosed.

IMPORTANCE OF DIAGNOSIS

It is important to make a diagnosis (Table 27.2) for a number of reasons:

- Urgent treatment may be life-saving, e.g. for malaria
- Unrecognised cases may act as a source of an outbreak, e.g. diseases
- The condition may be notifiable.

Table 27.2 Diagnostic clues in children returning from travel abroad with a fever

Symptom	Possible diagnoses
Sore throat ± skin lesions	Diphtheria and Lassa fever (both are very rarely imported to UK)
Jaundice	Hepatitis (usually A) Haemolysis, e.g. malaria
Neurological symptoms	Tick-borne diseases (e.g. Lyme disease, tick-borne and Japanese B encephalitis), typhoid, malaria and meningitis, including poliomyelitis
Respiratory symptoms	Tuberculosis, legionellosis, pneumonic plague, anthrax, acute respiratory distress syndrome secondary to falciparum malaria, typhoid, typhus, Q fever, *Entamoeba histolytica* infection and tropical pulmonary eosinophilia
Arthritis	Lyme disease, brucellosis, Reiter's syndrome, salmonellosis, yersiniosis and arbovirus infections
Lymphadenopathy	Visceral leishmaniasis, tuberculosis, trypanosomiasis, typhus and bubonic plague
Hepatosplenomegaly	Malaria, typhoid, visceral leishmaniasis, Q fever, brucellosis and the Katayama syndrome of schistosomiasis

TRAVELLERS' DIARRHOEA

The most common illness acquired abroad is travellers' diarrhoea, which occurs in up to a third of tourists. Causative organisms include bacteria (enterotoxigenic *Escherichia coli*, *Shigella*, *Salmonella*, *Campylobacter* and *Vibrio* species), viruses (especially rotavirus) and parasites (*Giardia lamblia*, *Entamoeba histolytica*, *Cyclospora cayetanensis* and *Cryptosporidium parvum*). The diagnosis is made on the basis of history and stool examination. Treatment should concentrate on rehydration and, as the condition is usually self-limiting, antimicrobial chemotherapy is not routinely indicated. Moderate to severe diarrhoea has been treated successfully with trimethoprim or ciprofloxacin. Remember that malaria may present with diarrhoea as a prominent feature.

OTHER INFECTIONS

Other infections typically present as a fever. If the itinerary has included any country where malaria is endemic, it is essential that this diagnosis is excluded by a blood film. This applies even if appropriate chemoprophylaxis has been taken. Resistance is common and increasing. *Falciparum* malaria can be rapidly fatal and is often not considered. Having excluded malaria, the history should include:

- Medical conditions antedating travel
- Nature and time of onset of symptoms
- The countries visited
- Living conditions and eating arrangements
- Activities pursued, including bathing in freshwater lakes and rivers, and forest walking
- Illness in travelling companions
- Details of immunisations and malaria prophylaxis.

A complete physical examination is important and should include careful examination of the skin.

All the usual 'home' causes of a fever should be considered as well as more exotic explanations. Combinations of symptoms with a fever may give a clue to the underlying cause (Table 27.2).

Rashes may also give a clue to the nature of an infection:

- A macular rash is found in typhus, typhoid, dengue and other arbovirus infections
- A haemorrhagic rash occurs with yellow fever and the viral haemorrhagic fevers
- Circinate erythema is found in early trypanosomiasis
- Erythema migrans may be present with Lyme disease
- Eschars are found in typhus and cutaneous anthrax.

A full blood count, and urine and stool microscopy and culture are essential in all returning travellers with an undiagnosed fever of more than a few days duration. An eosinophilia is a common finding (5–10%) and in approximately 50% will be due to a parasite. This is commonly intestinal but may be caused by other conditions, such as schistosomiasis. Haematuria may be the only indication of schistosomiasis. The index of suspicion should be high if the child has been in fresh water in an endemic area (mainly Africa but also in some parts of South America, south-east Asia and the Middle East). A schistosomal enzyme-linked immunosorbent assay (ELISA) should be performed and, if positive, further definitive tests will be necessary.

Further investigations will be dictated by the history and physical findings (see also Chapter 6). The following section gives an indication of the most likely infectious diseases depending on the itinerary. It must be used with caution, as not all possible infections are listed and some of those that are listed do not occur in all parts of the region. For features of the specific infections, reference should be made to Part Two of this book or to a specialised textbook.

NORTHERN AFRICA
Algeria, Egypt, Libya, Morocco and Tunisia

Arthropod-borne diseases are unusual but can occur. The main manifestation is fever possibly accompanied by neurological symptoms. Diarrhoeal diseases and hepatitis A are common as is typhoid fever in some areas. Schistosomiasis occurs mainly in close proximity to the Nile. Trachoma, rabies and poliomyelitis are other potential hazards.

SUB-SAHARAN AFRICA

Angola, Benin, Burkina Faso, Burundi, Cameroon, Cape Verde, Central African Republic, Chad, Comoros, Congo, Côte d'Ivoire, Djibouti, Equatorial Guinea, Eritrea, Ethiopia, Gabon, Gambia, Ghana, Guinea, Guinea-Bissau, Kenya, Liberia, Madagascar, Malawi, Mali, Mauritania, Mozambique, Niger, Nigeria, Réunion, Rwanda, São Tomé and Principe, Senegal, Seychelles, Sierra Leone, Somalia, Sudan, Togo, Uganda, Tanzania, Democratic Congo Republic, Zambia and Zimbabwe

Arthropod-borne diseases are common. *Falciparum* malaria and filariasis occur in most areas. Leishmaniasis, relapsing fever, typhus and forms of haemorrhagic fever can be found in many areas. Outbreaks of yellow fever happen periodically. Diarrhoeal diseases such as the dysenteries and giardiasis are common. Cholera is found in many areas. Hepatitis A, B and E are widespread. Polio, rabies and schistosomiasis are found in most parts of the region. The haemorrhagic fevers (Lassa, Marburg and Ebola), although present, are uncommon. Epidemics of meningococcal disease occur in the tropical savannah areas during the dry season.

SOUTHERN AFRICA

Botswana, Lesotho, Namibia, St Helena, South Africa and Swaziland

Malaria is only significant in certain areas. Other arthropod-borne diseases, although reported, are not a major problem to travellers. Amoebiasis and typhoid fever are common, as is hepatitis B. The area is polio-free but schistosomiasis is common in many areas.

NORTH AMERICA

Bermuda, Canada, Greenland, St Pierre and Miquelon and USA

Plague, rabies, Rocky Mountain spotted fever and arthropod-borne encephalitides occur but are uncommon. In the north-eastern USA and the upper Midwest, Lyme disease is endemic.

MAINLAND CENTRAL AMERICA

Belize, Costa Rica, El Salvador, Guatemala, Honduras, Mexico, Nicaragua and Panama

Cutaneous and mucocutaneous leishmaniasis and malaria are found in all countries but the latter's distribution is limited in Mexico, Costa Rica and Panama. Chagas' disease (American trypanosomiasis) is found in localised rural areas. Visceral leishmaniasis, onchocerciasis, filariasis, dengue fever and Venezuelan equine encephalitis are found to varying degrees in the region. Amoebic and bacillary dysentery, typhoid fever, helminth infections and animal rabies are common. Hepatitis A is common and cholera occurs in all countries.

CARIBBEAN CENTRAL AMERICA

Antigua and Barbuda, Aruba, Bahamas, Barbados, Cayman Islands, Cuba, Dominica, Dominican Republic, Grenada, Guadeloupe, Haiti, Jamaica, Martinique, Montserrat, Netherlands Antilles, Puerto Rico, St Kitts and Nevis, St Lucia, St Vincent and the Grenadines, Trinidad and Tobago, Turks and Caicos Islands and Virgin Islands (USA)

Malaria occurs only in Haiti and parts of the Dominican Republic. Cutaneous leishmaniasis, filariasis, human fascioliasis and tularaemia are found in small pockets. Dengue fever is also present. Bacillary and amoebic dysentery and hepatitis A are common.

TROPICAL SOUTH AMERICA

Bolivia, Brazil, Colombia, Ecuador, French Guiana, Guyana, Paraguay, Peru, Surinam and Venezuela

Malaria (*falciparum*, *vivax* and *malariae*), Chagas' disease and cutaneous and mucocutaneous leishmaniasis occur throughout the area. Yellow fever is found in forest areas of all countries except Paraguay and areas east of the Andes. Visceral leishmaniasis, onchocerciasis, filariasis, plague, dengue fever, viral encephalitis, bartonellosis and louse-borne typhus may be found in some parts. Amoebiasis, diarrhoeal diseases, helminth infections, hepatitis A and brucellosis are common. Cholera occurs in some countries. Hepatitis B and D are common in the Amazon basin. Schistosomiasis, rabies and hydatid disease are found in some countries. Epidemic meningococcal meningitis can be a major health hazard in Brazil.

TEMPERATE SOUTH AMERICA

Argentina, Chile, Falkland Islands (Malvinas) and Uruguay

Chagas' disease is widespread. Cutaneous leishmaniasis occurs in north-eastern Argentina and malaria in the north-west of the country. Salmonellosis, hepatitis A and intestinal parasitosis are common in Argentina, whereas cholera and typhoid are not. Tapeworm, typhoid, viral hepatitis and hydatid disease are found in the other countries of the area.

EAST ASIA

China, Hong Kong, Japan, Macao, Mongolia, North and South Korea

Malaria is found only in China. Filariasis, visceral and cutaneous leishmaniasis and plague may also be found in some areas of the country. Hantavirus, dengue fever, Japanese encephalitis and scrub typhus occur in many areas. Diarrhoeal diseases, hepatitis E and brucellosis are common in China. The oriental liver fluke (clonorchiasis) and oriental lung fluke (paragonimiasis) are reported in most countries. Hepatitis B is common whereas schistosomiasis is found mainly in the Yangtze river basin of China. Polio, trachoma and leptospirosis also occur in China.

EASTERN SOUTH ASIA

Brunei Darussalam, Cambodia, Indonesia, Laos, Malaysia, Myanmar, Philippines, Singapore, Thailand and Vietnam

Filariasis occurs in all countries and typhus in most. Malaria is endemic in all but Brunei and Singapore. Plague and melioidosis are found in Myanmar, Malaysia, Thailand and Vietnam. Dengue fever occurs in epidemics. Cholera, amoebic and bacillary dysentery, typhoid fever and hepatitis A and E are found in all countries. The giant intestinal fluke (fasciolopsiasis) and oriental lung fluke (paragonimiasis) are found in most countries, whereas the oriental liver fluke (clonorchiasis) and the cat liver fluke (opisthorchiasis) are found mainly in the Indochina peninsula. Schistosomiasis, polio and trachoma are found in some areas. Hepatitis B is common. Rabies is a potential hazard.

MIDDLE SOUTH ASIA

Afghanistan, Armenia, Azerbaijan, Bangladesh, Bhutan, Georgia, India, Iran, Kazakhstan, Kirgizstan, Maldives, Nepal, Pakistan, Sri Lanka, Tadzhikistan, Turkmenistan and Uzbekistan

Malaria is found in all countries except the Maldives. Filariasis, leishmaniasis, relapsing fever, typhus, dengue fever, Japanese encephalitis and various haemorrhagic fevers are found in many countries of the area. Cholera, dysentery, typhoid fever, hepatitis A and E and helminth infections are common. Brucellosis and hydatid disease are found in many countries. There are pockets of dracunculiasis in India and Pakistan. Hepatitis B and animal rabies are found in most countries. Urinary schistosomiasis is found in the south-west of Iran and meningococcal meningitis in India and Nepal. Polio is found all countries throughout the region, except for Bhutan and the Maldives.

WESTERN SOUTH ASIA

Bahrain, Cyprus, Iraq, Israel, Jordan, Kuwait, Lebanon, Oman, Qatar, Saudi Arabia, Syria, Turkey, United Arab Emirates and Yemen

Malaria is found in the rural parts of many countries of the area. Typhus and relapsing fever are present in some countries, as is visceral leishmaniasis. Cutaneous leishmaniasis is common. Typhoid fever, hepatitis A and brucellosis occur in most countries. Tapeworm and dracunculiasis are present in most countries. Hydatid disease, trachoma, animal rabies and polio occur in some countries.

NORTHERN EUROPE

Belarus, Belgium, Channel Islands, Czech Republic, Denmark, Estonia, Faeroe Islands, Finland, Germany, Iceland, Ireland, the Isle of Man, Latvia, Lithuania, Luxembourg, Moldova, Netherlands, Norway, Poland, Russian Federation, Slovakia, Sweden, Ukraine and the United Kingdom

Malaria is not a problem. Tick-borne encephalitis, Lyme disease and Crimean Congo haemorrhagic fever occur in the north. Hantavirus disease is present throughout the area. Infection with tapeworm, *Trichinella*, *Diphyllobothrium* and *Fasciola hepatica* and hepatitis A may occur in some areas. Diphtheria is a problem in some countries, especially in the former USSR. Polio is found in the Russian Federation and the Ukraine. Animal rabies is found in the rural parts of northern Europe except Finland, Iceland, Norway, Sweden and the UK.

SOUTHERN EUROPE

Albania, Andorra, Austria, Azores, Bosnia-Hercegovina, Bulgaria, Canary Islands, Croatia, France, Gibraltar, Greece, Hungary, Italy, Liechtenstein, Madeira, Malta, Monaco, Portugal, Romania, San Marina, Slovenia, Spain, Switzerland and Yugoslavia

Tick-borne encephalitis, Lyme disease and hantavirus disease are found in the south and east. Typhus, West Nile fever, cutaneous and visceral leishmaniasis and sandfly fever are found in countries bordering the Mediterranean. Bacillary dysentery and typhoid fever are common in the south-eastern and south-western parts of the area, where brucellosis may also be found. Hydatid disease occurs in the south-east. Hepatitis A and *Fasciola hepatica* infection are a problem in some parts of the area. Polio is present in parts of the former Yugoslavia. Hepatitis B is endemic in Albania, Bulgaria and Romania. Animal rabies is found in all countries of the area apart from Gibraltar, Malta, Monaco and Portugal.

AUSTRALIA, NEW ZEALAND AND THE ANTARCTIC

Communicable diseases are rarely more hazardous to tourists than in their country of origin. Mosquito-borne epidemic polyarthritis and viral encephalitis, and amoebic meningoencephalitis have been reported.

MELANESIA AND MICRONESIA–POLYNESIA

American Samoa, Cook Islands, Easter Island, Fiji, French Polynesia, Guam, Kiribati, Marshall Islands, Micronesia, Nature, New Caledonia, Niue, Palau, Papua New Guinea, Samoa, Solomon Islands, Tokelau, Tonga, Trust Territory of the Pacific Islands, Tuvalu, Vanuatu and the Wallis and Fortuna Islands

Malaria is endemic in some of the islands and dengue fever can occur in epidemics in most. Filariasis is widespread. Typhus has been found in Papua New Guinea. Typhoid fever, hepatitis A and helminth infections are common. Hepatitis B is endemic throughout the area. Trachoma is found in parts of Melanesia and polio in Papua New Guinea.

28 Refugees and internationally adopted children

POSSIBLE PROBLEMS

Refugees and children being adopted from abroad may have similar medical problems. Many of these will relate to lack of routine child health surveillance in the countries of origin, e.g. undetected defects of vision, hearing and speech, and omission of routine immunisations, whereas others will be infections acquired from the child's country of origin. The risk and type of infection depends upon the country from which the child has come. Children from the USA, western Europe and Australasia will be subject to the same level of care as in the UK and will suffer, broadly speaking, from the same infectious diseases (some arthropod-borne diseases may be more common in these countries). Children from some countries of eastern Europe may be at increased risk of diphtheria and tuberculosis. Enteric infections are also more common. Children who have lived in orphanages or received blood transfusions may have acquired human immunodeficiency virus (HIV) and/or hepatitis B infection, especially in Romania. Children from Africa, the Indian subcontinent and some parts of South America may have been exposed to numerous diseases not usually encountered in the West. Treatment for diagnosed diseases may have been suboptimal, suppressing the illness rather than eliminating the infection. Many infections may be asymptomatic at the time of entry to the country and some (e.g. schistosomiasis and liver flukes) may take years to become apparent. Recurrent fever due to chronic malaria is accepted as the norm in many countries.

MANAGEMENT AND SCREENING

In this section the management of asymptomatic children only is considered. The management of a child from abroad who has a fever or other symptoms is considered in Chapter 27 and relevant chapters in Part Two. For children being adopted from abroad an intercountry adoption form should be completed. This includes a thorough history and examination. All other children coming from abroad should, at least, answer a health questionnaire. Any omissions in routine child health surveillance or immunisations should be rectified. Whether or not to screen asymptomatic children from abroad for infections is unclear. In 1991, a study at the Hospital for Tropical Diseases, London, screened 1029 asymptomatic individuals (135 less than 14 years old) returning from a prolonged stay abroad. It was difficult to estimate in how many people the abnormalities that were found related to their stay abroad. Urine analysis of 830 cases showed abnormalities in 116. In none of these was the abnormality related to the stay abroad. Stool microscopy for cysts, ova and parasites showed abnormalities in 207 of 995 (20.8%). The most common finding was the presence of cysts of *Entamoeba histolytica* or *Giardia lamblia*. Almost all were treated, in spite of being asymptomatic. Out of 852 blood samples, 67 (7.9%) showed an eosinophilia. In 26 people this was associated with parasitosis (schistosomiasis in 18). The authors concluded that screening for tropical disease can be efficiently carried out by an informed health professional using structured history-taking and relevant laboratory tests. A survey of health authorities and boards in the UK, published in 1990, showed a wide variation in policy of screening children from abroad. The authors suggested the following procedure for children entering the educational systems in the UK after spending more than 8 weeks in Asia, the Far East, Africa and South America:

- The school nurse should interview the family before the child starts school and review the child's health. A Heaf test should be performed and, if negative, BCG should be given. Children already in school should be interviewed as soon as possible.
- If asymptomatic, the child can start school as soon as the interview has been completed.
- Immunisations should be completed (Table 28.1).*

Table 28.1 Immunisation of children previously unimmunised or with unknown immunisation status

Age	Primary immunisations required	Booster immunisations required subsequently
Under 12 months	DTP/Hib × 3 OPV × 3 Men C × 1†	As per schedule
12–48 months	DTP × 3 OPV × 3 Hib × 1 MMR × 2 Men C × 1†	DT + OPV after 3 years Td + OPV at age 15 years
4–10 years	DTP* × 3 OPV × 3 MMR × 2 Men C × 1†	Td + OPV at age 15 years Td at age 25 years
10–15 years	Td × 3 OPV × 3 MMR × 2 Men C × 1†	

* BCG should be given according to local policy. Acellular pertussis may be felt appropriate in older children as it has fewer side-effects than the whole-cell vaccine. † Two doses only required in children over 4 months old.
DTP = diphtheria/tetanus/pertussis; OPV = oral polio vaccine; Hib = *Haemophilus influenzae* type b; Men C = meningococcus C conjugate vaccine; MMR = measles/mumps/rubella; Td = tetanus/low-dose diphtheria.

* Unfortunately, immunisation schedules vary enormously between different countries, even in western Europe. They also vary from time to time and it is not possible to publish a guide to them as it would rapidly be out of date. Some information is available from websites of individual health departments and WHO.

- If the child does not already have a general practitioner, advice should be given on registering.

In the absence of evidence to the contrary, the above procedure is recommended. Consideration should also be given to voluntary confidential testing for children and adults from high-risk areas for HIV and hepatitis B infection. Screening for infectious diseases other than these and for tuberculosis cannot be justified.

29 Zoonoses

See also Chapter 33 concerning animals in school, animal bites and school visits to farms.

Zoonotic infections are those infections that are naturally transmissible between vertebrate animals and man. Many of the human communicable diseases described in detail in Part Two of this manual are zoonoses or, in the case of some of the infections, may be transmitted zoonotically from animals to humans. The zoonoses are a highly varied group of diseases and constitute an important public health problem. The organisms responsible may be bacteria, viruses, protozoa, helminths, chlamydias or rickettsias. Some are fortunately rare while others such as the food-borne infections are all too common. Many zoonotic infections are found in the UK, some may also be imported, while others such as the exotic or tropical infections are only likely to be encountered overseas. With the relaxation of quarantine on live animals coming into the UK (see Chapter 90) it is likely that the number and volume of imported zoonoses will increase. Some zoonoses may cause serious disease in humans; others produce apparently mild, nonspecific symptoms in some individuals but severe effects in others, while other zoonotic infections may cause no apparent signs or symptoms at all. Rabies, for example, though not endemic in Britain, is a life-threatening and usually fatal illness. Toxocariasis and toxoplasmosis, on the other hand, are usually asymptomatic, although in some circumstances they can cause severe disablement in affected humans. Cryptosporidiosis is effectively an acute self-limiting illness in healthy individuals, whereas in an immunocompromised patient the same infection may prove fatal. Other gastrointestinal zoonotic organisms such as salmonellas and *Campylobacter* can cause extensive morbidity and such human zoonotic infections may occur as local clusters or outbreaks that may be geographically widespread, both nationally and internationally affecting large numbers of people. Other zoonoses, such as hydatid disease, more often occur as single, apparently sporadic cases.

The variety of vertebrate animals from which humans may inadvertently acquire infections is as broad as the range of zoonotic infections themselves (Table 29.1). The animal types may be characterised within one of

Table 29.1 Some of the zoonotic infections that may be acquired by children in the UK and other parts of Europe

Disease/infection	Causative organism/ most common species	Common animal sources	Mode of spread/vector	Human epidemiology (England and Wales)*
Gastrointestinal infections				
Campylobacteriosis*	*Campylobacter jejuni*, *C. coli*	Cattle, poultry, pigs, sheep, birds, rodents, puppies and kittens	Ingestion of water contaminated by animal faeces; consumption of undercooked chicken, unpasteurised milk or contaminated foods; by the faecal–oral route direct from animals or person-to-person	There were over 50 000 indigenous and imported laboratory-reported infections in 1997 and numbers are rising; over 15% of these occurred in children. A major proportion of the infections are probably food-borne
Cryptosporidiosis*	*Cryptosporidium parvum*	Sheep, cattle, deer, goats, puppies and kittens	By the faecal–oral route direct from animals, or via contaminated water; consumption of contaminated milk; or by person-to-person	There are on average 4500–5000 indigenous and imported laboratory-reported cases each year; nearly two-thirds are in children
Giardiasis*	*Giardia lamblia*	Various wild and domestic animals	Direct by the faecal–oral route from animals or person-to-person; or ingestion of contaminated water	There are on average over 6000 indigenous and imported laboratory-reported infections each year; over a quarter are in children. Travel-associated cases and water-borne outbreaks have been reported

Table 29.1 continued

Disease/infection	Causative organism/ most common species	Common animal sources	Mode of spread/vector	Human epidemiology (England and Wales)*
Haemolytic uraemic syndrome/haemo-rrhagic colitis*	Escherichia coli O157/ verotoxin producing E. coli (VTEC)	Cattle	Consumption of raw or inadequately cooked beef; raw milk; unwashed fruit and vegetables contaminated with animal faeces; other contaminated foods; by the faecal-oral route direct from animals or person-to-person	Over 1000 isolates of VTEC O157 were confirmed in 1997; nearly half were in children. Several food-borne and animal-associated incidents have been recorded
Hymenolepiasis (dwarf and rat tapeworms)	Hymenolepis nana, H. diminuta	H. nana: house mice; dogs, cats and their fleas; H. diminuta: beetles; rats, and fleas; beetles	H. nana: direct ingestion of eggs passed in animal faeces, or by the faecal-oral route from person-to-person; H. diminuta: inadvertent ingestion of the infected insect	There are on average over 50 laboratory reports of human H. nana infections each year: over half are in children. H. diminuta infections are very rare
Salmonellosis*	Salmonella spp. (excluding S. typhi and S. paratyphi)	Poultry, cattle, sheep and pigs	Consumption of raw or inadequately cooked food from animals; raw milk; cross-contamination of cooked foods; by the faecal-oral route from animals or person-to person	There were over 32 000 indigenous and imported cases confirmed in 1997; nearly 30% were in children. Most are probably associated with food consumption
Yersiniosis*	Yersinia pseudo-tuberculosis and Y. enterocolitica	Wild and domestic animals	Infections may be food-borne, water-borne or possibly acquired by the faecal-oral route from animals or person-to-person	There were fewer than 200 laboratory-reported infections in 1997; around a quarter of these were in children. Food-borne infections from unpasteurised milk and cheese, for example, have occurred, as has an outbreak attributed to contact with an infected rabbit

Skin infections

Cowpox*	Cowpox virus	Cats and other felines, cattle and rodents	Direct contact between infected animals and abraded human skin	There are only a few laboratory reports each year in both children and adults
Dermatophytosis or ringworm*	*Trichophyton* spp., *Microsporum* spp.	Dogs, cats, cattle and horses		No data available but probably a common infection particularly among farmers, veterinarians, slaughtermen and those who work with horses, cattle and sheep
Mycobacteriosis*	*Mycobacterium marinum*	Fish and marine mammals	Direct transmission from infected fish, contaminated aquaria or marine mammal bites	On average around 20 laboratory-reported infections each year, mostly among tropical fish keepers
Orf–paravaccinia infection*	Orf–paravaccinia virus	Sheep and goats	Direct abraded skin contact with animal lesions, infected wool or hides, or contaminated pastures	There have been up to 25 laboratory reports each year (average around 15) including a few infections in children. It is probably an occupational hazard affecting mainly shepherds, veterinarians, slaughtermen and butchers
Pasteurellosis	*Pasteurella multocida* and *P. haemolytica*	Dogs and cats	Direct transmission via animal bites, scratches and licks	There are on average around 250 laboratory-reported infections each year but only a small proportion occur in children

Ta+ble 29.1 continued

Disease/infection	Causative organism/ most common species	Common animal sources	Mode of spread/vector	Human epidemiology (England and Wales)*
Respiratory tract infections				
Q fever	Coxiella burnetii	Sheep, cattle, goats and ticks	Inhalation of dust contaminated by placental tissue and fluids; direct contact with animals or animal products; consumption of contaminated milk; or possibly tick bites	Fewer than 100 laboratory reports of indigenous and imported infections each year, but very rarely in children. Cases have been reported in farmers, veterinarians, slaughtermen and tannery workers
Chlamydiosis, ornithosis or psittacosis	Chlamydia psittaci	Avian strain: psittacine and other birds including ducks, turkeys, pigeons; Ovine strain: sheep and possibly goats and cattle	Avian strain: inhalation of aerosols or dust contaminated by infected bird faeces or nasal discharges; ovine strain: inhalation of aerosol or dust contaminated by the products of gestation or abortion	There are on average 400 laboratory reported indigenous and imported infections annually but very few occur in children. Cases have occurred in poultry processing, aviary, quarantine station and pet-shop workers, bird keepers and veterinarians
Systemic/other infections				
Capnocytophaga canimorsus infection	Capnocytophaga canimorsus (CDC group DF-2)	Dogs	Direct transmission via bites or licks	Reports of this infection are rare (there were two in 1997) and it occurs infrequently in children
Cat-scratch disease	Uncertain – Bartonella henselae,	Cats/kittens	Direct transmission via scratches, bites and licks	There are very few reported cases
Variant Creutzfeldt– Jakob disease	Prion	Cattle with BSE	Probably by ingestion of contaminated bovine (cattle) products	85 cases by late 2000 in the UK, 3 in children

Disease	Organism	Animal source	Transmission	Notes
Hydatid disease (echinococcosis)	*Echinococcus granulosus* (known as '*E. multilocularis*' in Continental Europe	Dogs; sheep	Ingestion of tapeworm eggs that are passed in infected dog faeces from the contaminated environment, dog hairs or unwashed salads/vegetables	There are an average of 20 laboratory reports each year but rarely in children. Many infections are probably acquired overseas
Leishmaniasis* (cutaneous and visceral)	*Leishmania* spp.	Wild animals such as rodents and canines, and domestic dogs	Transmitted by sandfly bites from infected animals or from human to human	Between 10 and 20 laboratory reports of imported infections occur annually, occasionally in children
Leptospirosis including Weil's disease	*Leptospira interrogans* serovars *hardjo* and *icterohaemorrhagiae* (Weil's disease)	*L. hardjo:* cattle; *L. icterohaemorrhagiae:* rats and other rodents	Organisms are excreted in the animals' urine and transmission may occur through inhalation of aerosols; or through abrasions, wounds or mucous membranes	There are 20–50 cases of leptospirosis, mainly in adults, confirmed each year although there is likely to be under-diagnosis of *L. hardjo* infections. An average of around 15 cases of Weil's disease are confirmed annually, mostly in farmers and those in contact with inland waters
Listeriosis*	*Listeria monocytogenes*	Various domestic and wild animals	Direct transmission from animals; ingestion of contaminated food; or direct from mother to unborn infant in utero or during birth	On average around 100 infections are reported each year and about 20% are associated with pregnancy. A variety of foods such as cheese and pate have been implicated as the source of infection in some cases
Lyme disease*	*Borrelia burgdorferi*	Deer, wild rodents and ticks	Tick bites	Over 150 indigenous and imported infections were reported in 1997, mostly in adults. More may be clinically diagnosed and treated without recourse to laboratory confirmation. Those at risk include foresters, deer farmers and residents in or visitors to endemic areas

Table 29.1 continued

Disease/infection	Causative organism/ most common species	Common animal sources	Mode of spread/vector	Human epidemiology (England and Wales)*
Systemic/other infections				
Rabies*	Rabies virus	Wild and domestic animals such as dogs, foxes or bats	Transmission via saliva through bites, scratches or abrasions; person-to-person spread via corneal transplants has been recorded	Reports are rare in both adults and children; the last recorded imported case was in 1996
Toxocariasis*	Toxocara canis, T. cati	Dogs/puppies, foxes and cats	Ingestion of worm eggs from the environment contaminated with infected animal faeces	There have been up to 40 laboratory reports annually, around half of which are in children; many more infections probably go unrecognised or undetected
Toxoplasmosis*	Toxoplasma gondii	Cats/kittens, and rodents or birds; or sheep, pigs, cattle and goats	Ingestion of cysts from soil or water contaminated with infected cat faeces; ingestion of tissue cysts in raw or undercooked meat or goats' milk; through transplantation of organs or blood from an infected person; or transplacentally from mother to fetus	Around 500 infections are reported on average annually; many more probably go unrecognised or undiagnosed. About 10% of infections are in children

* See chapters in Part Two. BSE = bovine spongiform encephalopathy.
Sources of data: laboratory reports to the PHLS Communicable Disease Surveillance Centre (CDSC) and cases confirmed by the PHLS Reference Laboratories, 1997 or average 1990–1997 and Creutzfeld–Jakob disease (CJD) surveillance unit.

three groups. First, there are domestic pets or 'companion animals' as the veterinary profession now describes them, such as cats and dogs. These live in close proximity to their owners and may transmit gastrointestinal and skin infections as well as toxoplasmosis and toxocariasis. Rabbits have been known to transmit yersiniosis. The second group includes all live- stock and infections that may be acquired through direct contact either with infected live animals or with dead carcases or through the consump- tion of infected or contaminated meat. Examples include skin and gas- trointestinal infections such as orf–paravaccinia virus, cryptosporidiosis and salmonellosis. Finally, the last group comprises all wild or exotic ani- mals. Some of these may come into the first group; for example, psittacine birds such as parrots are kept as pets and are known to transmit psittaco- sis, turtles may transmit salmonellosis, and tropical fish, *Mycobacterium marinum* infections. Other diseases usually associated with wild or exotic animals include imported infections such as leishmaniasis.

The transmission characteristics of human zoonotic infections are an interesting feature in the epidemiology of these infections. Zoonoses may be transmitted via direct or indirect means and there may be several routes within each of these. Direct transmission includes the consumption or ingestion of undercooked or raw meat or other food derived from ani- mals that may contain pathogenic organisms, e.g. salmonella in poultry, fresh eggs and untreated milk. Other direct means of transmission are via the faecal–oral route; for example, *Cryptosporidium* is a common infection in calves and lambs suffering from diarrhoea and may be transmitted to humans following direct contact. Similarly, *Campylobacter* enteritis may be acquired directly from infected puppies. The inhalation of organisms in respiratory aerosols is another direct route of transmission; the cattle form of leptospirosis (*Leptospira hardjo*) or psittacosis may be acquired by this route. And finally, transplacental or vertical transmission of infec- tions from a pregnant mother to her fetus may occur with some zoonoses such as toxoplasmosis. Indirect routes of transmission include the con- sumption of food, or ingestion of or contact with water that has been con- taminated by zoonotic organisms; for example, there have been food- borne outbreaks of *Campylobacter* infection, water-borne incidents of cryptosporidiosis, and Weil's disease (*Leptospira icterohaemorrhagiae*) is transmitted through contact with natural waters contaminated with infect- ed rats' urine. Psittacosis may also be acquired through the inhalation of dust contaminated by discharges from infected birds, or the ovine form of this disease may be acquired from clothing contaminated by the products of gestation from aborting sheep suffering from EAE (enzootic abortion of ewes). Finally, certain zoonoses may be transmitted to man by other, invertebrate animals; for example, Lyme disease (*Borrelia burgdorferi*) is acquired from infected animals via tick bites.

However, it must be remembered that this relatively simple classifica- tion of transmission routes for zoonotic infections may be complicated by those diseases that may be acquired via more than one route, some of which may not necessarily be zoonotic. For example, cryptosporidiosis may be transmitted directly by the faecal–oral route from infected farm animals to man, by the consumption of raw milk from infected animals or by ingestion of contaminated water. Alternatively, it may also be transmitted between humans by the faecal–oral route, e.g. during outbreaks among nursery school children. Another example is toxoplasmosis, which may be acquired by: the consumption of undercooked meat such as lamb containing *Toxoplasma* cysts; the inadvertent ingestion of oocysts excreted by infected felines; inadequate washing of salads and vegetables contaminated by infected cat faeces; or direct transmission from infected pregnant women to their fetuses, which may result in symptomatic congenital toxoplasmosis. There are other examples of zoonotic diseases that have more than one route of transmission, such as salmonellosis and listeriosis, although it is often difficult to determine the relative importance of each with respect to prevention and control of infections.

In spite of the large number of human zoonotic infections, many only very rarely come to the attention of paediatricians, particularly those associated with occupational exposure. For example, certain streptococcal infections such *Streptococcus suis* meningitis and bacteraemia are usually found in butchers, abattoir workers and pig farmers. However, many children are raised on farms or in rural environments and many more have contact with household pets, with whom they invariably have close contact. Children playing in parks and other public areas are also at some risk from acquiring infections from animals either through direct contact or from the contaminated environment. Objects from gardens, parks and elsewhere may be picked up, handled and sucked by infants, dirty fingers often end up in their mouths and pica may also result in the transmission of zoonotic infections. Hand washing and drying may be infrequent and inadequate, and usually require adult supervision. Schoolchildren are increasingly likely to visit zoos, farms and other sites of recreational and educational interest where they are often encouraged to make close contact with the animals and participate in grooming, feeding and other such activities. Some children who live in or visit rural areas may be more likely to encounter zoonotic infections such as Lyme disease, usually endemic where deer are present, or hydatid disease, associated with sheep farming areas, although such indigenous infections in children appear to be rare. Children may often be bitten or scratched by animals and thus acquire infections such as pasteurellosis. Many now travel overseas with their parents, sometimes to exotic places, and may be exposed to a wide range of infections for which there is no preventative measure apart from avoidance of direct contact with certain animals, the consumption of undercooked or raw meat, untreated water and unwashed salads or vegetables, and the adoption of general hygienic precautions.

The zoonoses are a complex and intriguing group of diseases. They have received much media and public health attention in recent years and it seems unlikely that the current interest will wane. However, there are many unanswered questions in the epidemiology of these infections and further research is required if progress is to be made in their prevention, treatment and control. Those working in public health as well as the general public should be kept informed, but not alarmed, of the possible risks of acquiring infection from animals, whether at home or abroad. Simple hygienic measures such as the careful washing and drying of hands before eating and drinking, the adequate cleansing of wounds inflicted by animals and the covering of cuts and abrasions are all important measures in preventing the acquisition of many zoonotic infections. The likelihood of acquiring a serious infection from animals needs to be put into perspective. Education is an important factor in the prevention and control of zoonoses and it should be remembered that contact with animals can be as beneficial to an individual's health as it may be harmful (see Chapter 33 pp. 219–221).

FURTHER READING

Bell JC, Palmer SR, Payne JM (1988) The zoonoses. Infections transmitted from animals to man. Edward Arnold, London.

Palmer SR, Soulsby EJL, Simpson DIH (eds) (1998) Zoonoses. Biology, clinical practice, and public health control. Oxford University Press, Oxford.

30 Laboratory diagnosis of infection

INTRODUCTION

The laboratory diagnosis of infection is entirely dependent on the clinical acumen of the paediatrician in recognising the possibility that the child might be infected. Laboratory tests are not a substitute for clinical diagnosis but a necessary adjunct to confirm the diagnosis, to identify the microorganism and to aid treatment. In order for this to be maximally efficient there must be good communication between clinician and laboratory and it is essential that well-taken appropriate samples are sent, together with as much relevant information as possible.

In order to interpret microbiological tests it is necessary to understand what is normal and what is abnormal. In particular, humans have a rich and varied normal flora.

NORMAL FLORA

Of the 10^{14} cells in man only 10^{13}, 10%, are human. The remainder (9×10^{13}) constitute the normal flora. The normal flora is composed of bacteria, fungi and some protozoa and multicellular organisms. In addition some viruses are 'normally' present within the body and excreted from body surfaces. The colonisation is not uniform throughout the body (Table 30.1); for example, the respiratory tract below the vocal cords is normally sterile whereas the oropharynx and gastrointestinal tract have a rich and varied normal flora. It is important to know which sites have a normal flora

Table 30.1 Normal flora

Sites normally colonised (no. bacteria)	Sites normally sterile
Mouth and nose (c. 10^8–10^9/mL)	Trachea and lungs
Pharynx (c. 10^6–10^8/mL)	Blood
Oesophagus and stomach (10^2–10^3/mL)	Cerebrospinal fluid
Small intestine (10^2/mL)	Bone and joints
Large intestine (10^{10}–10^{12}/mL)	Urinary tract above anterior urethra
Vagina (10^8/mL)	Liver, gall bladder and peritoneal cavity
Skin (10^1–10^4/cm^2)	Pleural space
Anterior urethra (10^2–10^3/cm^2)	Middle ear and sinuses

and which microorganisms can be found at a particular site in order to interpret the results of laboratory tests.

Viruses

Following initial infection, each of the human herpesviruses (HHV1–HHV8) remains with the host for life. All except varicella-zoster (HHV-3, VZV) are excreted asymptomatically for the rest of the individual's lifetime. Adenovirus (in particular type 1) tends to persistently infect lymphoid tissue and can be excreted for long periods in saliva and faeces. Other viruses (HIV, hepatitis B and C, G and TTV viruses) persist for long periods asymptomatically but may eventually cause symptomatic disease.

Bacteria

The vast majority of the normal flora is composed of bacteria. Thus the large intestine contains large (c. 10^{12}/mL) numbers of anaerobic bacteria (bacteroides, clostridia, eubacteria, fusobacteria) and lesser numbers of aerobic bacteria such as *Escherichia coli* (10^7/mL) and *Staphylococcus epidermidis* (10^3/mL). The naso-oropharynx has a rich normal flora and potential respiratory or meningeal pathogens (*Streptococcus pneumoniae* in 20–40%, *Haemophilus influenzae* in 40–80%, *Streptococcus pyogenes* in 5–10%, *Staphylococcus aureus* in 10–20% and *Neisseria meningitidis* in 5–20% of individuals) can be found. Thus isolation of these organisms from a throat swab or nasopharyngeal aspirate does not necessarily mean that they are causing disease. In contrast, detection of bacteria in normally sterile areas (providing the sample has been taken correctly) indicates infection.

Fungi

Yeasts such as *Pityrosporon ovale* can be readily detected on skin and *Candida albicans* as part of the normal flora of the mouth, large intestine and vagina. Dermatophytes may be found on the skin in the absence of overt infection.

Parasites

Protozoa such as *Entamoeba coli*, *Endolimax nana* and even *Giardia lamblia* and *Entamoeba histolytica* can be present in the intestine in the absence of disease. Infestation with the adult worms of *Taenia solium* or *T. saginata* is rarely symptomatic, as is that of the whipworm (*Trichuris trichiura*). Finally, a large proportion of the population will harbour the arthropod *Demodex folliculorum* (follicle mite), especially in the hair follicles and the sebaceous glands of the face.

DIAGNOSTIC TESTS

In general, the procedures available for diagnosis of infection are:

* nonspecific tests to help to determine whether infection is present
* specific tests that will determine the nature and antimicrobial susceptibility of the pathogen (Table 30.2).

NONSPECIFIC TESTS

These tests will only act as pointers to or confirmation of the presence of an infection. They are neither 100% sensitive nor 100% specific.

Table 30.2 Laboratory tests for infection

Nonspecific tests: is infection present?
* White cell count and differential (Nitroblue tetrazolium test)
* Acute phase proteins (ESR, C-reactive protein, orosomucoid, α-antitrypsin)
* Cytokines (tumour necrosis factor, interleukins 1, 6)
* Endotoxin (*Limulus* lysate for Gram-negative bacteria)
* CSF lactate, protein and glucose estimations

Specific tests: what is the pathogen?
* Rapid (20 min–4 h)
  - *Visualisation*
    Light microscopy, electron microscopy, immunofluorescence microscopy
  - *Antigen detection*
    ELISA, latex particle agglutination (LPA), radio-immunoassay (RIA) Counter-immunoelectrophoresis (CIE)
  - *Genome detection*
    DNA hybridisation, polymerase chain reaction or other nucleotide amplification methods
  - *Toxin detection*
    Vibrio cholerae heat-labile toxin, *Clostridium difficile* toxin
* Conventional (slower: minimum of 18 h)
  - Viral culture (not available for all viruses, expensive)
  - Bacterial culture (most pathogenic bacteria are cultivable within 24 h)
  - Fungal culture (can take up to 1 week depending on fungus)
  - Antimicrobial susceptibility (by culture takes about 18 h usually).
* Antibody detection
  Except for certain infections (e.g. hepatitis A), serological tests are of greater value for epidemiological rather than diagnostic purposes.

White cell count

In general, the peripheral white cell count will be raised with a neutrophilia, often with a left shift in bacterial infection and lymphocytosis in viral infection. Severe bacterial infection may also induce thrombocytopenia. Exceptions to this include neutropenia in severe bacterial infection (e.g. meningococcal septicaemia and particularly in sepsis neonatorum) and lymphocytosis in pertussis. A very high neutrophil count usually indicates a collection of pus.

Acute phase proteins

During acute infection due to bacteria or fungi the liver produces a variety of acute phase proteins, which result in an increased plasma viscosity and raised erythrocyte sedimentation rate. Perhaps the most useful measurement is of C-reactive protein (CRP). Levels can be estimated in blood or in cerebrospinal fluid (CSF). During acute bacterial infection levels rise from < 1 mg/L to 100 mg/L or more, and remain raised for several days. Viral infection does not lead to a large rise in CRP levels.

Cytokines

The cytokines tumour necrosis factor (TNF), interleukin-1 (IL-I) and interleukin 6 (IL-6) are produced in particular by macrophages, neutrophils and monocytes in response to bacterial infection; indeed, they contribute to the pathogenesis of sepsis. The value of measuring these cytokines as markers of infection has still to be completely evaluated.

Endotoxin

This is an integral constituent of the outer membrane of Gram-negative bacteria. It is released either spontaneously (e.g. by meningococci) or when the bacteria die. Its measurement in blood is difficult but can provide evidence of infection by Gram-negative bacteria.

SPECIFIC TESTS

Rapid

To be of most value in management of infection tests should be sensitive, specific and, if possible, rapid.

Direct visualisation

This can be by light microscopy using stained or unstained material. In general, the sensitivity of this method is a minimum of 10^3-10^4 organisms/mL. It is simple and rapid to carry out and is useful for detecting, for example, protozoa (*Cryptosporidium*, *Giardia*) in faeces, bacteria in CSF or pathogens in wounds. It is less useful for detecting bacteria in blood (the numbers are too small) or for detecting bacterial pathogens where there is a rich normal flora (e.g. stool samples).

Negative stain electron microscopy is a rapid and specific test and is used primarily to detect viral enteropathogens in stool or virus in skin lesions, although it has also been used to detect viruses in respiratory secretions. To be visualised, there must be a minimum of 10^6 virus particles in a sample. The above methodologies are 'catch-all' techniques that will detect the pathogen no matter what it is. The remaining techniques are all directed to detecting an individual pathogen: thus, if there are five potential pathogens for a particular infection, five separate tests must be carried out.

Immunofluorescence antigen detection (IFAT) employs fluorochrome tagged antibodies against, for example, respiratory viruses. Since such tests are detecting viral antigens on infected cells it is important that the sample (usually a nasopharyngeal aspirate) is transported to the laboratory on ice as quickly as possible. Using this technique it is possible to detect measles, respiratory syncytial, influenza or parainfluenza virus infections with relatively high sensitivity and specificity.

Antigen detection

A variety of antigen detection tests employing diverse technologies (e.g. ELISA, LPA, RIA, CIE) has been developed. Their speed of operation, sensitivity and specificity depend upon the sample tested and the technology used. Examples include detection of bacterial antigens such as capsular polysaccharides of meningococci, pneumococci and *H. influenzae* type b, viral antigens such as rotavirus, respiratory syncytial virus and Norwalk agent, and fungal antigens such as the capsular antigen of *Cryptococcus neoformans*. The use of urinary antigen detection in diagnosis remains unclear, especially since it is known for example that urinary excretion of *H. influenzae* type b capsular antigen can be detected in throat carriers or following Hib immunisation.

Genome detection

These are potentially the most sensitive diagnostic tests. For example, it is possible for genome amplification using the polymerase chain reaction (PCR) to detect just one infective particle. This high sensitivity can be a disadvantage in producing false positives. A number of amplification techniques have now been introduced into diagnostic microbiology laboratories in kit form. These include genome amplification formats such as polymerase chain reaction and ligase chain reaction (LCR) and formats where the detection system, when bound to a specific DNA sequence, is amplified, such as branched chain DNA (bDNA) or hybrid capture assay.

In PCR a sequence (200–500 base pairs) of double-stranded genomic DNA is identified as specific for a particular organism. Oligonucleotide primers (15–20 bp) are synthesised which are complementary to the 5' ends of the sense and antisense DNA strands. These act as starters or primers for synthesising the new DNA strands. This is done enzymically using a DNA polymerase. The reaction is carried out in a thermal cycler at temperatures between 50°C and 98°C, so a thermostable DNA polymerase was sought. It was obtained from a bacterium discovered in hot springs (it is able to grow at high temperatures). The bacterium is *Thermus aquaticus* and the enzyme Taq. In PCR the reagents, target DNA, primers, Taq and solutions of the individual nucleotides are mixed in a buffered solution and heated to

95°C. This melts the target DNA, i.e. separates the two DNA strands. The mixture is then cooled to 55°C, this allows the primers (which are in great excess), to bind to the target sense and antisense DNA strands. The temperature is then raised to 70°C, to allow the Taq polymerase to sequentially add bases to the primers as directed by the target DNA. This three-step cycle is repeated over and over again and at each cycle the target DNA (between the primers) doubles in quantity. At the end of 30–40 cycles there will be sufficient target DNA (amplicon) to be detected by gel electrophoresis or ELISA. The technology is very sensitive (e.g. 10–20% more sensitive than culture or antigen detection in detecting *Chlamydia trachomatis*). However great care must be taken to prevent cross-contamination from samples or, more importantly, from the amplicons. For this reason it is advisable to have separate rooms for sample and reagent preparation and the thermal cyclers.

PCRs are commercially available for the detection of HIV, HBV, HCV, HPV, HHV-1, HHV-2, HHV-5 (cytomegalovirus) and *C. trachomatis*, and many more are under development. Whether they will fully replace cultural techniques is uncertain. The problems are their extreme sensitivity (which is a soluble problem), they are pathogen specific (this can be overcome by multiplex PCR or, for bacteria, by PCR of 16S rRNA operons and sequencing), cost and determination of antimicrobial susceptibility. Another use for PCR is in quantification. This is used to monitor progress, initiate therapy and assess results of therapy in infection with human immunodeficiency virus (HIV) and hepatitis C virus (HCV).

Antibody detection

For the most part, antibody detection is not useful for the immediate diagnosis of infection since it usually requires acute and convalescent (approximately 2 weeks later) samples. However, there are some sensitive specific IgM assays (e.g. for hepatitis A) that will provide diagnosis at clinical presentation.

Conventional

This involves culture of samples from infected sites. It thus requires that the microorganisms remain viable until they can be cultured (i.e. should be taken to the laboratory as quickly as possible). Some samples may require transport media; for example, samples for virological culture are placed in iso-osmotic media containing protein and antibiotics (to prevent bacterial overgrowth). For interpretation of bacteriological culture it is necessary to know what is normal and what is abnormal at a particular site. The major disadvantage of cultural techniques is the time taken; for example, most aerobic bacteria will require 18–24 h incubation for colonies to appear and some anaerobes will take longer. The major advantages are that the organism is available for determination of antimicrobial susceptibility, epidemiological purposes and medicolegal purposes.

The potential pathogens, samples required, precautions of transport and time taken for detection of agents causing infection by organ system are shown in Tables 30.3–30.10.

Table 30.3 Laboratory investigation of CNS infection

	Potential pathogens	Samples required	Transport	Nonspecific tests	Specific tests	Time taken
Meningitis, neonate	E. coli, group B strepto-cocci, Listeria, other Gram-negative bacilli	CSF, blood (for culture)	Rapid	CSF: protein, WCC, glucose, CRP Blood: WCC, CRP	CSF: Gram film, antigen-detection (group B strep.. E. coli K1) culture	1–24 h
	HSV	CSF, saliva, blood	VTM		Virus culture, PCR	24–36 h
Meningitis, older children	N. meningitidis, S. pneumoniae, H. influenzae type b M. tuberculosis	CSF, blood (for culture) Throat swab	Rapid, BTM	CSF: protein, WCC, glucose, CRP Blood: WCC, CRP	CSF: Gram film, antigen detection, culture Blood: culture, antigen detection	1–24 h (NB. for TB up to 6 weeks)
	Enteroviruses, mumps	CSF, throat swab, faeces, serum	VTM		Virus culture, PCR Serology: CSF, serum	24–48 h
Meningoencephalitis	Mumps, enteroviruses, HSV, lymphocytic choriomeningitis	CSF, throat swab, faeces, serum	Rapid, VTM	Blood: WCC, CRP CSF: WCC, protein, CRP	Virus culture, PCR Serology: blood, CSF	24–48 h
Cerebral/spinal abscess	S. aureus, S. milleri, S. pneumoniae, oral anaerobes (Bacteroides, Fusobacterium), H. influenzae	Pus, blood for culture	Rapid, BTM (put some pus in blood culture bottle)	Blood: WCC, CRP	Gram-stained film, culture	18–72 h

BTM = bacterial transport medium; CRP = C-reactive protein; CSF = cerebrospinal fluid; HSV = herpes simplex virus; PCR = polymerase chain reaction; WCC = white cell count; VTM = viral transport medium.

185

30 Laboratory diagnosis

Table 30.4 Laboratory investigations of gastrointestinal infection

	Potential pathogens	Samples required	Transport	Nonspecific tests	Specific tests	Time taken
Hepatitis	Hepatitis A virus Hepatitis B virus Hepatitis C virus Hepatitis D virus Hepatitis E virus	Serum	No special precautions except to prevent infection of hospital staff	Liver function tests	HAV IgM ELISA HBsAg, HBeAg, HBcAb (IgM) HCVAb, HCV genome (RT-PCR) HDVAb HEV IgM, IgG	1–4 h but since tests are expensive often batched
Gastritis	*Helicobacter pylori*	Gastric biopsy serum, saliva	Rapid, BTM	–	Histology ('gold standard'), rapid urease, culture, serology (serum and saliva)	5–7 days
Diarrhoeal disease	**Viruses** Rotavirus, astrovirus, adenovirus 40/41, calicivirus, Norwalk agent	Faeces, vomit	No special precautions	Stool pus cells	Electron microscopy, ELISA, LPA	1–8 h
	Bacteria *Salmonella, Shigella, Campylobacter, E. coli*	Faeces, vomit	Rapid	Stool pus cells	Culture	24–48 h
	Protozoa *Cryptosporidium, Giardia, Cyclospora*	Faeces, vomit	No special precautions	Stool pus cells	Microscopy of stained smears	1–2 h

BTM = bacterial transport medium; ELISA = enzyme-linked immunosorbent assay; LPA = latex particle agglutination; RT-PCR = reverse transcription-polymerase chain reaction.

Table 30.5 Respiratory tract infection

	Potential pathogens	Samples required	Transport	Nonspecific tests	Specific tests	Time taken
Otitis media/sinusitis	H. influenzae, S. pneumoniae, M. catarrhalis, anaerobes	Pus from cavity, blood culture	Rapid, BTM	Blood: WCC, CRP	Gram film, antigen detection, culture	18–48 h
Tonsillitis/pharyngitis	Viruses (most common), e.g. adenovirus, EBV	Throat swab, serum	VTM	Blood: WCC and film for EBV	Virus culture, serology	1–3 days
	S. pyogenes (A or C), C. diphtheriae	Throat swab	BTM	–	Gram film, culture	18–24 h
Epiglottitis	H. influenzae type b	Blood culture, swab (with care), urine	BTM	Blood: WCC, CRP	Culture, antigen detection in urine	18–24 h
Laryngotracheo-bronchitis, croup	Parainfluenza 1–4, influenza A, B, C, RSV, adenovirus	Nasopharyngeal aspirate, serum	Rapid, on ice	–	IFAT Virus culture, serology	< 8 h 24–72 h
Pneumonia	**Viruses** Parainfluenza, RSV, influenza, adenovirus, measles	Nasopharyngeal aspirate, serum	Rapid, on ice	–	IFAT Virus culture, serology	< 8–48 h
	Bacteria S. pneumoniae, H. influenzae type b, S. aureus, M. pneumoniae, C. psittaci, C. pneumoniae, L. pneumophila	Blood (for culture), sputum, transtracheal aspirate, evoked sputum (if possible), serum, urine	Rapid	Blood: WCC, CRP	Blood: culture Sputum: Gram film, culture, antigen detection Urine: antigen detection	18–24 h
Pertussis	B. pertussis, B. parapertussis	Pernasal swab, serum, saliva	Rapid, BTM	WCC – lymphocytosis	Bacterial culture, serology	24–48 h
	Adenovirus	Nasopharyngeal aspirate, serum	Rapid, VTM		IFAT Virus culture, serology	< 8 h

BTM = bacterial transport medium; CRP = C-reactive protein; EBV = Epstein–Barr virus; IFAT = immunofluorescence antigen detection; RSV = respiratory syncytial virus; WCC = white cell count; VTM = viral transport medium.

Table 30.6 Laboratory diagnosis of exanthems and enanthems

	Potential pathogens	Samples required	Transport	Specific tests	Time taken
Maculopapular erythematous rash	**Viruses** Measles, enteroviruses, EBV, parvovirus, rubella, HHV-6	Throat swab, nasopharyngeal aspirate, serum	VTM	Virus culture, IFAT, serology. IgM, rise in titre	4–72 h
	Bacteria N. meningitidis (septicaemia), S. pyogenes	Blood culture, throat swab	Rapid, BTM	Blood culture, serum antigen	18–24 h
Petechial purpuric rash	**Viruses** Enteroviruses, adenoviruses	Throat swab, faeces, serum	VTM	Virus culture, serology	24–72 h
	Bacteria N. meningitidis, other Gram-negative bacteria	Blood culture, lesion scrape	BTM	Gram film, culture	18–24 h
Vesicular/pustular rash	HSV1 and 2, varicella-zoster virus, enterovirus (hand, foot and mouth disease)	Vesicle fluid, serum, throat swab, faeces	VTM	Electron microscopy, virus culture, serology	1–72 h
	S. aureus (impetigo)	Lesion swab or pus	BTM	Gram film, bacterial culture	18–24 h
Nodules	Human papilloma virus, molluscum contagiosum, cowpox, parapox	Needle sample of lesion	No special precautions	Electron microscopy	1 h

BTM = bacterial transport medium; HHV-6 = human herpesvirus 6; HSV = herpes simplex virus; IFAT = immunofluorescence antigen detection; VTM = viral transport medium.

Table 30.7 Laboratory diagnosis of genitourinary tract infection

	Potential pathogens	Samples required	Transport	Nonspecific tests	Specific tests	Time taken
Urinary tract	E. coli, Proteus spp., Klebsiella spp., S. epidermidis, P. aeruginosa	MSSU, suprapubic aspirate, catheter specimen, bag (least useful)	Rapid or keep cool	Blood: WCC, CRP Urine: WCC (> 10/mm³)	Quantitative bacterial culture (> 10⁵ cfu/mL in pure culture) (NB. Catheter or suprapubic aspirate should be sterile unless there is infection)	18–24 h
Genital tract, vulvovaginitis	Candida albicans, group B streptococci.	Swab or, better still, discharge	Rapid, BTM	–	Gram film, culture	18–24 h
	Enterobius vermicularis	Cellophane tape slide	Rapid, BTM		Examination of slide for ova	1 h
Genital tract, sexually transmitted	**Viruses** Herpes simplex virus Human papilloma virus	Discharge/swab Sample of wart	VTM		Virus culture, electron microscopy	1–24 h
	Bacteria N. gonorrhoeae, C. trachomatis, T. pallidum	Discharge/swab Blood for serology	Rapid, BTM		Bacterial culture Cell culture, ELISA, IFAT Dark ground microscopy Serological tests for syphilis	18–48 h 6–72 h 1–4 h
	Protozoa Trichomonas vaginalis	Discharge/swab	TTM		Culture and microscopy	18–24 h

BTM = bacterial transport medium; CRP = C-reactive protein; ELISA = enzyme-linked immunosorbent assay; IFAT = immunofluorescence antigen detection; MSSU = midstream specimen of urine; TTM = *Trichomonas* transport medium; VTM = viral transport medium.

Table 30.8 Laboratory diagnosis of skin and soft tissue infections

	Potential pathogens	Samples required	Transport	Nonspecific tests	Specific tests	Time taken
Skin						
Carbuncle, furuncle	S. aureus	Pus	2–3 h	–	Gram film, culture	18–24 h
Vesicle	HSV-1, HSV-2, VZV, enterovirus	Vesicle fluid	Rapid	–	Electron microscopy, culture	2–24 h
Impetigo	S. aureus, S. pyogenes	Pus, vesicle fluid or crust	2–3 h	–	Gram film, culture	18–24 h
Nodules	Molluscum contagiosum, papillomavirus (warts), cowpox, orf	Sample of nodules	2–3 h	–	Electron microscopy (culture)	2–24 h
Granuloma	M. tuberculosis, M. marinum, M. avium	Sample of tissue	2–3 h	–	Histology, acid-fast stain, culture	2 h–6 weeks
Cellulitis	S. pyogenes, H. influenzae (b), anaerobes (necrotising fasciitis)	Samples of tissue or exudate	Rapid	–	Gram film, culture	2–48 h
Ringworm	Microsporum, Trichophyton, Epidermophyton	Skin, nail scraping, hair	–	Wood's light	Microscopy (KOH), culture	2 h–5 days
Intertrigo	Candida spp.	Sample of lesion	–	–	Gram film, culture	2–24 h

Scabies	Sarcoptes scabiei	Clinical or sample of lesion from burrow	–	Microscopy	2 h
Orbital cellulitis	H. influenzae type b	Samples from lesion, blood culture	Rapid	Bacterial culture	18–24 h
Lice	Pediculus capitis	Hair	–	Microscopic examination (nit = egg)	2 h
Lymph gland					
Lymphoadenitis*	S. pyogenes, M. tuberculosis, M. avium/intracellulare, Bartonella henselae (cat-scratch disease)	Pus from gland	–	Gram or acid-fast film, culture	2 h–6 weeks
Eyes					
Conjunctivitis	Adenovirus (3, 7, 8, 19), enterovirus (70), Coxsackie virus (A24), HSV	Swab from conjunctivae	Rapid, VTM	Electron microscopy, virus culture, immunofluorescence, PCR	18–48 h
	H. influenzae, S. pneumoniae, N. meningitidis, N. gonorrhoeae, C. trachomatis	Swab of pus and conjunctivae	Rapid, BTM

Chlamydia transport | Gram film culture, Giemsa (poor)

ELISA, IFAT, culture | 18–24 h

4–72 h |

BTM = bacterial transport medium; ELISA = enzyme-linked immunosorbent assay; IFAT = immunofluorescence antigen detection; KOH = potassium hydroxide; PCR = polymerase chain reaction; VTM = viral transport medium; VZV = varicella-zoster virus.

Table 30.9 Laboratory diagnosis of infections of bone, joint and muscle

	Potential pathogens	Samples required	Transport	Nonspecific tests	Specific tests	Time taken
Bone						
Acute osteomyelitis	S. aureus, H. influenzae	Blood culture, pus from bone	Rapid	WCC, CRP	Gram film, culture	18–24 h
Chronic osteomyelitis	M. tuberculosis P. aeruginosa, coliforms	Pus	–	WCC, CRP	Acid-fast film, culture Gram film, culture	2 h–6 weeks 18–24 h
Joint						
Acute arthritis	S. aureus, H. influenzae, Salmonella spp., N. meningitidis, N. gonorrhoeae	Joint fluid, blood culture	Rapid, BTM	WCC, CRP	Gram film, culture	2–24 h
Reactive arthritis	Immune reaction to: N. meningitidis, N. gonorrhoeae, C. trachomatis, Salmonella spp., Campylobacter spp.	Blood, joint fluid	–	WCC, CRP, HLA-typing (HLA B27)	Culture (should be –ve), PCR (is +ve)	–

Muscle

Pyomyositis	S. aureus (tropical), S. pyogenes	Pus, tissue, blood culture	Rapid, BTM	WCC, CRP	Histology, Gram film, culture	2–24 h
Gas gangrene	C. perfringens	Tissue, blood culture	Rapid, BTM	WCC, CRP	Histology, Gram film, culture	2–48 h
Necrotising fasciitis	S. pyogenes	Tissue	BTM	–	Gram film, culture	18–24 h
Synergistic gangrene	S. aureus and anaerobes	Tissue	Rapid, BTM	–	Gram film, culture	18–72 h

BTM = bacterial transport medium; CRP = C-reactive protein; HLA = human leukocyte antigen; WCC = white cell count.

Table 30.10 Infection of the cardiovascular system

	Potential pathogens	Samples required	Transport	Nonspecific tests	Specific tests	Time taken
Infective endocarditis	'Viridans' streptococci, coagulase-negative staphylococci, *Haemophilus aphrophilus*, *Enterococcus* spp., *Candida* spp., *Aspergillus* spp., *Coxiella burnetii*, *Salmonella* spp., *S. aureus* (acute)	Blood culture (4–5 samples)	–	WCC, CRP	Culture	18–72 h (may be much longer)
Pericarditis	Coxsackie B virus	Faeces, pericardial fluid, blood	Rapid, VTM	WCC, CRP, ECG	Virus culture, serology, PCR	24–72 h
	Haemophilus influenzae, *S. pneumoniae*, *S. pyogenes*, *S. aureus*, *N. meningitidis*, *M. tuberculosis*	Blood culture, pericardial fluid	BTM	WCC, CRP, ECG	Gram film, culture	18–24 h
Myocarditis	Coxsackie A and B viruses, echo virus, mumps	Faeces, throat swab, blood	Rapid, VTM	WCC, CRP, ECG	Virus culture, serology	24–72 h
	N. meningitidis, *S. aureus*, *S. pyogenes*	Blood	–	WCC, CRP, ECG	Culture	24–48 h

BTM = bacterial transport medium; CRP = C-reactive protein; PCR = polymerase chain reaction; WCC = white cell count; VTM = viral transport medium.

31 The use of antibiotics and antivirals

ANTIBIOTICS

Antibiotics or antimicrobials are one of the few examples of drugs administered to a patient not for their direct effect on the patient (although this does occur as a consequence of their action) but in order to kill infecting microorganisms. Antibiotics are the most frequently used and arguably the most frequently abused agents in the pharmacopoeia.

In designing a new antibiotic the aim is to produce an agent that is maximally toxic for the microorganisms and minimally toxic to man. This is achieved by targeting sites or pathways that are unique to the bacterium. Unfortunately this is not always successful and all antibiotics produce human toxicity to varying degrees.

The therapeutic index (maximum tolerated dose divided by the minimum effective dose) provides a numeric expression of this. Some antibiotics, such as penicillins, are very safe and thus have a very high therapeutic index. Others, such as gentamicin, have a low maximum tolerated dose and thus a therapeutic index that is low. A further complication is that bacteria, which under optimal conditions have a doubling time of 20 minutes, have boundless opportunities to mutate to circumvent an antibiotic's activity. Furthermore the genes for antibiotic resistance may be disseminated promiscuously among bacterial genera by means of plasmids and transposons ('jumping genes'). Our production of new antimicrobials is only just exceeding the development of resistance.

Another unwanted side-effect of antimicrobials is in altering the host's normal flora (see Chapter 30). Some antibiotics, e.g. ampicillin, erythromycin and co-amoxiclav, are re-excreted into the gastrointestinal tract (or just poorly absorbed) and affect the predominantly anaerobic normal flora of the large bowel. This may result in antibiotic-associated diarrhoea or at its worse promote colonisation by *Clostridium difficile* resulting in pseudomembranous colitis. The intestinal flora may also act as a sink for development and dissemination of antibiotic resistance genes.

Antibiotics can be bactericidal (actively kill dividing bacteria) or bacteriostatic (prevent bacteria from dividing). Although these divisions are not immutable (e.g. chloramphenicol is cidal for meningococci but static for *Escherichia coli*), in general it is better to use bactericidal antibiotics for severe life-threatening infection, especially if the host is immunoincompetent.

Antimicrobial agents can act at various sites within the microorganisms (Table 31.1).

Cell wall replication

By possessing a thick peptidoglycan cell wall, bacteria are able to survive both severe changes in osmotic pressure and many host degradative enzymes. This represents a target unique to bacteria and antibiotics acting at this site should theoretically be less toxic to humans.

Table 31.1 Antibiotics by mode of action

Inhibition of:	Spectrum of activity	Cidal	Routes of administration	Volume of distribution (L/kg)	Toxicity	Need to monitor levels	How eliminated	Used in neonates
DNA replication								
5-flucytosine	Fungi	+	Oral, i.v.	0.7–1	M*, GI,	+	U	+
Griseofulvin	Fungi	–	Oral, i.v.	1.2–1.4	Mild	–	H	–
Metronidazole	Anaerobes, protozoa	–	Oral, i.v.	0.76–1.02	Mild	–	H	+
Nitrofurantoin	GNB	+	Oral	0.6	Mild	–	U	NL
Quinolones	Bacteria (broad)	+	Oral, i.v.	1–2.5	Mild	–	U	–
Sulphonamides	Bacteria (broad)	+	Oral, i.v.	0.2–0.8	D*M*S*R*	–	H, U	+
Trimethoprim	Bacteria (broad)	+	Oral, i.v.	1–1.5	Mild	–	U	–
Co-trimoxazole	Bacteria (broad), fungi, *Pneumocystis*	+	Oral, i.v.	–	Principally to sulphonamide	–	U	–
Para-amino salicylic acid	Mycobacteria	+	Oral, i.v.	0.8	Mild, S	–	U	–
Transcription								
Rifampicin	Bacteria (broad), mycobacteria	+	Oral, i.v.	1	L*S*	–	H	+
Translation								
Aminoglycosides	Bacteria (broad)	+	i.v., topical	0.2–0.3	R* O*	+	U	+
Chloramphenicol	Bacteria (broad)	+/–	Oral, i.v.,	0.25–1.99	M*	+	H	–
Fusidic acid	GPB	+	Oral, i.v., topical	0.2	L, GI,	–	H	+

Macrolides	GPB, mycobacteria	–	Oral, i.v., topical	0.75	L*, S*, O	–	H	+
Tetracyclines	Bacteria (broad)	–	Oral, i.v., topical	1.3	Teeth	–	H	–
Streptogramins	GPB	+	Oral, i.v.	NA	?	–	H	–
Oxazolidinones	GPB	–	Oral	NA		–	U	–

Cell wall replication

Bacitracin	GPB	+	Topical	NA	R*S*	–	NA	+
β-lactams	Bacteria (broad)	+	Oral, i.v.	0.2–0.7	Rare S	–	U	+
Glycopeptides	GPB	+	i.v.	0.6	S* R (rare)	+	U	+
Cycloserine	GPB, mycobacteria	+	Oral, topical	0.8	N, P	–	U	–

Cell membranes

Amphotericin B	Fungi	+	i.v., topical		R*, M	–	U	+
Nitroimidazoles	Fungi	–	Oral, i.v., topical		H*	–	H	+
Nystatin	Fungi	+	Topical		Rare	–	NA	+
Polymyxins	GNB	+	Topical		R*, S	–	U	+
Isoniazid	Mycobacteria	+	Oral		Rare L*, N	–	U	–
Ethambutol	Mycobacteria	–	Oral		Optic neuritis	–	U	–

Key: * = severe; D = dermatological; GI = gastrointestinal disturbance; GNB = Gram-negative bacteria; GPB = Gram-positive bacteria; H = hepatic metabolism; i.v. = intravenous; L = liver; M = marrow suppression; N = neurotoxic; NA = not applicable; NL = not licensed in UK but used; O = ototoxicity; P = psychiatric; R = renal; S = hypersensitivity; U = urinary excretion.

Bacitracin

This is a very toxic antibiotic obtained from a strain of *Bacillus licheni-formis* isolated from a wound of a patient named Tracy. It is not absorbed orally and when given parenterally is highly nephrotoxic. Its main use is as a topical agent in combination with other antibiotics. Although there are generally few problems when it is applied topically, hypersensitivity reactions are possible and, if applied to extensive areas of inflammation, significant absorption can occur. Bacitracin is active against most Gram-positive bacteria.

Glycopeptides

Vancomycin and teicoplanin are both glycopeptide antibiotics and are active against most Gram-positive bacteria, principally staphylococci. They are not absorbed when given orally. Vancomycin is given by a slow intravenous infusion or intraventricularly; teicoplanin can be given as a bolus. Glycopeptides are occasionally nephrotoxic. The major problem is of hypersensitivity and allergic reactions, in particular the 'red man' syndrome. This apparently occurs less readily with teicoplanin, is more likely to occur if the infusion is too rapid and can be managed with antihistamines. Vancomycin is indicated for severe infections due to multidrug-resistant Gram-positive bacteria in neonates or older children. Levels should be monitored.

β-lactams

This is the largest and most widely used group of antibiotics. Within this group there are three major subdivisions: the penicillins, the cephalosporins and the monobactams. Each has a β-lactam ring as the active moiety and inhibits transpeptidation, the final stage in assembly of peptidoglycan.

benzylpenicillin, the first penicillin used in man, is still effective against streptococci, pneumococci and meningococci, although varying prevalences of resistance occur in many parts of the world. *Staphylococcus aureus* is resistant by virtue of producing β-lactamase enzymes. The penicillinase-resistant penicillins, flucloxacillin (for oral administration) and cloxacillin (for intravenous administration) were developed to counter this problem. Staphylococci resistant to these agents (MRSA) have now emerged (permeability mutants). Ampicillin was developed to broaden the spectrum to cover Gram-negative as well as Gram-positive bacteria. Now, however, many enterobacteria produce β-lactamases that render them resistant to ampicillin. Clavulanic acid, a β-lactamase inhibitor, is added to ampicillin (co-amoxiclav) to overcome this problem. New β-lactamases not susceptible to inhibition by clavulanic acid have already emerged. The ureido penicillins such as azlocillin were developed to extend the spectrum to cover *Pseudomonas aeruginosa*.

The penicillins are among the safest antibiotics available. Hypersensitivity reactions ranging from skin rashes to anaphylactic shock are the main but rare side-effects. Their incidence seems to be overestimated. There is a 10% chance that a penicillin-allergic patient will also be cephalosporin-allergic.

Cephaloridine was the first cephalosporin; it should not be used now since it is toxic and is easily hydrolysed by Gram-positive and Gram-negative β-lactamases. In general, the second-generation cephalosporins such as cephradine, cefuroxime and cefaclor have a broad spectrum of activity. Cefaclor and cefuroxime have useful activity against *Haemophilus influenzae* but no cephalosporin is active against *Listeria monocytogenes*. They are likely to be hydrolysed by Gram-negative β-lactamases.

The third-generation cephalosporins such as ceftazidime, cefotaxime and ceftriaxone must be given parenterally, have high intrinsic activity, are less likely to be inactivated by Gram-negative β-lactamases but are less likely to be active against *S. aureus*. Enterococci are resistant to third-generation cephalosporins and production of extended-spectrum β-lactamases by *Proteus*, *Serratia* and *Enterobacter* spp. has now appeared in *E. coli* and *Salmonella* spp. The cephamycins cefoxitin and moxalactam are also active against most anaerobic bacteria. Their use should be avoided in neonates since they interfere with vitamin K metabolism.

Aztreonam is the only monobactam available for clinical use. It is active only against Gram-negative bacteria, must be administered parenterally and has been little used in paediatric practice.

The new carbapenems such as imipenem and meropenem, which have a very broad spectrum of activity, have been used in children with cystic fibrosis and their use in neonates has still to be fully evaluated.

The β-lactams are a very useful and nontoxic group of antibiotics. Their use will depend upon the particular infection and prevalence of resistance in the locality.

Cell membrane disruption

Amphotericin B

This is the principal antifungal drug available for treating systemic mycoses. It is fungicidal for yeasts (*Candida*, *Cryptococcus*), dimorphic fungi (*Histoplasma*, *Blastomyces*, *Coccidioides*), dermatophytes (*Trichophyton*, *Microsporum*, *Epidermophyton*) and moulds (*Aspergillus*, *Penicillium*). Fungal resistance is not yet a problem. It is not absorbed through skin or mucous membranes when given topically. For systemic mycoses it must be given as a slow infusion. The main side-effects are hypotensive reactions and nephrotoxicity, the earliest sign of which is hypokalaemia. A test dose should be given. Liposomally entrapped amphotericin B is less toxic. Combination with 5-flucytosine is useful.

Nystatin

Nystatin is a polyene antifungal drug. It is fungicidal for a variety of fungi but is used most often in candidiasis. It is applied topically and must not be given parenterally since it is particulate and not a solution. Development of resistance is rare. Both nystatin (discovered in New York State) and amphotericin B chelate sterols in the fungal membrane.

Nitroimidazoles

These inhibit the production of ergosterol in the fungal cell membrane. In general, they are fungistatic. They are absorbed well orally. Miconazole is given orally or topically and ketoconazole (which is hepatotoxic) can also be given intravenously. Both affect a wide spectrum of fungi but are excreted poorly in urine. The newer imidazoles, fluconazole and itraconazole are fungicidal and have been used in place of amphotericin B for systemic mycoses, although there are no paediatric trial data.

Polymyxins

Polymyxins bind to the lipid A portion of lipopolysaccharide of Gram-negative bacteria and cause membrane disruption. Most Gram-negative bacteria (except *Proteus*, *Neisseria* and *Brucella*) are susceptible but their main use has been in treating severe *Pseudomonas* infections. Polymyxin B and colistin (polymyxin E) can both be given intravenously but both have been superseded to a large extent by less toxic antibiotics. They cause nephrotoxicity, neurotoxicity and hypersensitivity. When used topically, it is usually in combination with other antibacterials for superficial infections.

DNA replication

Most microorganisms are rapidly and continually replicating and thus need a continuous supply of nucleic acids for chromosomal replication.

5-flucytosine

This is a nucleoside analogue used for treating systemic fungal infections (*Candida*, *Cryptococcus*, *Torulopsis*). It can be given by the oral or intravenous route. Resistance develops rapidly both in vitro and in vivo and 5-flucytosine is often combined with amphotericin B with synergistic effects. High dosage (peak greater than 100 mg/L) is associated with bone marrow toxicity with reversible thrombocytopenia and leukopenia. It can be used in neonates, providing levels are monitored.

Griseofulvin

This is an antifungal drug that inhibits mitosis by affecting microtubules. It is fungistatic for common dermatophytes (*Microsporum*, *Epidermophyton*, *Trichophyton*). It is given orally, is concentrated in keratinised tissue and is thus used for treating ringworm, onychomycosis and tinea capitis. It is generally nontoxic but is contraindicated in neonates and should only be used for severe childhood infections.

Metronidazole

Metronidazole is active against obligate anaerobes and some protozoa (*Trichomonas*, *Entamoeba*, *Giardia*). Under anaerobic conditions it is converted to a nitrosamine, which causes DNA fragmentation and inhibits DNA synthesis. It can be administered orally, rectally or intravenously. Although mutagenic for bacteria it is not associated with carcinogenesis. It has an Antabuse-like effect and high doses may cause central nervous system effects and peripheral neuropathy. It is used prophylactically in large intestinal surgery.

Nitrofurantoin

This is used for treating urinary tract infections due to Gram-negative bacteria. It causes DNA fragmentation in *E. coli* but resistance can develop readily. It is administered orally and can be used for both therapy and prophylaxis. It is inactive under alkaline conditions and is not useful for treating urinary tract infection due to *Proteus* spp. The most serious side-effect is an allergic pneumonitis, which is fortunately rare. In patients with glucose-6-phosphate dehydrogenase (G-6-PD) deficiency, nitrofurantoin produces haemolytic episodes. It should not be used in neonates.

Quinolones

Quinolones prevent DNA replication by inhibiting bacterial DNA gyrase. The first quinolone, nalidixic acid, is used solely for the treatment or prophylaxis of urinary tract infection and is administered orally. It is active only against Gram-negative bacteria and resistance develops easily. It should not be used in infants under 3 months or in G-6-PD deficiency. Currently, the 'newer' quinolones such as ciprofloxacin or ofloxacin are not licensed for use in those under 18 years since they induce cartilage damage in weightbearing joints of young beagle dogs. They are very useful agents with a large volume of distribution and a broad spectrum of activity, and are bactericidal. For these reasons they have been used in paediatric practice for severe infection, including those in neonates and patients with cystic fibrosis, with little or no evidence of induction of arthropathy. They are also used in the chemoprophylaxis of meningococcal disease. New fluoroquinolones such as levofloxacin, grepafloxacin and moxifloxacin have been developed that also have activity against streptococci (the major deficit in the spectrum of the others). Serious reactions (anaphylactoid) are rare but they should not be administered with theophylline since quinolones inhibit the metabolism of methylxanthines. Resistance to these quinolones is developing slowly and plasmid-encoded resistance has been encountered. They can be administered orally or intravenously.

Sulphonamides

These are structural analogues of para-amino benzoic acid and competitively inhibit the bacterial synthesis of folic acid. Bacteria have an absolute requirement for folic acid to produce new nucleotides. Because of relatively high prevalence of resistance (which can be plasmid encoded) and of side-effects, sulphonamides are little used in paediatric practice. Sulphonamides are a frequent cause of rashes and can cause Stevens–Johnson syndrome. They may also cause crystalluria and renal failure, bone marrow suppression, and haemolytic anaemia in G-6-PD deficiency. They may precipitate kernicterus in neonates. Some sulphonamides, e.g. silver sulphadiazine, are used topically in the treatment and prophylaxis of infection in patients with burns.

Trimethoprim

Trimethoprim inhibits bacterial dihydrofolinic acid reductase and this prevents synthesis of folic acid. It has a broad spectrum of antibacterial activity, is bactericidal and has a large volume of distribution. High-level resistance to trimethoprim (> 1000 mg/L) is increasing and is usually plasmid-encoded. The drug can be administered by the oral or intravenous routes. It is generally well tolerated with no serious side-effects. If administered to neonates, folate supplementation may be necessary.

Co-trimoxazole

Co-trimoxazole is a combination of sulphamethoxazole and trimethoprim. It was considered that this combination, by blocking two steps on the same pathway, might prevent the development of resistance. This expectation has not been realised. Most of the toxicity of co-trimoxazole results from the sulphamethoxazole. Absolute indications for the use of co-trimoxazole (rather than trimethoprim) are *Pneumocystis carinii* pneumonia, brucellosis and nocardiosis.

Transcription

Rifampicin

Rifampicin is a rifamycin, which is the only class of antibiotics to inhibit DNA-dependent RNA polymerase. It can be administered orally or intravenously. It has a broad-spectrum antibacterial activity, a large volume of distribution, and is bactericidal. Unfortunately, resistance (a one-step event) develops readily. The main indications for use are for treating tuberculosis, leprosy and atypical mycobacteria, and in prophylaxis of meningococcal or *H. influenzae* type b disease. It has also been used (usually in combination) to treat brucellosis, legionellosis and severe or multiresistant staphylococcal (coagulase-positive or -negative) infections, including endocarditis and central nervous system shunt infection. Rifampicin should not be given to patients with liver damage. The most severe side-effect is hypersensitivity. It induces liver microsomal enzymes and may decrease the efficacy of drugs (e.g. corticosteroids or warfarin) that are conjugated by such enzymes. It colours urine and tears pink or red.

Translation

Aminoglycosides

Aminoglycosides prevent binding of peptidyl tRNA to polysomes and inhibit protein synthesis. They are derived from *Streptomyces* spp. (end in -mycin) or *Micromonospora* spp. (end in -micin). They are rapidly bactericidal broad-spectrum antibacterials. They have no activity against anaerobes, streptococci and intracellular pathogens. There are varying prevalences of resistance to the individual aminoglycosides among aerobic Gram-negative bacilli (least frequently to amikacin). This resistance is frequently plasmid-encoded. Aminoglycosides are poorly absorbed orally and thus must be given intravenously (some, e.g. gentamicin, can be given intrathecally). Penetration into cerebrospinal fluid (CSF) or bronchial secretions is poor. They are most useful for treating septicaemia in children or neonates, complicated urinary tract infection and bacterial endocarditis. They are also used prophylactically for abdominal surgery. They have a low therapeutic index and levels must be monitored. Toxicity is particularly associated with prolonged high trough levels.

Aminoglycosides are ototoxic (tinnitus, deafness and vestibular disturbances), nephrotoxic (usually reversible) and may promote neuromuscular blockade. Diuretics (such as frusemide) and cephaloridine interact with aminoglycosides to potentiate nephrotoxicity. Some aminoglycosides (e.g. neomycin) are used topically, in combination with other antibiotics, in eye drops, ear drops and ointments.

Aminoglycosides have also been administered by nebuliser to children with cystic fibrosis.

Chloramphenicol

This drug inhibits peptide bond formation and mitochondrial NADH oxidase. It is administered orally, intravenously or topically in ointments and eye drops. It is bactericidal for *H. influenzae*, *Neisseria meningitidis* and *Streptococcus pneumoniae* but bacteriostatic for aerobic Gram-negative bacilli such as *E. coli*, salmonellas and *Klebsiella pneumoniae*. It has a wide volume of distribution and penetrates well into CSF. It used to be the mainstay of treatment for bacterial meningitis and still is in low-income countries. Because of concerns over toxicity, bacterial resistance and efficacy it has largely been superseded by third-generation cephalosporins such as cefotaxime or ceftriaxone. It is still indicated for initial empirical treatment of brain abscesses, melioidosis and rickettsial infection (e.g. Rocky Mountain spotted fever) where tetracycline cannot be used. It can produce dose-related marrow suppression and a rarer dose-independent irreversible aplastic anaemia. It should not be used in neonates because of the risk of 'grey-baby syndrome' (pale cyanotic skin, hypotension, metabolic acidosis followed by cardiovascular collapse).

Tetracyclines

These prevent access of aminoacyl tRNA to acceptor sites on the mRNA-ribosome complex. They are broad-spectrum, bacteriostatic antibiotics with a large volume of distribution. They should not be used in children under 8 years or in pregnant women, because they are deposited in immature teeth, which may become soft and discoloured, and in bone. They may be indicated for treatment of infection due to erythromycin-resistant strains of *Chlamydia psittaci*, *Rickettsia* spp., *Mycoplasma* spp., *Ureaplasma* spp. and in relapsing fever (*Borrelia recurrentis*) and Lyme disease (*Borrelia burgdorferi*). They may be administered intravenously, orally (absorption may be unpredictable) or topically. The topical administration is usually for conjunctivitis or infected eczema.

Macrolides

Macrolides are a group of antibiotics that affect bacterial peptide chain initiation. They are bacteriostatic or bactericidal for anaerobic and aerobic

Gram-positive bacteria, *Mycoplasma* spp. and *Chlamydia* spp., depending on the organism, the macrolide and the dosage. Erythromycin may be given orally or intravenously and is the most frequently used macrolide. It penetrates into most sites except for brain and CSF. The newer macrolides azithromycin and clarithromycin have much higher potency. Macrolides are indicated for the treatment of infection due to *Chlamydia* spp., *Mycoplasma* spp., atypical mycobacteria and Gram-positive bacteria or for prophylaxis of bacterial endocarditis in patients who are penicillin-allergic. Erythromycin has been used to eliminate carriage of *Bordetella pertussis* and is the drug of choice for legionellosis. Clindamycin is used for treating deep staphylococcal sepsis. Erythromycin can cause hepatotoxicity and, rarely, Stevens–Johnson syndrome. Lincomycin should not be given to neonates and clindamycin can induce ventricular fibrillation. Spiramycin is used for prevention of transmission of toxoplasmosis from mother to fetus and treatment of congenitally infected infants. It has also been used for treating cryptosporidiosis in immunocompromised children but controlled trials have not demonstrated efficacy.

Fusidic acid

This prevents binding of aminoacyl tRNA to the ribosome. It is bactericidal for both aerobic and anaerobic Gram-positive bacteria but is used principally to treat staphylococcal (coagulase-positive and -negative) infections. It penetrates well into bone, joints and burn crusts but poorly into CSF. It can be administered orally, intravenously or topically but resistance develops readily both in vitro and in vivo. Its main indications for use are in osteomyelitis, arthritis and endocarditis but is often used in combination with other antistaphylococcal antibiotics. Fusidic acid produces phlebitis when given into peripheral veins and should be given through a central line. It is generally a safe drug but can cause hyperbilirubinaemia and jaundice.

Streptogramins

These bind to ribosomes and inhibit peptidyl transferase activity. Synercid is a combination of two pristinomycin derivatives, quinupristin and dalfopristin. It has been introduced because of increasing concern over vancomycin- and methicillin-resistant *S. aureus* (VMRSA), vancomycin-resistant enterococci (VRE) and multidrug-resistant coagulase-negative staphylococci. It has a Gram-positive spectrum of activity (but is also active against *H. influenzae* and *Moraxella catarrhalis*), is bactericidal and can be given orally. Streptogramins are excreted in bile. Resistance has already developed.

Oxazolidinones

These are synthetic antimicrobials that inhibit protein synthesis in Gram-positive bacteria and have activity against *Mycobacterium tuberculosis*.

ANTIVIRAL AGENTS

Compared to antibacterials, there is a paucity of antiviral agents. The major reason for this is that, as obligate intracellular pathogens, viruses subvert the host cell's biosynthetic machinery to replicate themselves. Thus drugs that might inhibit viral replication are likely also to be toxic, and this was certainly the case for the earlier agents. Most antivirals are nucleoside analogues but others directed against different targets (e.g. protease inhibitors, neuraminidase inhibitors) are gradually being developed (Table 31.2).

Table 31.2 Antiviral agents

Agent	Viral target	Administration	Resistance described
Nucleoside analogues			
Idoxuridine	HHV 1, 2, 3	Topical	−
Trifluorothymidine	HHV 1, 2, 3	Topical	−
Aciclovir	HHV 1, 2, 3	Topical, oral, i.v.	+
Penciclovir	HHV 1, 2, 3, HBV	i.v.	+
Adenine arabinoside	HHV 1, 2, 3	i.v.	−
Ganciclovir	HHV 5	Oral, i.v.	+
Cidofovir	HHV 5	i.v.	−
Zidovudine (AZT)	HIV	Oral, i.v.	+
Stavudine (D4T)	HIV	Oral, i.v.	+
Didanosine (DDI)	HIV	Oral, i.v.	+
Zalcitabine (DDC)	HIV	Oral	+
Lamivudine (3TC)	HIV, HBV	Oral	+
Ribavirin	Paramyxoviruses, HCV, HIV, Hantavirus, arenaviruses	Nebulised, i.v.	+
Prodrug nucleoside analogues			
Famciclovir	HHV 1, 2, 3	Oral	+
Valaciclovir	HHV 1, 2, 3	Oral	+
Non-nucleoside reverse transcriptase inhibitors			
TIBO	HIV	Oral	+
Nevirapine	HIV-1	Oral	+
Delavirdine	HIV-1	Oral	+
Protease inhibitors			
Saquinavir	HIV	Oral	+
Ritonavir	HIV	Oral	+
Indinavir	HIV	Oral	+
Nelfinavir	HIV	Oral	+
Other			
Foscarnet	HHV 1, 2, 3, 5	Oral, i.v.	+
Amantadine (rimantidine)	Influenza A	Oral	+
Zanamivir	Influenza	Oral	−
Pirodavir	Picornaviruses	Oral	−

HBV = hepatitis B virus; HCV = hepatitis C virus; HHV = human herpesvirus; HIV = human immunodeficiency virus; i.v. = intravenous.

Nucleoside analogues

Idoxuridine and trifluorothymidine were among the earliest antiviral drugs to be discovered. Both are extremely toxic but can be used topically, especially on ocular and skin lesions of herpes simplex viruses I and II (HHV 1 & 2) and varicella-zoster virus (HHV-3). Trifluorothymidine is the treatment of choice of HSV-keratoconjunctivitis.

Aciclovir

Aciclovir (ACV) is structurally related to guanosine but lacks a complete deoxyribose ring (hence 'acyclo'). In order to accumulate in cells it must be phosphorylated in three steps from mono- to di- and then to triphosphate. It is a poor substrate for cellular enzymes and thus does not accumulate. However the herpesviruses (HHV-1, 2, 3) encode a thymidine kinase that efficiently converts ACV to the monophosphate, which can be further phosphorylated to the di- and triphosphate. Thus ACV only accumulates in and is toxic for herpesvirus-infected cells. The ACV is added to the herpesvirus genome in place of guanosine but since it does not possess the cyclic deoxyribose moiety the next nucleoside in the chain cannot be added. Thus chain termination occurs, new viral DNA synthesis is stopped and the infection is cured.

ACV is effective in both primary and recurrent mucocutaneous herpesvirus infections in immunocompromised hosts, in primary and recurrent genital herpes and in life-threatening infection such as herpes encephalitis and neonatal disease. It is useful in treating shingles, if given early and in some countries (but not the UK), is used for treating chickenpox. Unfortunately, aciclovir is also available as an ointment as an 'over the counter' medication for applying to cold sores. Resistance has developed. The mutant virus has become resistant by stopping production of thymidine kinase (TK⁻ mutant). These have arisen predominantly in immunocompromised hosts. Penciclovir has a similar structure and mode of action to ACV and valaciclovir and famciclovir are esters (prodrugs) of ACV and penciclovir respectively.

Aciclovir and derivatives have largely replaced the use of adenine arabinoside (vidarabine), which inhibits the herpesviral DNA polymerase. It is poorly soluble and must be given with large amounts of intravenous fluid.

Ganciclovir

Ganciclovir has a similar structure to ACV. It has activity against HHV-1, 2 and 3 but is primarily used against HHV-5 (cytomegalovirus), which interestingly does not possess thymidine kinase. It is, however, phosphorylated by a novel viral enzyme to a monophosphate, which then inhibits viral DNA polymerase. There is little experience of its use in children. It is used for treating cytomegalovirus (CMV) infection in AIDS and immunosuppressed transplant patients. There are some uncontrolled studies of its use in congenitally and symptomatically infected neonates with some benefit. This must be balanced against its bone marrow suppressive activity.

Zidovudine

Zidovudine (azidothymidine, AZT) inhibits HIV reverse transcriptase (RT). To be active it is converted to the triphosphate by cellular kinases. Resistance develops easily because HIV is so mutable (it is estimated that during acute infection 10^9 new HIV particles are produced per day and 10^6 of these are mutant) and involves alterations in RT. AZT does exhibit synergistic or additive effects with a number of other antiretrovirals but antagonism with ribavirin and stavudine. AZT has been given in pregnancy and to neonates, infants and children. Its major toxic effects are bone marrow suppression, myopathy and hepatic damage.

Stavudine

Stavudine (D4T) is a potent inhibitor of HIV RT but the host cellular thymidine kinase has greater affinity for AZT than for stavudine, which may explain why the combination is antagonistic. Resistance can develop with mutations in the RT gene. Some mutations give cross-resistance to AZT and some to zalcitabine. Peripheral neuropathy is the major dose-limiting toxicity but it is less myelotoxic than AZT.

Didanosine

Didanosine (DDI) is also an RT inhibitor that also has activity against AZT-resistant HIV. Resistance to DDI does develop but less frequently and profoundly than to AZT. It is also phosphorylated intracellularly. Its major toxicity is pancreatitis but also causes reversible, dose-related peripheral neuropathy. In general it is well tolerated in children.

Zalcitabine

Zalcitabine (DDC) is also an RT inhibitor that is dependent on intracellular phosphorylation. It exhibits synergy with AZT and some protease inhibitors. Resistance in HIV develops less readily than to AZT. It causes a dose-related peripheral neuropathy.

Lamivudine

Lamivudine (3TC) has a potency similar to AZT in inhibiting HIV-1 and HIV-2 RT. Resistance occurs rapidly during monotherapy and a number of mutations in the RT gene have been described. Combination therapy with AZT does not delay the development of lamivudine-resistance but does that of AZT resistance. Lamivudine is also active in suppressing chronic hepatitis B virus (HBV) replication and in trials produced significant improvement in chronic hepatitis. Resistant HBV has, however, emerged. The major side-effect is headache.

Ribavirin

This is a guanosine analogue with a wide spectrum of activity against RNA and DNA viruses. In respiratory syncytial virus (RSV) bronchiolitis it is administered as an aerosol but its use is controversial, with different studies giving opposite results. It is useful in treating persistent paramyxovirus infections in immunocompromised hosts. It is also being examined as treatment for Lassa fever and other arenavirus infections, hantavirus and hepatitis C virus (in combination with interferon). Its value in treating HIV infection is also controversial.

Nevirapine

This is a non-nucleoside reverse transcriptase inhibitor active only against HIV-1. Resistance to it develops rapidly so it is given as part of combination therapy. It is associated with headache, rash, fever and mouth ulcers.

Delavirdine

This is also active only against HIV-1 RT and shows antagonism with nevirapine. Resistance develops early and it is used in combination therapy. It causes maculopapular rashes, mild headache, nausea and fatigue.

Protease inhibitors

During HIV replication the products of the *pol*, *env* and *gag* regions of the genome are produced as long polyproteins (e.g. gp 160 from the *env* region). As the virus is assembled these are cleaved by an HIV-specific aspartate protease (e.g. to gp 120 and gp 41 from gp 160). The protease inhibitors are targeted against the specific HIV-encoded protease.

Saquinavir

This drug is active against both HIV-1 and HIV-2 and shows additive or synergistic activity with AZT, zalcitabine, stavudine and lamivudine. Resistance arises slowly by an accumulation of changes in the protease gene. Some give cross-resistance to other protease inhibitors. In general, saquinavir is well tolerated, with nausea and diarrhoea occurring in only 5% of subjects.

Ritonavir and indinavir

These are metabolised in the liver by the p450 pathway and induce its activity and may thus interfere with other drugs utilising this pathway or be affected by them. Both are associated with nephrolithiasis.

Other antivirals

Foscarnet

Foscarnet is phosphonoformate and is active against HHV-1, 2, 3, 4, 5, 6 and 8. It inhibits viral DNA polymerase. Its major clinical use is in CMV infections. Its safety and efficacy has not been established in children. Its major toxicity is in the kidney and in inducing electrolyte disturbances.

Amantadine (and rimantadine)

These inhibit the cellular uptake of influenza-A virus, although not all strains are sensitive. Its major indication is for prophylaxis in influenza but central nervous system side-effects are reported in 11–33% of young adults, including nervousness, insomnia, slurred speech, tremor, depression, confusion and hallucination.

Pirodavir

Pirodavir is a member of a family of substituted phenoxy-pyridazinamine compounds that are active against picornaviruses (rhinoviruses, polioviruses and enteroviruses). It works by binding to hydrophobic pockets in the canyon floor of the picornavirus surface and inhibiting viral uncoating.

Zanamivir

This is a new class of antiviral that inhibits the neuraminidase of influenza virus. In recent trials it was therapeutically highly effective. It has not yet been used in children.

CLINICAL USAGE OF ANTIBIOTICS AND ANTIVIRALS

The decision on which antibiotics to use will depend upon the likely pathogen, the current resistance patterns of the pathogen, the site of infection and the toxicity of the agent.

Some pathogens have remained predictably sensitive to antibiotics (e.g. in the UK all meningococci are sensitive to penicillin or cefotaxime). For others the situation is much more fluid. For example, Gram-negative enteric bacteria such as *E. coli*, klebsiellas and salmonellas are able to acquire plasmids conferring resistance to aminoglycosides and third-generation cephalosporins with great ease. The incidence of such resistance varies from hospital to hospital and even from ward to ward. It is thus of great importance for units such as neonatal intensive care or oncology to have information on their local antibiotic resistance patterns. Antibiotics may be used prophylactically or therapeutically.

Prophylactic use

There are few absolute indications for the prophylactic use of antimicrobials and this is one area where misuse is common. Examples of indications for prophylaxis include rifampicin or ciprofloxacin for close contacts of cases of meningococcal or *H. influenzae* type b invasive disease (only less than 5 years old), metronidazole and gentamicin prior to colonic surgery and amoxycillin (or erythromycin) prior to dental treatment in children with cardiac valvular defects.

Examples of misuse include giving antibiotics to children with viral respiratory tract infections to prevent bacterial superinfection or giving antibiotics to prevent infection in children with urinary catheters.

Therapeutic use

In general antibiotics may be administered when:

1. infection is suspected but not proven on clinical grounds (pre-emptive)
2. infection is proven, pathogen suspected or unknown (empirical)
3. infection is proven, pathogen and antimicrobial susceptibility known.

In paediatric practice situations 1 and 2 are the most commonly encountered and 3 applies 24–48 hours after initial administration of antibiotics. At this stage the antimicrobial chemotherapy should be reviewed and rationalised.

For initiation of pre-emptive therapy there will be varying levels of suspicion that trigger its administration. For example, in premature neonates, because the signs of infection are so nonspecific but the results of infection potentially catastrophic, therapy with broad-spectrum antibiotics is frequently initiated. On subsequent review in approximately only 10% of such episodes is infection actually present. Hence rationalisation of therapy after 48–72 hours is important.

For empirical therapy there will be good evidence that an infection is present and it may be possible to predict likely pathogens and even their antimicrobial chemotherapy. For example, urinary tract infection is usually caused by *E. coli*, which currently is usually susceptible to trimethoprim, cephradine or co-amoxiclav. Again, it will be possible to rationalise the therapy according to the microbiology results. Paediatricians should not be afraid to change therapy to optimise chances of recovery from infection. All hospitals will have local guidelines to aid treatment, which will be based on local patterns of infection and antibiotic resistance.

Antiretroviral therapy

Use of single antiretroviral drugs led rapidly to the development of HIV resistant to the drugs. This has led to the concept of combining two, three or even four different antiretrovirals. The aim of this has been to suppress HIV replication completely, thus preventing or curing AIDS and preventing the development of antiviral resistance. Some even had the expectation that, as the HIV-infected lymphocytes, macrophages, etc. died without allowing HIV replication, HIV would be completely eliminated from the patient. It is too early to assess these expectations completely, but they seem unlikely. Combination therapy, sometimes called highly active antiretroviral therapy (HAART), involves giving mixtures of nucleoside and non-nucleoside RT inhibitors and protease inhibitors. They undoubtedly have a synergistic or at worst additive effect (providing the correct mixture is chosen) but do have the disadvantage of increasing the chance of toxicity and drug interactions. There are few trial data available in children; thus guidelines are mostly extrapolated from adult experience. The guidelines are modified by experience (BHIVA, 1998) but the major questions (Table 31.3) are when to treat, with what to treat, how to monitor therapy and for how long should treatment continue?

HAART has been highly successful in adult populations and should be as effective in children. In some studies, fluctuations in CD4 counts have been encountered despite low HIV loads. Ominously, strains of HIV have emerged that are resistant to more than three different antiretrovirals.

FURTHER READING

BHIVA Guidelines Writing Committee (1998) 1998 Revision to the British HIV Association guidelines for antiretroviral treatment of HIV-seropositive individuals. Lancet 352: 314–316.

Table 31.3 Antiretroviral therapy

When to treat	Benefits of treatment outweigh risks
	CD4 count greater than 350 cells/mL (i.e. immune system salvageable)
	Viral load (high enough to be associated with risk of disease progression)
	Patient or guardian agrees to treatment
With what to treat	**< 50 000 RNA copies/mL**: Two nucleoside analogues plus either a non-nucleoside RT inhibitor or protease inhibitor
	> 50 000 RNA copies/mL: Two nucleoside analogues plus one or two protease inhibitors
How to monitor therapy	Plasma viral load (should be < 500 RNA copies/mL and preferably less than 50 RNA copies/mL by week 24 of the therapy)
How long to continue	Unknown – may be for life, but will be limited by adverse reactions and perhaps by emergence of resistance

32 Infection control in hospital

See also sections on Universal precautions (blood spills, etc.) on page 219, Vulnerable children (page 221) Protecting pregnant staff (page 221) and Needlestick injuries (page 222) in Chapter 33.

Nosocomial or hospital-associated infections are those infections that occur as a result of the patient being admitted to hospital. The pathogens are acquired during the hospital stay and may present during hospitalisation or after discharge to home. In contrast, community-acquired infections are caused by pathogens acquired outside hospital. Nosocomial infections have been targeted as one of several potentially preventable health problems.

SIZE OF THE PROBLEM

Most of the data on the incidence of paediatric nosocomial infection come from North America. It is not possible to extrapolate data from surveys of adult nosocomial infection to paediatric populations. Paediatric infection rates from North America range from 1.2 to 10.3 per 100 discharges. The reported rate is higher in children's hospitals (mean 4.1/100 discharges, range 2.8–10.3) than that for paediatric wards within general hospitals (mean 1.2/100 discharges, range 1.2–5.5). A prevalence survey undertaken in 1980 in 43 district general hospitals in the UK indicated that 22% of paediatric patients had community-acquired infection and 6.3% hospital-acquired infection. In contrast, 16.8% of patients in neonatal intensive care units (NICU) had hospital-acquired infection.

There are no specific data on the overall morbidity, mortality and financial costs of paediatric nosocomial infection. However, in 1987 in the USA it was estimated that nosocomial infection, taking all age groups, resulted on average in 4 days extra stay in hospital, caused an estimated 30 000 deaths each year and added an extra $3–10 billion to hospital costs. Clearly, there are major benefits in decreasing hospital-associated infection. In order to do this there must be an understanding of the major sites of infection, the pathogens involved, their pathogenesis and which services are most likely to experience nosocomial infection.

WHICH PATIENTS AND WHICH SERVICES?

In most surveys the majority of nosocomial infections present in NICU, haematology/oncology and neonatal surgery. This is not surprising since patients on these wards are the most likely to be immunoincompetent and are exposed to the greatest risk. A Canadian study showed that nosocomial infection rates for NICU, infant neurosurgery, haematology/oncology, neonatal surgery and paediatric ICU were 14.0%, 12.3%, 11.7%, 9.1% and 6.0% respectively. In contrast, infection rates in ophthalmology, isolation wards and orthopaedics were 0.2%, 1.3% and 2.9% respectively.

In general, the younger the child the higher the nosocomial infection rate (NIR). Thus those less than 23 months had an NIR of 11.5%, those aged 2–4 years 3.6% and those over 5 years 2.6%. The patterns of infection also changed with age.

SITES OF INFECTION

Although there are wide differences between different surveys, respiratory tract (16–24% of infections), gastrointestinal tract (17–35%) and bacteraemia (10–21%) are the three most frequent nosocomial infections. This contrasts with adult nosocomial infection, where urinary tract infection is the commonest. In paediatric hospitals urinary tract infection accounts for 6–9% of nosocomial infection. It has been shown that the median stay in hospital prior to the development of nosocomial infections was 8.4 days, 10.7 days, 12 days, 19 days and 24.9 days for meningitis, wound infection, gastrointestinal infection, urinary tract infection and bacteraemia respectively. This may of course be an underestimate if patients discharged home have subsequently developed a hospital-associated infection.

PATHOGENS INVOLVED

This is another area of difference from adult nosocomial infection. Children are of course at greater risk of viral infection and surveys of paediatric nosocomial infection that do not include viruses will underestimate rates. Outbreaks of nosocomial respiratory tract infection due to respiratory syncytial virus and adenovirus, of gastrointestinal tract infection due to rotavirus and hepatitis A virus and of varicella zoster in NICU are well-described. In most surveys bacteria account for between 65–70% (Gram-positive 50%, Gram-negative 18%) of paediatric nosocomial infection, viruses for up to 25% (the majority gastrointestinal infection) and fungi for 5%. The distribution of pathogens varies according to the paediatric service, the age of the patient and the site of infection. For example, coagulase-negative staphylococci (e.g. *S. epidermidis*) are particularly associated with implant infections (most often intravascular catheters) and infections related to intravascular catheters are responsible for 5–6% of paediatric nosocomial infection.

PATHOGENESIS OF NOSOCOMIAL INFECTION

Nosocomial infections can occur as outbreaks or epidemics or as sporadic cases. Although the outbreaks of infection are the most highly visible and worrying, numerically, sporadic infections are far more important. In order to prevent both epidemic and sporadic nosocomial infection it is necessary to understand the pathogenesis of infection, modes of transmission and portals of entry.

Infections can be divided into exogenous and endogenous. In exogenous infection the pathogen gains direct access to the patient from the environment (animate or inanimate) and initiates disease. Endogenous infections are derived from the patient's own microflora (see Chapter 30). Endogenous infections may be subdivided into primary endogenous, in which the pathogen is derived from the patient's own normal flora, and secondary endogenous, in which the pathogen colonises the patient, becoming part of the 'normal' flora, and subsequently causes infection. Examples of exogenous infection are secondary cases of bronchiolitis due to respiratory syncytial virus (RSV) and gastroenteritis due to *Salmonella* spp. or rotavirus. Exogenous nosocomial infections can be sporadic but have a propensity to result in outbreaks. Examples of primary endogenous infections include abdominal abscesses due to *Streptococcus milleri* following appendectomy or cerebrospinal fluid (CSF) shunt infections due to *S. epidermidis*. Primary endogenous infections are always sporadic. Secondary endogenous infection can appear either sporadically or in outbreaks; examples include cases of multidrug-resistant *Klebsiella pneumoniae* colonising neonates in NICU resulting in septicaemia and meningitis in a proportion of those colonised. It can be seen that different methods are needed to control exogenous and primary and secondary endogenous infections.

MODES OF SPREAD

Although there are numerous possibilities for spreading potential pathogens in hospital, in general nosocomial infections are transmitted by contact, vehicles, air or vectors. Of the above, person-to-person transmission on the hands of hospital staff or even patients is undoubtedly the most important mode. The incidence of nosocomial infections rises when staffing levels are inadequate, since this leads to a decrease in hand-washing by overburdened staff and staff have contact with an increased number of patients. It has been shown that hands are an important mode of spread even of respiratory pathogens such as RSV and adenovirus, which were previously considered to be spread by air. Overcrowding on wards also increases the likelihood of transmission of pathogens by air or by contact.

Vehicles of transmission of nosocomial infection could be food (e.g. *Salmonella* spp.), water (e.g. *Cryptosporidium*), contaminated intravenous solutions (e.g. *Klebsiella*, *Serratia* or *Enterobacter* spp.) or blood and blood products (e.g. hepatitis B or C virus, human immunodeficiency virus, cytomegalovirus). Of equal importance are items of medical equipment. For example, there have been outbreaks of infection due to contaminated rectal thermometers (*S. eimsbuettel*), breast-milk pumps (*K. pneumoniae*) and gastroscopes (*Helicobacter pylori*).

Airborne spread of pathogens can occur: examples include varicella-zoster virus in neonatal units and *Aspergillus* spp. in oncology units. Nevertheless this is of secondary importance in comparison to hand transmission. Although rodents and cockroaches can be found in hospitals, there is little evidence that they are important vectors of infection.

HOST FACTORS

The variations in hospital-associated infection rates in the different paediatric services are to a large extent a reflection of the immunocompetence and thus susceptibility to infection of the patients. Thus patients in NICU have defects in nonspecific (poor temperature control, no established normal flora, poor inflammatory response, impaired phagocytosis) and specific (IgG reflecting maternal IgG, no IgA, low IgM, depressed T-cell function) immunity, which are more evident the more premature the neonate. In haematology/oncology wards patients are immunosuppressed both by their disease and by chemotherapy or radiotherapy (see also Chapter 22).

CONTROLLING NOSOCOMIAL INFECTIONS

From the foregoing it is apparent that controlling nosocomial infections is of major importance. It is also apparent that the interactions between microorganisms in patients, hospital staff and the hospital environment that result in nosocomial infection are complex and that infection control measures must extend into many facets of the paediatric hospital or ward. The aims of effective infection control are:

- To prevent patients from acquiring infection in hospital
- To provide adequate hospital care for patients entering hospital with a community-acquired infection while preventing its dissemination to others
- To prevent transmission of infection to or from hospital staff and visitors
- To prevent nosocomial infections being disseminated in the community.

In order to do this it is essential that each hospital should have an infection control team.

Role of the infection control team

The infection control team (ICT) normally consists of the infection control doctor (ICD), infection control nurse(s), a medical microbiologist (if not the ICD) and a representative of the hospital management team. This team should report to an infection control committee (ICC), which should comprise the ICT, the consultants in communicable disease control, an occupational health physician, a paediatrician with an interest in infectious diseases, a paediatric surgeon and a nurse manager, The committee may co-opt as necessary representatives from the Central Sterile Supply Department, Laundry Services, Building Services, Catering, Pest Control, Pharmacy and operating theatres.

The ICT should be responsible for the day-to-day control of nosocomial infection. It will be responsible for formulation and application of infection control policies (including involvement in formulation of policies on antibiotic usage, isolation, immunisation, disinfection and sterilisation, commissioning and decommissioning theatres and medical equipment). It will be responsible for surveillance of nosocomial infection and providing regular reports to the ICC. It will be responsible for liaising with the community over problems of infection. Finally and most importantly, the ICT has an educative role for hospital staff to present information on how nosocomial infection occurs and how best to prevent it. Such education will require repeated reinforcement.

In addition to general infection control the ICT will be responsible for initiating the correct responses for notification, investigation and curtailment of outbreaks of infection. Each hospital should have structures (policies and action group) to manage major or minor outbreaks of infection.

Methods for infection control

It is beyond the scope of this chapter to give detailed description of infection control policies. Each paediatric hospital and, under certain circumstances, each ward (e.g. NICU) will need to draw up its own policy, taking into account local problems and facilities. The policy will need to encompass areas such as preadmission infection screening (for booked admissions), precautions to be taken with infected patients, methods and degrees of patient isolation and hand-washing between handling patients. Isolation policies should balance the risk of transmission of infection with the difficulty of treating patients in isolation and the psychological problems posed to a child by isolation. Examples of types of isolation and precautions are shown in Table 32.1.

The NICU is an area of particular risk for development of nosocomial infection. Extra attention focused on NICU can yield great benefit. As in other areas, hand-washing is of prime importance in preventing transmission of microorganisms that can either cause exogenous or secondary endogenous infection. Unlike in most other areas the inanimate environment may also be a source of infection; for example, outbreaks of bacteraemia and meningitis have been associated with strains of *K. pneumoniae* colonising blood gas analysers and breast-milk pumps. It is therefore advisable to wash hands prior to handling as well as after handling the

Table 32.1 Examples of isolation and precautions for infection control

	Diseases/pathogen	Methods
Strict isolation	e.g. Diphtheria, plague, rabies	Single room, gown, gloves, mask. Strict hand-washing prior to leaving room. Articles contaminated bagged, labelled, decontaminated or incinerated
Contact isolation	e.g. Bronchiolitis, conjunctivitis, impetigo, MRSA	Single room (? cohort for RSV), masks for close contact, gowns if soiling likely, gloves if touching infected area. Strict hand-washing. Contaminated articles bagged, labelled, decontaminated or incinerated
Respiratory isolation	e.g. Measles, meningococcal disease, whooping cough	Single room, masks for close contact. Gloves not indicated. Strict hand-washing. Contaminated articles bagged, labelled, decontaminated or incinerated
Enteric isolation	e.g. Rotavirus, shigellosis, cryptosporidiosis; all patients with diarrhoea unless proven to be noninfective	Single room (? cohort for rotavirus). No masks, gown if soiling likely, gloves if handling infective material. Strict hand-washing. Contaminated article bagged, labelled, decontaminated or incinerated
Blood/ body fluid precautions	e.g. Hepatitis B, HIV	Isolation not indicated, no masks, gloves for handling blood or body fluid. Gowns if soiling likely. Contaminated articles, bagged, labelled, decontaminated or incinerated. Avoid needlestick or sharps injury. Clean spills with 0.5% sodium hypochlorite
Protective isolation	Immunosuppressed patients (e.g. bone marrow transplant)	Single room, positive pressure. Gowns, gloves, masks. Sterilised food and drink. Aims to prevent access of potential pathogen to patient

neonates or their intravenous lines or ventilators. There is no evidence that gowning prevents infection unless the neonate is to be directly handled. Masks are usually used only for special procedures such as siting umbilical artery catheters. Gloves are used when handling infants with diarrhoea or draining wounds. They do not replace hand-washing. The use of overshoes is to be discouraged. It is an ideal way of transferring microorganisms from shoes to hands.

Control of infection in hospital requires an enthusiastic, able and vigilant team that is prepared to educate and convince hospital staff that nosocomial infection is important and that its impact can be lessened by application of effective methods.

FURTHER READING

Garner JJ, Simmons BP (1983) CDC guidelines for isolation precautions in hospitals. Infection Control 4: 245–325.

Hospital Infection Control (1988) Guidance on the control of infection in hospitals prepared by the joint DHSS/PHLS Hospital Infection Working Group.

Wenzel RP (1992) Prevention and control of nosocomial infection, 2nd edn. Williams & Wilkins, Baltimore, MD.

33 Infection control in the community

PRIMARY PREVENTIVE PRACTICES IN THE DAY CARE, NURSERY AND PRIMARY SCHOOL SETTINGS, IN COMMUNITY SETTINGS AND IN THE HOME

The following practices are recommended to reduce the incidence and transmission of infection in child care and other community settings. Many of the practices are applicable elsewhere and, where practical, will also reduce disease incidence and transmission in the home. They can be used as a basis for 'enteric precautions' in specific diseases.

Reducing risks of faecal–oral transmission of infection

- Day care facilities should have written policies for preventing and managing child and staff illness.
- Toilets and toilet training equipment should be well maintained and cleaned daily. Nappy-changing surfaces should be nonporous and cleaned between use. If disposable paper coverings are used they must be discarded after each use and the surface underneath cleaned if damp or soiled.
- Soiled disposable nappies or soiled wiping cloths should be discarded in a secure, plastic-lined container operated by a foot pedal so that hand contact can be minimised.
- Faeces should be placed in a toilet. Nappies should not be rinsed in sinks but may be placed to soak prior to washing in a sterilising solution such as Napisan.
- Nappy-changing areas should never be located in, or open directly on to, food preparation areas; similarly, nappy changing should never take place where food is prepared.
- The use of child-sized toilets, or access to steps and modified toilet seats, should be encouraged as early as practical. The use of potties should be discouraged. When they have to be used, e.g. with younger toddlers, they should be emptied into a toilet, cleaned in a sink (not used for food preparation) and disinfected after each use. Potties, flush toilets and nappy-changing areas should be cleaned with a freshly prepared solution of household bleach.

- Written procedures for hand-washing in day-care, nursery and primary school facilities should be established and enforced. Hand-washing sinks should be adjacent to each nappy-changing and toileting area. These sinks should be washed and disinfected at least daily and when soiled; they must not be used for food preparation or for rinsing soiled clothing or cleaning potties.
- Children should have access to height-appropriate sinks, soap dispensers and disposable paper towels.
- Spills of vomit, urine and faeces should be cleaned using a bleach-containing commercial cleaner. Gloves should always be worn when handling bleach.
- Optimally, toys that are placed in children's mouths or otherwise contaminated by body secretions should be cleaned with water and detergent, disinfected and rinsed before handling by another child. All frequently touched toys in rooms that house infants and toddlers should be cleaned and disinfected daily. Toys in rooms for older children (no nappy users) should be cleaned weekly and when soiled. The use of shared soft, nonwashable toys in infant/toddler areas of child care programmes should be discouraged.
- Food should be handled in a safe and careful manner to prevent the growth of microorganisms. Tables and counter tops used for food preparation and food service should be cleaned between uses, and before and after eating. No one who has signs or symptoms of illness, especially vomiting, diarrhoea and infectious skin lesions that cannot be covered, or who is infected with potential food-borne pathogens, should be responsible for food handling. Hands should be washed using soap and water before handling food. Staff who work with children with nappies, whenever possible, should not prepare food. Carers who prepare food for infants should be especially aware of the importance of careful hand-washing.
- Unpasteurised milk or milk products should not be served.
- Food, particularly chicken and comminuted meat products (beefburgers, sausages, etc.), should be well cooked and eggs should not be used without cooking or pasteurisation (e.g. in cake icing, fillings or mayonnaise).
- Hands must be washed after touching an infected child or possibly contaminated material (e.g. nappies, soiled bedding).
- Articles contaminated by vomitus or faecal material should be discarded (if disposable) immediately into a plastic bag or placed in a secure container before washing.
- Disposable gloves may be used for touching infected articles in institutional settings (e.g. day care centres) where infectious illnesses are concerned. Masks and gowns are not usually used outside hospital.

Universal precautions for preventing transmission of blood-borne infection

- Written hygiene policies and procedures should include cleaning and disinfecting floors, play tables and spills of blood, body fluids and wound or tissue exudates.

- **For spills of blood or blood-containing body fluid, and of wound and tissue exudates**, the procedures are as follows:
  - Hands, skin or mucous membranes exposed to another person's fluids should be washed promptly and thoroughly.
  - Disposable gloves are to be used throughout and any cuts, abrasions or inflamed areas kept covered by waterproof plasters. Gloves should be securely disposed of afterwards.
  - The spill should be cleaned with freshly diluted household bleach (1 in 10 dilution, i.e. 1 part of bleach to 10 parts water). Gloves must be worn. The bleach should be poured gently over the spill and covered with paper towels. If possible the bleach should then be left for 30 minutes before wiping up with more paper towels. More solid spillages contaminated with body fluids, such as bloody vomit or faeces, can be scooped up into a bucket of hot soapy water and the scoop cleaned or disposed of as contaminated waste.
  - Contaminated materials and gloves should be discarded in a sealed bag.
  - Hands should be washed afterwards.
- Tooth brushes and flannels should not be shared.
- When a child with a blood-borne infection (e.g. a child who is hepatitis-B-antigen-positive or HIV-infected or HIV indeterminate status) is cared for at home, carers should be supplied with disposable gloves and cleaning fluids.

PREVENTING EXPOSURE TO ZOONOSES

Animals in schools

Pets should be kept in enclosed spaces, which should be kept clean of waste. All animals should be handled by children only under close staff supervision. Hands should be washed after handling animals or animal wastes. Dogs and cats should be kept away from child play areas. This guidance applies as much to home as at school. However, special precautions need to be taken in schools. There are good educational reasons for having animals in school. Caring for the animals teaches responsibility, their presence is useful for teaching an appreciation of nature and living things and they help children to learn skills of observation.

However there can be health risks and the rules above need to be adhered to. Certain animals are notoriously liable to carry infection, notably reptiles, which have been implicated in outbreaks of *Salmonella* infection. Their presence in school is difficult to justify. Birds of the parrot family can carry psittacosis and others can be infected with histoplasmosis. That does not rule out birds, but they must come from a reputable dealer and donations of pet birds should be accepted on condition of a veterinary check. Handling of animals should be avoided except by children who are looking after animals. Even the most docile hamster or gerbil will bite if held roughly (see Animal and human bites, below) and rabbits and guinea pigs can transmit ringworm to humans. Concern sometimes arises when a school pet dies. However necropsy is hardly ever indicated.

Farm visits

In recent years many farmers have opened their farms to the public and encouraged children and schools to visit. Many thousands of children visit farms safely; however, these are workplaces and there are hazards, including potential exposure to zoonoses. Some serious incidents have taken place involving infection with *E. coli* O157, *Listeria*, *Salmonella*, etc. These animal infections can be acquired from the farm environment, i.e. children do not have to touch animals to acquire the infections. There are now codes of practice issued by the Health and Safety Executive that farms have to adhere to. In addition, there are simple precautions that all schools and parents should follow when visiting farms.

Precautions for school visits to farms

- Check that the farm is well managed and that the grounds and public areas are as clean as possible. Note that manure, slurry and sick animals present a particular risk of infection and animals must be prohibited from any outdoor picnic areas.
- Check that the farm has washing facilities adequate and accessible for the age of the children visiting, with running water, soap (preferably liquid) and disposable towels or hot-air dryers. Any drinking water taps should be appropriately designated in a suitable area.
- Explain to children that they cannot be allowed to eat or drink anything, including crisps, sweets, chewing gum, etc., while touring the farm or to put their fingers in their mouths because of the risk of infection.
- If children are in contact with or feeding farm animals, warn them not to place their faces against the animals or taste the animal feed.
- Ensure that all pupils wash and dry their hands thoroughly after contact with animals and particularly before eating and drinking.
- Meal-breaks or snacks should be taken well away from areas where animals are kept and pupils should be warned not to eat anything that may have fallen to the ground.
- Any crops produced on the farm should be thoroughly washed in drinking water before consumption.
- Ensure that pupils do not consume unpasteurised produce, e.g. milk or cheese.
- Ensure that all children wash their hands thoroughly before departure and that footwear is as free as possible from faecal material.

Animal and human bites (see also Chapter 12, p. 62)

This is a frequent cause of consultation and often the possibility of infection is raised. Bites should always be promptly cleaned and irrigated with a large amount of water or saline, cleaning away any debris. If the wound is extensive the child should be referred promptly to an Accident and Emergency Department. Tetanus immunisation status should be revived and immunisation given as necessary (see Chapter 101). There is no need to take cultures unless consultation has been delayed and there is evidence of infection. Prophylactic antibiotics are rarely needed but may be considered when there is a puncture wound, especially into a delicate area such as a joint, the hand or the face. Infections that have followed bites are:

- **From cats and dogs***: Staphylococci and streptococci, *Pasteurella*, *Capnocytophaga canimorsus* and various anaerobes
- **From humans**: Staphylococci and streptococci, various anaerobes, hepatitis B.

Co-amoxiclav or azithromycin are suitable agents.

Where an animal bite has taken place abroad the issue of rabies must be considered (see Chapter 90). Children with major educational difficulties have spread hepatitis B through biting and it is important that they and those caring for them are immunised against this infection (see Chapter 64).

VULNERABLE CHILDREN

Some children have medical conditions that make them especially vulnerable to infections that would rarely be serious in most children. Such children include those being treated for leukaemia or other cancers, children on high doses of steroids by mouth and children with conditions that seriously reduce immunity. Usually, schools or nurseries are made aware of such children through their parents or the carers of the School Health Service.

Such children are especially vulnerable to chickenpox or measles. If they are exposed to either of these infections parents/carers should be informed promptly so that they can seek further medical advice as necessary (see Chapters 22 and 23).

IMMUNISATION STATUS

- Those responsible for the health care of the child in the centre/school/nursery should have access to and renew their immunisation records. If any child is underimmunised, this should be rectified at the earliest opportunity.
- The health status of all employees must be checked before entering employment, with special attention to screening for tuberculosis and immunisation status.

PROTECTING PREGNANT STAFF IN SCHOOLS, NURSERIES AND HEALTH-CARE SETTINGS

Infection control practices are not that different for pregnant and non-pregnant staff coming into contact with children (teachers, nurses, doctors, assistants, etc.). All should be subject to pre-employment screening.

Particular issues arise with regards to chickenpox, rubella and parvovirus, all of which very occasionally harm the unborn child. If a pregnant woman is exposed to chickenpox in the first 20 weeks of pregnancy or right at the end of pregnancy (within 3 weeks of her expected date of delivery) she should be seen promptly by the doctor responsible for her antenatal care as she will probably need to have her blood tested to check she is already immune (see Chapter 42). All pregnant women should have had their rubella immunity checked. However, if there is exposure to rubella, a pregnant woman in any but the latest stages of

---

* While infections from other animals (hamsters, mice, etc.) are possible, they are not mentioned in the literature and must be very rare.

pregnancy (last trimester) should promptly contact the doctor giving her antenatal care.

Parvovirus is more difficult as the interventions to prevent damage of the fetus are not easy to give but, again, if a woman is exposed in the first half of pregnancy she should seek prompt medical advice (see Chapter 83). Cytomegalovirus (CMV) presents a risk but not one that can be easily dealt with. A number of children, especially younger ones, excrete CMV at some time and may pose a risk to the unborn child of their carer but since it cannot easily be predicted which child is excreting, and even prior infection does not guarantee immunity in the adult, this seems an inevitable hazard of caring for children (see also Further reading, below).

NEEDLESTICK INJURIES

A common source of anxiety, both parental and medical, is cases where a child has come into contact with a discarded needle found in the community. For the parents, often the immediate concern is that the needle came from a drug injector and that therefore there is a threat of HIV. In fact, the risk of this is usually vanishingly small: the level of HIV in drug injectors is often low, far lower than for hepatitis B infection, HIV does not survive for long outside the body and it is known that, even where there is a fresh needlestick injury in a hospital (e.g. where a doctor or nurse injures him/herself with a needle that has come out of a person known to be HIV-infected), the risk of actual transmission is only around 1 in 300.

A careful history must be taken. Quite often this reveals that in fact there has not been any actual injury. The risks of transmission of any infection if there has been an injury are small. The least small is with hepatitis B virus (HBV) because the virus can survive outside the body and the risk of transmission is far higher than for HIV. Usually it is justified to give a short course of HBV immunisation (see Chapter 64), to take some blood for testing for HBV markers (to make sure that the child was not already immune) and to store blood in the very unlikely event that the child is found later to have HIV or HCV infection and it needs to be shown whether this came from the needle exposure or was pre-existing. Although hepatitis C is quite transmissible, cases of HCV infection through this type of scenario are seemingly rarer than for hepatitis B, perhaps because hepatitis C does not survive well outside the body. There is no treatment to prevent HCV infection.

Of course, needlestick injuries are far more common in hospital, where care needs to taken over where and how needles are discarded. Children can squeeze their hands into the holes at the top of some types of sharps bins (this has happened!), so that these must not, for example, be placed on the floor or at toddler height.

PROTECTING CHILDREN FROM INFECTIONS IN STAFF

Essentially, the rules here are the same for excluding children (see Appendix V). Two exceptions to this concern hepatitis B (health-care staff) and tuberculosis. All health-care staff coming into direct contact with patients must have their hepatitis B immunity status checked, have complete immunisation and be shown to be immune. This is as much for their own protection as for that of children and older patients. All persons caring for children, including nurses, teachers and nursery nurses, require pre-employment screening for tuberculosis as there have been a number of cases of teachers passing their infection on to children.

MAKING PARENTS AWARE

- Upon a child's entry to nursery/school, parents must be made aware of the need to share information about illnesses that might be of a readily communicable nature in the educational setting, in the child or in any member of the immediate household.
- **When children are known to have been exposed to an important communicable disease**, e.g. meningococcal infection, the head of the centre, nursery or school should, following consultation with medical advisors, inform parents, preferably in writing, of any action to be taken.

CONSULTATION – SEEKING HELP AND ADVICE

The circumstances when consultation should occur cannot be strictly defined; however listed in Table 33.1 are conditions for which consultation and action may be required if they occur, or are strongly suspected, in a child, the family of a child, or a staff member. If in doubt it is always safer to promptly consult the local relevant health authorities, i.e. the Medical Officer for the centre/nursery/school, the Consultant in Communicable Disease Control (CCDC), the Environmental Health Department, who should be notified promptly (ie by phone that day) about cases of communicable diseases involving children or care providers in the child care setting. Action that may need to be taken is detailed under the sections for individual conditions in Part Two. Some recommendations for exclusion periods are contained in Appendix V; however, it is important that these should not be interpreted rigidly but following consultation.

Table 33.1 Infectious conditions requiring urgent medical consultation should they appear in the children, staff or families of children in a day nursery or school

Campylobacter	Hepatitis A or B	Ringworm (tinea)
Cryptosporidiosis	Impetigo	Rotavirus
Diphtheria*	Influenza	Rubella
E. coli	Measles	Salmonellosis
Food poisoning	Meningococcal disease	Shigella
Giardiasis	Pertussis	Tuberculosis
Haemophilus influenzae (type b) infection	Respiratory syncytial virus (bronchiolitis)	Typhoid and paratyphoid fevers

* Rare but very important when it occurs.

OUTBREAK CONTROL

Definition

An outbreak of infection may be defined either as two or more linked cases of the same illness, or as the situation when the observed number of cases unaccountably exceeds the expected number.

Objectives of control

The objectives in controlling an outbreak are:

- To reduce to a minimum the number of primary cases of illness – this involves the prompt recognition of the outbreak and identification and control of the source of the infection or contamination
- To reduce to a minimum the number of secondary cases of infection, by identifying cases and taking appropriate action to prevent any spread
- To prevent further episodes of illness by identifying continuing hazards and eliminating them or minimising the risk they pose

While outbreaks in schools and day care centres pose the greatest risk because of the potential for rapid and large-scale transmission of infection it needs to be remembered that family outbreaks affecting members of a single household account for the majority of outbreaks. And therefore most cases of infection seen in schools or nurseries will represent household or community transmission rather than transmission in the institution itself. However, this does not remove the responsibility of staff and their medical advisers in preventing secondary transmission occurring in the school.

The role of the Consultant in Communicable Disease Control (or equivalent public health doctor) is crucial. Their remit is the surveillance, prevention and control of all communicable disease among the population of the district. As such they work closely with microbiologists, other medical specialists, including paediatricians, and environmental health officers employed by the local authority.

Coordinated outbreak control plans should have been drawn up by health and local authorities in consultation with the CCDC, the Chief Environmental Health Officer, the Public Health Laboratory Service, local NHS Trusts and other bodies (e.g. water companies) as appropriate. These plans can be adapted to different types of outbreaks and are put into operation when the disease poses a health hazard to the local population, there are a large number of cases or the disease is unusual or poses a particular hazard. When an outbreak occurs or is suspected the PHLS Communicable Disease Surveillance Centre (020 8200 6868) or the Scottish Centre for Infection and Environmental Health (0141 300 110) should be informed. Both provide advice on a 24-hour basis and can provide personnel if invited.

FURTHER READING

Department of Health (1994) Management of outbreaks of foodborne illness. HMSO, London.

Mirza A, Wyatt M, Begue RE (1999) Infection control practices and the pregnant health care worker. Paediatr Inf Dis J 18: 18–22.

Part Two: Specific infections

Notifiable if dysenteric

ORGANISM

A protozoan parasite, *Entamoeba histolytica* exists as pathological potentially invasive trophozoites and a hardy infective cyst, which can exist for
many months in a moist environment. There are pathogenic and nonpathogenic strains identifiable by different isozymes. Nonpathogenic forms are
sometimes referred to as *E. dispar*.

EPIDEMIOLOGY

The organism is found worldwide; the major reservoir is man. Prevalence
is higher where sanitation is poor. It can act as a commensal or the parasite may invade from the gut but most infections are asymptomatic.
Infection is unusual in preschool children, especially infants, although when
infection occurs in young children it can be severe. Other factors predis-
posing to severe infection are immunosuppression and malnutrition.

Transmission

Contaminated water, faecal–oral route and by raw fruit and vegetables
exposed to contaminated water. Cysts pass through the stomach
unharmed and then form trophozoites in the small intestine, which go on
to affect the colon. Adults can have chronic infection and pass cysts for
years, although this is usually confined to nonpathogenic strains. Sexual
transmission has been recorded between adults by oral/anal sex.

Incubation period

Usually this is 2–4 weeks but it can be shorter and seemingly also occasionally extends to years.

NATURAL HISTORY AND CLINICAL FEATURES

Most infection is asymptomatic. Symptoms can be mild with constipation or
loose stools and abdominal distension, although amoebiasis is an unusual
cause of such presentations in children. Severe disease can be dysenteric
or nondysenteric. The dysenteric form (acute amoebic colitis) presents with
fever, abdominal pain, diarrhoea with blood and mucus and can proceed to
peritonitis. Nondysenteric amoebiasis is milder with intermittent diarrhoea
and abdominal pain. Invasion of the liver occurs rarely, causing abscesses.
Invasive disease is commonest in young adults rather than children.

Diagnosis

Fresh stool specimens (or specimens preserved in 10% formalin) will
often reveal trophozoites or cysts on microscopic examination in colonic
disease. However a single specimen may be insufficient to detect infection. Where there is diagnostic difficulty a rectal biopsy may be useful to
demonstrate invasive trophozoites. These will require specialist viewing

by an experienced microbiologist. Extraintestinal amoebiasis may also be difficult to detect or diagnose. When it is suspected, specialist advice should be sought and serology (fluorescent antibody test or ELISA) is often helpful. Liver abscess may be identified by ultrasound or computed tomography scan supplemented by serology.

MANAGEMENT

Asymptomatic carriage is treated with diloxanide furoate. Amoebic dysentery is treated with oral metronidazole, as is extragastrointestinal amoebiasis, where tinidazole can also be used. Rehydration may be required.

PREVENTION OF CASES

Water supplies should be treated to remove or kill cysts and foods that may have been contaminated, such as lettuces and other salads, should be washed carefully with treated water before consumption (see Chapter 26, p. 154). Enteric precautions (see Chapter 22, p. 214 for when hospitalised and Chapter 33, pp. 217–218, for when in the community) are indicated for patients with symptomatic or asymptomatic infection. Household contacts should be investigated for asymptomatic infection.

35 Aspergillosis

ORGANISM

Aspergillus fumigatus, *A. flavus* and other *Aspergillus* species. These are spore-bearing fungi.

EPIDEMIOLOGY

These species are ubiquitous in the environment. Spores in the atmosphere seem to be particularly prevalent at the sites of building works, farm buildings and aviaries. Pulmonary aspergillosis mainly affects individuals who are immunocompromised or have pre-existing lung disease such as cystic fibrosis or bronchiectasis. *Aspergillus* spp. may produce a fungal ball (aspergilloma) in those with lung cavities or cysts. Invasive *Aspergillus* infections almost exclusively affect immunocompromised individuals. Low-grade infection in sinuses and in the external auditory canal may occur in those with normal immunity.

Allergic bronchopulmonary aspergillosis mainly affects atopic individuals, particularly asthmatics. It can complicate cystic fibrosis but is relatively rare in childhood.

Transmission

This is by inhalation of spores. Individuals undergoing severe immunosuppression, as in bone marrow transplantation, may also develop aspergillosis associated with invasion of the organism from previously colonised sinuses.

Incubation period

Unknown.

NATURAL HISTORY AND CLINICAL FEATURES

Allergic bronchopulmonary aspergillosis presents with episodic wheezing. Brown sputum may be produced and sometimes there is a low-grade fever.

Infection with *Aspergillus* as a cause of exacerbation of symptoms in children with lung disorders such as cystic fibrosis is rare, although it is common to find the organism in the sputum. If it occurs it is likely to present with cough, increased sputum and haemoptysis. Aspergillomas may be asymptomatic and be found incidentally on chest X-ray or they may lead to haemoptysis, which is occasionally life-threatening.

Invasive aspergillosis affects patients undergoing prolonged myelosuppression as occurs in patients receiving intensive cytotoxic chemotherapy or bone marrow transplantation. It also occurs in patients with neutrophil function disorders such as chronic granulomatous disease. The infection most commonly enters through the lung, producing symptoms of cough, haemoptysis and fever with or without the clinical signs of pneumonia. Invasion of the blood stream results in disseminated infection, which may affect the brain, bones, liver and kidneys. Mortality is extremely high in disseminated disease.

Diagnosis

The finding of *Aspergillus* species in sputum in children with chronic lung disease has to be interpreted carefully in the context of the clinical picture. The diagnosis of invasive disease depends on the demonstration of characteristic fungal hyphae in tissue specimens with or without culture of the organism in Sabouraud's or other suitable medium. Antibody tests have proved disappointing in the diagnosis, possibly because patients with significant disease are usually immunocompromised.

In bronchopulmonary aspergillosis the chest X-ray shows flitting opacities, particularly in the perihilar regions. There is usually a marked eosinophilia in the blood, with a raised total IgE level. *Aspergillus*-specific IgE can be demonstrated using a radioallergosorbent test (RAST) or skin prick test.

MANAGEMENT

Allergic bronchopulmonary aspergillosis is treated with systemic corticosteroids. Maintenance inhaled corticosteroids may be required.

Invasive aspergillosis should be treated with systemic antifungals and the treatment of choice is amphotericin B (for further details see Chapter 24).

In view of the difficulties in confirming a diagnosis of invasive fungal infection, early empirical treatment with amphotericin is often initiated in immunosuppressed patients who develop fever with or without pneumonitis.

Surgical excision is the treatment of choice for aspergilloma and may sometimes have a role in the management of other forms of invasive disease.

PREVENTION OF CASES

Patients undergoing prolonged myelosuppressive treatment should, where possible, be cared for in facilities with filtered air to reduce spore exposure. This is particularly important if building works are nearby. In older children who are to undergo bone marrow transplantation, it is important to check for evidence of chronic sinus infection that might harbour *Aspergillus* species. Prophylactic regimens includes the use of low-dose systemic amphotericin given during periods of intense immunosuppression. Itraconazole given orally is also increasingly used in this context and for longer-term use in chronic granulomatous disease. There are as yet no published clinical trial data on these approaches. Oral itraconazole has variable bioavailability. An intravenous preparation as well as newer imidazole agents (e.g. voriconazole) are under evaluation.

FURTHER READING

Walmsley S, Devi S, King S et al (1993) Invasive aspergillosis in a pediatric hospital: a ten year review. Pediatr Infect Dis J 12: 673–682.

36 Botulism (infant and food-borne botulism)

ORGANISM

Clostridium botulinum is an anaerobic, spore-forming bacillus that produces neurotoxins. On the basis of the serological characteristics of the toxins there are seven types (A–G). Cases of botulism are occasionally caused by neurotoxins produced by other *Clostridium* species. The *C. botulinum* bacterium and its toxins are sensitive to boiling but spores require higher temperatures to ensure their destruction. The toxin irreversibly binds to the synaptic membrane of cholinergic nerves, preventing the release of acetylcholine and blocking neuromuscular transmission. This results in flaccid paralysis and autonomic dysfunction. As such, botulism is the opposite of tetanus, as this toxin is trophic for inhibitory neurones, causing spasm.

EPIDEMIOLOGY

There are three types of botulism; infant botulism, food-borne botulism and wound botulism. Infant botulism is due to the ingestion of *C. botulinum* or its spores, leading to colonisation of the gut and local production of neurotoxin (the young infant's gut is peculiarly susceptible to such colonisation). Food-borne botulism is a form of food poisoning or intoxication due to ingestion of food in which *C. botulinum* has produced toxin. It rarely affects children because the foods most commonly contaminated are rarely eaten by children. Wound botulism is due to the local production of toxin by the organism growing in wounds. It has been seen recently among injecting drug users in some countries. Most cases of infant botulism are due to neurotoxin type A or B while food-borne botulism is usually due to toxin types A, B or E, and occasionally types F or G.

C. botulinum is ubiquitous in the environment in that it has a spore-forming stage. Spores can be found in dust, soil, untreated water, the digestive tracts of animals and fish and occasionally in a number of foods. However food-borne botulism does not occur unless circumstances permit the growth of organisms and production of toxins. All three types of botulism are uncommon in industrialised countries. Wound botulism is exceptionally rare and has not been reported in the UK. Over 1000 cases of infant botulism have been reported worldwide but only five cases in the UK. Some 90% of cases are in infants less than 6 months old and 50% in infants under 3 months of age. Honey and corn syrup have been implicated as the dietary source in some cases in the USA, where spores have been found occasionally in honey. However no spores of *C. botulinum* were found in a survey of honey in the UK. Infant botulism in the USA has also been attributed to importation into homes of dust on clothes.

Cases of food-borne botulism often occur as outbreaks, which can involve considerable numbers through large-scale contamination of food stuffs. An important source of cases in the USA is from inadequately performed home preserving of meats, fish and vegetables. This has not been a recent source of cases in the UK, where there have been 32 cases (all ages), including three deaths, since 1977.

Transmission

Infant botulism is due to the ingestion of spores or bacteria while food-borne botulism arises from ingestion of preformed toxin in contaminated food. Person-to-person spread cannot take place.

Incubation period

In infant botulism there may be a period of between 3 days and 2 weeks between colonisation and symptoms appearing. In food-borne botulism symptoms appear rapidly, within 12–36 hours if toxin levels are high. Longer periods have been described (up to a week) when intoxication is light.

NATURAL HISTORY AND CLINICAL FEATURES

Infant botulism

Signs of intoxication in infants are nonspecific. The first sign is usually constipation followed by lethargy, poor feeding, drooling, hypotonia and general weakness. There is often a descending symmetrical weakness starting in the muscles innervated by the bulbar centres leading to a number of signs including decreased cry, poor suck and gag reflexes and loss of facial expression and eye control, followed by loss of deep tendon reflexes. Sudden apnoea and respiratory failure are the major life-threatening complications. However, with meticulous care prognosis is good, although recovery is slow as it requires sprouting of new terminal motor neurones to reinnervate muscle fibres and relapses can occur. Infant botulism is a rare but important differential diagnosis for the 'floppy baby syndrome'. It has also been implicated as a rare cause of sudden infant death syndrome (SIDS).

Food-borne botulism

Vomiting, diarrhoea or constipation and abdominal cramps may be initial features. However clinical features are mostly caused by toxin affecting the nervous system. In older children and adults cranial nerve palsies predominate, causing, among other bulbar signs, dysphonia, ptosis and double vision. Mental function and sensation are generally well-preserved. A generalised weakness and descending paralysis is ominous and death may occur at all ages because of respiratory failure or superinfection. The differential diagnosis includes myasthenia gravis, which will respond to an endrophonium test. Acute inflammatory polyneuropathies (such as Guillain–Barré syndrome) usually show sensory changes, develop areflexia early and rarely begin with cranial nerve signs. Patients with polio are usually unimmunised (for polio) and have a history of a febrile illness.

In both food-borne and infant botulism the condition may last for 6–8 months. However, the condition is potentially self-limiting and with meticulous supportive care a complete recovery can be achieved.

Diagnosis

Because of the nonspecific clinical features, demonstration of toxin (from food, serum and faeces) or culture of the organism from food is essential for diagnosis for all types of botulism. Once the diagnosis is suggested clinicians and microbiologists should take specialist advice and refer specimens for testing.* All samples, including the suspect food, should be sent urgently if the diagnosis of botulism is considered likely. For infant botulism the specimens of choice are stools and enema fluid as they may be the only specimens containing *C. botulinum* or its toxin. Stool specimens may be difficult to obtain because of constipation, in which case a rectal wash-out may be justified.

MANAGEMENT

The course of both infant and food-borne botulism is often prolonged. Specialist advice is essential with all but the mildest cases being managed in intensive care until the severity of intoxication can be ascertained. Much of the treatment is supportive and includes careful attention to respiratory status, hydration and nutrition. In infant botulism, elective ventilation is preferable to awaiting the development of apnoea and ventilatory failure.

In food-borne botulism an equine-based antitoxin is available and its use should be considered for symptomatic cases†, at an early stage as application of antitoxin is ineffective after the toxin has fixed to tissues.

---

* In the UK the Food Hygiene Laboratory, Central Public Health Laboratory, 61 Colindale Avenue, London NW9 5HT, tel. 020 8200 4400, provides specialist testing and advice.
† Small stocks of the antitoxin are currently (2000) held at centres around the country. Details of current centres are available from the Food Hygiene Laboratory (see above).

However, antitoxin should be given with great care because of the high incidence of adverse reactions produced by the equine-based serum. Antibiotics are only used to treat secondary infection.

In infant botulism, antibiotics are also only used to treat secondary infections, e.g. pneumonias. Antitoxin is not recommended for infant botulism because of the high incidence of adverse reactions and the lack of evidence of any efficacy in the face of ongoing toxin release.

PREVENTION OF FURTHER CASES

Prevention of botulism is by meticulous attention to instructions in food preparation, especially in home-preserving. All toxin is inactivated by heating at 80°C for 30 minutes and spores are destroyed by heating to over 120°C for 2 minutes. However not all foodstuffs are suitable for such treatment. Once a case of infant or food-borne botulism is suspected, the Consultant in Communicable Disease Control or the Director of Public Health must be contacted immediately so that other persons who have shared the food can be identified, along with other food that may also be contaminated. The Communicable Disease Surveillance Centre and the Food Hygiene Laboratory, Central Public Health Laboratory must also be informed (see above, p. 231) and the latter will assist in diagnosis.

FURTHER READING

Brett M (1994) Infant botulism. Quarterly Communicable Disease Review. J Publ Hlth Med 16: 361–363.

Midura TF (1996) Update: infant botulism. Clin Microbiol Rev 9: 119–125.

37 Brucellosis

ORGANISM

These are Gram-negative coccobacilli and include *Brucella melitensis*, *B. suis*, *B. abortus* and *B. canis*.

EPIDEMIOLOGY

Infection occurs in cattle, sheep, pigs, goats and humans. The rare cases seen in the UK are usually acquired in the Mediterranean.

Transmission

Person-to-person infection does not occur. Although infection in adults usually results from occupational exposure (slaughterhouses) the disease does occasionally occur in children as a result of ingestion of infected milk.

Incubation period

Difficult to determine, but thought to be 2–3 months.

NATURAL HISTORY AND CLINICAL FEATURES

This is often a mild infection, particularly when caused by *B. abortus*. A more serious illness is caused by *B. melitensis*, with fever, chills, weight loss and arthralgia. Clinical signs include hepatomegaly and splenomegaly. Occasionally, meningoencephalitis is present.

Diagnosis

Culture of blood, bone marrow or urine. Prolonged culture is needed and serological tests are available.

TREATMENT

Oral doxycycline for 3–6 weeks is the treatment of choice for older children and adults. In children under 12 years co-trimoxazole 60 mg/kg/day (maximum 3g/day) in divided doses for 3–6 weeks is used. Addition of rifampicin may redice the relapse rate. In severe disease gentamicin should be added to make a triple combination.

PREVENTION OF FURTHER CASES

Eradication of brucellosis in cattle, swine and other animals and avoidance of unpasteurised milk. The local Consultant in Communicable Disease Control (or their public health equivalent) and veterinary officials should be alerted to any cases.

38 Burkholderia

ORGANISM

These Gram-negative bacilli are in rRNA group II of the family Pseudomonadaceae. Pathogens include *Burkholderia cepacia*, *B. pseudomallei* and *B. mallei*.

EPIDEMIOLOGY

B. cepacia is an important opportunist pathogen, especially in patients with cystic fibrosis (CF) and chronic granulomatous disease. It is also a soil saprophyte and a plant pathogen (causing onion rot). Certain strains (or genomovars) are able to spread much more readily between CF patients and are able to cause fatal disease. One lineage (ET-12: Edinburgh Toronto electrophoretic type 12), emerged in the 1980s and affected CF units throughout the world. There is evidence that infection/colonisation with a less virulent *B. cepacia* does not prevent superinfection and death with *B. cepacia* ET-12. It is a late (usually in adolescence and early adulthood) coloniser in CF but does spread from person to person. Transmission can also occur via fomites.

B. pseudomallei causes melioidosis, which is most often acquired in south-east Asia and northern Australia but cases have been reported from India, Central America, Turkey and Africa. Infection can be acquired both as a zoonosis and from the environment but the latter is much more important. Infection can be acquired by inhalation or through cuts and abrasions. The age–distribution curve shows two peaks, one at 9 years and the other at over 65 years. Disease can occur years after initial infection and it appears that *B. pseudomallei* remains dormant in macrophages. There is a strong association between developing disease and having diabetes mellitus. *B. mallei* causes glanders, which is a zoonosis acquired in particular from horses.

NATURAL HISTORY AND CLINICAL FEATURES

In CF, acquisition of a pathogenic strains of *B. cepacia* is associated with diminishing lung function and poor weight gain. It may also progress to the fatal cepacia syndrome where the bacterium causes severe pneumonia and bacteraemia.

The clinical spectrum of melioidosis is very broad – up to 60% will have bacteraemia and community-acquired sepsis syndrome. There can be multifocal metastic abscesses, meningitis or, if acquired by inhalation, pneumonia. Parotitis is present in a third of paediatric cases.

Diagnosis

Diagnosis is by detection of the bacteria by culture, although nonculture detection (polymerase chain reaction) is also available. The bacteria can be difficult to identify. *B. pseudomallei* requires category III containment when grown.

TREATMENT

B. cepacia can be resistant to most available antibiotics and can prove very difficult to treat. Treatment should be guided by the sensitivity pattern of the particular isolate and nebulised or intravenous administration of antibiotic combinations may be necessary.

B. pseudomallei also tends to be multidrug-resistant. Intravenous ceftazidime with or without co-trimoxazole decreases mortality rates by about 50% (i.e. from 74% to 37%). Treatment should be given for at least 2 weeks.

PREVENTION OF FURTHER CASES

For *B. cepacia* a policy of segregating infected from noninfected patients in hospital and at social events (camps, etc.) has greatly decreased the incidence of new cases.

There is no vaccine for *B. pseudomallei* and prevention is by avoiding contact with the bacteria.

ORGANISM

Campylobacters are motile, non-spore-forming Gram-negative rods. *Campylobacter jejuni* is a Gram-negative bacillus (some other campylobacters – such as *C. lari* – also cause diarrhoea and *C. fetus* is also an important cause of neonatal meningitis or septicaemia).

EPIDEMIOLOGY

Infection with campylobacters represents a worldwide zoonosis and the main reservoir of infection is in the gastrointestinal tract of wild and domesticated animals and birds, although the main source of human infections is thought to be from farm stock. Many infected animals and birds develop a lifelong carrier state and meat from slaughtered animals and poultry is frequently contaminated from intestinal contents. Numbers of reported cases of *Campylobacter* infection in humans have been rising steadily in recent years in the UK so that they are now a more important source of food poisoning reports than *Salmonella* species. Undercooked chickens and unpasteurised milk are a source of outbreaks. Cats and dogs may also act as a source, with puppies and kittens being more likely to transmit infections to children. In humans, gastroenteritis due to *C. jejuni* occurs in all ages worldwide and is also a common cause of travellers' diarrhoea. Child-to-child spread occurs in families but seems rare in day-care centres. In the UK there is often a summer peak of infection. In low-income countries asymptomatic infection seems to be more common. *C. jejuni* may be transmitted perinatally, causing a neonatal gastroenteritis, while *C. fetus* will more often result in a severe infection in the baby, which may be fatal.

Transmission

Transmission to humans is usually by ingestion of contaminated foods (including unpasteurised milk, improperly cooked poultry and contaminated water) or direct contact with young animals (puppies and lambs on farm visits), but the main source of infection has yet to be clarified. An unexpected source of infection has been wild birds (typically magpies) raiding and contaminating milk bottles on doorsteps. Person-to-person spread is uncommon but does occur. Organisms are excreted while patients are symptomatic but excretion may also continue for several weeks after the start of the illness. Appropriate antibiotic treatment rapidly terminates excretion.

Incubation period

Usually 3–5 days with a range of 1–10 days.

NATURAL HISTORY AND CLINICAL FEATURES

For *C. jejuni* this is variable and asymptomatic infections occur. Principal features are those of an acute enteric infection: diarrhoea, fever, malaise, abdominal pain, nausea and vomiting. The stool may show mucus, blood and pus. The illness is over in a few days and may be mild. However, infection may also mimic acute appendicitis and it can also be severe and prolonged, especially in older children and adults. Febrile convulsions can occur. In prolonged cases it may be mistaken for ulcerative colitis. Uncommon manifestations include reactive arthritis, meningitis and Reiter's and Guillain–Barré syndromes.

Diagnosis

Rapid presumptive diagnosis can be achieved by microscopic examination (darkfield or Gram staining) of stool smears; however, the technique is not easy and laboratories may need to be notified that the infection is suspected. Definitive diagnosis is by culture of *C. jejuni*. The organism may also be isolated from blood in systemic infections, as can *C. fetus*.

MANAGEMENT

For infection with *C. jejuni*, treatment is symptomatic in most cases (see Chapter 18). Enteric precautions should be applied, although they are less crucial than for other, more infectious gastrointestinal infections. Severely affected children and adults should be given a 5–7-day course of antibiotics such as erythromycin, with ciprofloxacin as an alternative although the latter is not licensed for use in children in the UK. Also, ciprofloxacin resistance is increasing in *C. jejuni* so early assessment of response and antimicrobial sensitivity testing are important.

PREVENTION OF FURTHER CASES

When more than one case occurs, the Consultant in Communicable Disease Control or Director of Public Health should be informed in case a common source outbreak is occurring. See also Chapter 33.

Pasteurisation of milk, provision of clean water, proper cooking of poultry and deterring wild birds from raiding 'doorstep' milk will prevent many cases. Children visiting farms need to be supervised to ensure that hand-washing precautions should be applied (see Chapter 33). Enteric precautions need to be applied for managing symptomatic cases; however, if these are well-applied to affected hospital workers and infected food handlers they need not be excluded.

40 Candidiasis (thrush, moniliasis)

For systemic candidiasis, see Chapter 24

ORGANISM

Candida albicans, a yeast, is the most common pathogen, but C. *tropicalis* and others can be important in immunocompromised individuals.

EPIDEMIOLOGY

The organism is found worldwide. It colonises the skin and mucous membranes. Colonisation is increased by the use of broad-spectrum antibiotics. Oral and perineal thrush is common in neonates, and vaginitis in women of childbearing age. It can be sexually transmitted. Chronic mucocutaneous candidiasis may be associated with endocrine disorders or immunodeficiency. Systemic candidiasis is very unusual in normal hosts. Premature babies, immunodeficient patients and those with indwelling catheters may develop fungaemia with multi-organ disease or extensive superficial disease.

Transmission

Transmission is via person-to-person contact and contaminated feeding bottles, dummies, etc.

Incubation period

This is variable and poorly documented, but probably 2–5 days for oral thrush.

NATURAL HISTORY AND CLINICAL FEATURES

Oral thrush presents as white areas on the mucous membranes of the mouth. They may look like milk patches but leave a raw area when scraped off. The mouth may be sore, making it difficult to feed. In the immunocompromised patient there may only be raw areas rather than white patches. In the napkin region there is a clearly demarcated edge to the area of inflammation and satellite lesions are common.

Diagnosis is usually clinical. The organism is so common on mucous membranes and skin that isolation of the organism from suspect lesions in these sites cannot be taken as diagnostic. However when *C. albicans* invades tissue it produces pseudohyphae and detection of these by direct microscopy and Gram-stained smears is a valuable adjunct to clinical diagnosis.

MANAGEMENT

Topical nystatin is first-line therapy. Miconazole can also be used. In perineal disease in infants, oral treatment should be given in addition to topical treatment of the lesions. Hygiene is also very important. Strict disinfection of feeding bottles and dummies is essential and wet napkins should be changed as soon as possible. Once inadequate hygiene has been excluded, recurrent candidiasis should raise the possibility of an impairment of immunity and the appropriate investigations should be undertaken (see Chapter 21). Systemic treatment with fluconazole may be useful for recurrent or persistent infection.

PREVENTION OF FURTHER CASES

Dummies, feeding bottles and other objects destined for a baby's mouth must not be shared. Where eradication is difficult, sterilisation by boiling may be necessary. Treatment of *Candida* on the breastfeeding mother's nipples may be necessary to prevent reinfection of the baby. Prophylactic treatment with nonabsorbable agents or fluconazolis used in patients undergoing intensive myelosuppressive treatment (see Chapter 22).

41 Cat-scratch fever

ORGANISM

A small bacterium – *Bartonella henselae*.

EPIDEMIOLOGY

This is an uncommon infection but it occurs worldwide.

Transmission

It is believed that this occurs when a cat (usually a kitten) scratches a human. There is no evidence of person-to-person infection.

Incubation period

A papule appears 3–10 days after the scratch. Lymphadenopathy follows 2–6 weeks later.

NATURAL HISTORY AND CLINICAL FEATURES

The presenting complaint is lymphadenopathy, which may progress to suppuration. Usually there is a history of a cat scratch followed by the appearance of a small papule. Fever and malaise may not occur. A small number of cases with hepatosplenic granulomata have been described. These were seen in children with persistent fever both with and without an external lymphadenopathy and cat scratch or superficial papule.

Diagnosis

From the history and presence of necrotising granuloma on lymph node biopsy.

Cat-scratch disease may be confused with atypical tuberculosis. In some cases, microorganisms are identified on the Warthin–Starry silver stain. The bacterium can be cultured on simple media.

Management

Aspiration of lymph nodes except as a diagnostic procedure is not indicated. Rifampicin and azithromycin have been used in some cases of abdominal granulomas and was probably effective. In most cases of lymphadenitis recovery occurs without treatment.

42 Chickenpox and herpes zoster (varicella zoster)

ORGANISM

Varicella-zoster virus (VZV) is also known as human herpesvirus 3 (HHV-3); it is an enveloped DNA virus. There is only one serotype.

EPIDEMIOLOGY

Humans are the only reservoir of infection. The disease occurs throughout the year but is commoner in spring and winter. Chickenpox is highly infectious, with an attack rate of up to 90%. The majority of individuals become infected in early or middle childhood and remain immune into adulthood. In the UK and the USA, in the past 20 years, first infections have increasingly been taking place in older age groups. As the likelihood of severe morbidity and even mortality (estimated at 1 per 50 000 cases in children and 1 per 4000 cases in adults) increases with age of occurrence, this secular change is of significance. However, more morbidity results from herpes zoster (recrudescence of infection), with a lifetime risk of about 25%. In England and Wales there are estimated to be 3000 admissions to hospital for chickenpox (60% are children) and 6000 admissions for herpes zoster.

Though varicella infection in childhood is normally benign it may be severe in the immunosuppressed child, in the newborn infant when infection develops in the mother close to the time of delivery and in those with severe dermatological problems such as Ehlers–Danlos syndrome. It can give rise to the fetal varicella syndrome when a nonimmune pregnant woman (c. 5% of the population) becomes infected in the first half of pregnancy. The disease is more severe in males.

Transmission

Transmission is by direct contact, by droplet infection or through recently soiled materials such as handkerchiefs. The period of infectivity is from 1–2 days prior to eruption of the rash (when infectivity is maximal) and until 5 days after onset in an immunocompetent individual. In immunocompromised patients the course of the illness (and infectiousness) is prolonged, and patients should be considered infectious as long as new lesions (vesicles) continue to appear on the skin.

Incubation period

From 11 days to 20 days, with the commonest period 14–17 days. The incubation can be prolonged in someone given varicella-zoster immune globulin. The period is somewhat shorter in the neonate infected perinatally, with the usual period between appearance of the rash in the mother and clinical signs in the neonate being 8–16 days; shorter periods have been recorded.

NATURAL HISTORY AND CLINICAL FEATURES

Primary infection with VZV results in chickenpox. There may be a short (less than 24 hours) coryzal prodrome followed by fever and an itchy, vesicular rash. Severity varies and asymptomatic infections occur. Crops of vesicles, sparser on the limbs than on the trunk, appear over 3–5 days. The most common complication is staphylococcal infection of the skin. Other complications are unusual in immunocompetent children but are protean, including hepatitis, thrombocytopenia, arthritis, glomerulonephritis, bacterial superinfection (staphylococcal and pneumococcal pneumonias sometimes associated with empyema and pleural effusion), cerebellar ataxia, hemiplegia, postinfective polyneuropathy and encephalitis. Aspirin given during the illness is thought to increase the risk of Reye's syndrome. Recurrences are unusual but have been described in immunocompetent children.

Following chickenpox the virus persists as a latent infection in the dorsal root ganglia and may reappear following reactivation of the virus as herpes zoster (shingles), a painful vesicular rash in the dermatome of the affected nerves (see Plate 2). Zoster occurs in immunocompetent children but is more common in adults. Zoster may occur in children who have not had chickenpox themselves, if their mothers had chickenpox during pregnancy.

In adults the acute illness of varicella, fever and constitutional disturbance is more severe and pneumonia is a more common complication than in children. Immunosuppressed children have continued cropping of lesions, generalised zoster, encephalitis, pancreatitis, hepatitis and pneumonia.

Infection in pregnancy (see also pp. 28–29)

Chickenpox in a pregnant woman, especially in the third trimester, is frequently severe for the woman, with a considerably raised risk of chickenpox pneumonia and other complications. Regardless of whether this occurs there are also risks for the fetus.

There is heightened risk of spontaneous abortion in early pregnancy and intrauterine death later. Infection during the first 20–25 weeks of pregnancy may result in varicella embryopathy (the 'fetal varicella syndrome'). The risk is greatest in weeks 13–20 (around 2–3%) and lower before this (around 0.4%). Such congenital varicella has not been seen after the 20th week of pregnancy. There are many signs, including the following. Cicatricial skin lesions tend to follow a dermatomal pattern. Bone and muscle hypoplasia, normally in one limb, results in atrophy, and there may also be neurological, ophthalmological, gastrointestinal and genitourinary abnormalities. Low birth weight is almost invariable. The condition may be difficult to diagnose prenatally but is seen in only 2% of infants whose mothers acquired infection in the first 20 weeks of pregnancy. Exposure to VZV late in pregnancy or shortly after birth in a nonimmune mother puts the neonate at risk of severe, overwhelming varicella with a particularly high mortality from varicella pneumonia. The risk rises from 7 days before birth and seems to be greatest if the mother develops a rash in the period from 5 days before birth to 2 days after. The attack rate is high and there is a substantial neonatal mortality.

Diagnosis in the infant is usually made on clinical features. Virus isolated from vesicle fluid can be identified by electron microscopy, virus culture and specific monoclonal antibodies. Anti-VZV antibodies can be confirmed by enzyme immunoassay but such tests are usually used to demonstrate immunity in an individual exposed to VZV. Some laboratories may have access to polymerase chain reaction (PCR).

MANAGEMENT

Varicella-zoster immunoglobulin (VZIG) may be given to high-risk individuals to prevent infection and aciclovir may be used if infection has already occurred.

Treatment of the infected neonate

High-dose intravenous aciclovir (10–20 mg/kg/8 h) for 14 days at the first sign of any symptoms.

Treatment of infected immunocompetent children

Symptomatic treatment only is required in childhood but **aspirin should never be used as an antipyretic**. Children with chickenpox should not be admitted to hospital unless absolutely necessary because of the risk to immunosuppressed patients. Those hospitalised with proved or suspected varicella should be barrier-nursed in isolation. Children may gain relief from itching by use of local antipruritics.

The infected child with deficient cell-mediated immunity

Intravenous aciclovir should be given at the first sign of infection. Secondary bacterial infections of the skin or lungs may need specific treatment. *Staphylococcus aureus* is one of the commonest pathogens in such circumstances.

PREVENTION OF FURTHER CASES

Exposed immunosuppressed children

The immunosuppressed child (see Chapter 22 for definition) should be given VZIG if known to be varicella-seronegative and in close contact with a case of chickenpox or shingles. This includes children on systemic steroids and children infected with human immunodeficiency virus. If VZIG is not available, commercial normal intravenous immunoglobulin may be used (see Appendix VI).

Pregnant women
(See also Chapter 3.)

Exposure in early and mid-pregnancy
Pregnant women exposed to varicella will usually be VZV-immune and there is almost always an opportunity to test for anti-VZV antibodies before having to give VZIG. The risk of varicella syndrome seems highest in the second trimester (2–3% risk) and lower in the first trimester (around 0.4% risk). It is unclear whether VZIG given following exposure will protect the fetus against varicella syndrome; however, if the woman is susceptible and in the first 20 weeks of pregnancy VZIG is usually given and is likely to be successful in at least modifying the maternal disease. Herpes zoster in pregnancy seems to confer little risk to the fetus and does not justify intervention. Although there is less evidence that VZIG is needed later in pregnancy, it may also be given to women between 21 and 36 weeks gestation.

Exposure in late pregnancy
If the woman is susceptible and near term (within 4 weeks), then VZIG should be given. Although it may not prevent infection, it will usually ameliorate the severity of infection when given up to 10 days after contact.

Exposed neonates
Varicella-zoster immunoglobulin should be given to the newborn if the mother has developed varicella or herpes zoster in the 7 days before or after birth. VZIG should also be given to any exposed premature neonate (prior to 30 weeks or under 1 kg birth weight) even if the mother is immune, because maternal antibody is poorly transferred to the preterm fetus. Intravenous aciclovir is sometimes used prophylactically in the mother and in her baby where maternal infection occurs just before delivery.

Hospital outbreaks
A number of hospital occupational health departments enquire routinely about prior chickenpox in staff and test those without a history for antibody to VZV. Susceptible staff (history and anti-VZV-negative) can sometimes then be excluded from contact with vulnerable patients from 8–21 days after exposure and may monitor their own condition for varicella.

Immunisation
A live attenuated vaccine is available on a named patient basis from SmithKline Beecham Pharmaceuticals (Mundells, Welwyn Garden City, Herts, AL7 1EY). From 9 months up to and including 12 years one dose of 0.5 ml is required. For those older, two doses separated by at least 6 weeks are necessary. It is thought to give at least 6 years of immunity in immunocompetent individuals. In the USA the vaccine is now included as part of the universal immunisation programme and is given at the same

time as the first dose of MMR. The vaccine is not licensed at present (2000) and cannot be recommended as part of the routine schedule in the UK. As the vaccine is live, specialist advice should be sought when it is given to immunocompromised children and it may be necessary to stop immunosuppressive therapy for a time (see also Chapter 5).

43 Chlamydial infections

C. trachomatis ophthalmia neonatorum is notifiable

Chlamydia species are obligate intracellular parasites which are a delineated group of bacteria distinct from other eubacteria. *C. trachomatis* and *C. pneumoniae* only have human hosts while *C. psittaci* is also found in domestic animals and birds.

CHLAMYDIA TRACHOMATIS

ORGANISM

C. trachomatis. Some serotypes (A–C) cause endemic trachoma and others (D–K) sexually transmitted infections. Type L causes lymphogranuloma venereum.

EPIDEMIOLOGY

This is the commonest cause of treatable sexually transmitted infection in the UK and other industrialised countries. In the UK, prevalence surveys among sexually active women under age 35 years frequently find prevalences of infection to be around 3–4%, with higher prevalences (6–8%) among women having terminations or attending STD clinics. Prevalence is highest among younger sexually active women (16–19-year-olds) and is often asymptomatic. If the mother is infected, up to 50% of infants develop conjunctivitis after delivery and almost half of untreated infants with conjunctivitis will develop pneumonia. *C. trachomatis* ophthalmia is more common than that due to the gonococcus and is notifiable. Identification in the genital tract of older children implies sexual abuse or early sexual intercourse. In low-income countries, infection with *C. trachomatis* is a very important cause of trachoma and blindness.

Transmission

The neonate acquires infection during passage through the birth canal; adults through sexual intercourse. In low-income countries, eye infection occurs through close person-to-person contact.

Incubation period

Neonatal chlamydia develops a few days to several weeks after birth (see below). Adult sexually acquired infection seems to appear about a week after intercourse with an infected person.

NATURAL HISTORY AND CLINICAL FEATURES

In infants a purulent neonatal conjunctivitis may develop 5–14 days after birth and cannot be distinguished on clinical appearances from gonococcal or other infections. Inadequate treatment, e.g. with chloramphenicol, may result in recurrence and, rarely, in corneal scarring. Pneumonia may develop 4–6 weeks after birth and is associated with poor feeding, a cough and tachypnoea. The chest X-ray shows hyperinflation and generalised patchy shadowing. Pneumonia, although requiring treatment, is often self-limiting but the outcome may be more serious in the preterm infant with coexistent chronic lung disease (bronchopulmonary dysplasia). Infection in the adolescent male often leads to nonspecific/nongonococcal urethritis and in the female to salpingitis, chronic pelvic inflammatory disease and possible infertility.

Diagnosis

A Gram stain should be performed quickly on the exudate in all cases of purulent conjunctivitis, to exclude gonococcal infection. Because *C. trachomatis* is an intracellular bacterium the specimen should include cells from the conjunctivae collected by firmly drawing a cotton-wool swab over the everted lower eyelid. Rapid diagnostic tests detecting antigen using monoclonal antibodies (direct fluorescent antibody – DFA) have been introduced and allow diagnosis of *C. trachomatis* from a smear on a microscopic slide. An enzyme-linked immunosorbent assay (ELISA) and acid-based tests (PCR, LCR) are also available and increasingly used. The rapid diagnostic tests may be too insensitive to detect organisms in nasopharyngeal or tracheal aspirate for diagnosis of pneumonia but are recommended for use in conjunctivitis.

For infections in adolescents and adults noninvasive amplification tests, polymerase chain reactions (PCR) and ligase chain reaction (LCR) use urine specimens. These are highly sensitive but all these tests, including the ELISA, may yield false-negative results. The definitive tissue-culture test should be performed when there is a suspicion of sexually transmitted disease in children following sexual abuse (see Chapter 20).

Management

A topical eye preparation (e.g. tetracycline) is used in combination with oral erythromycin in the treatment of chlamydial ophthalmia. Oral erythromycin must be given to reduce the risk of relapse of conjunctivitis when a topical preparation is discontinued and to prevent development of pneumonia. Erythromycin is used for treatment of pneumonia and there is good evidence that it can be used alone in management of ophthalmia. Children with genital infections should be treated with erythromycin, and adolescents with tetracycline or doxycycline. Azithromycin is increasingly being used among adults with genital infection because it is effective as a single dose. Parents of infants with neonatal ophthalmia should be investigated and treated in a genitourinary medicine clinic.

PREVENTION OF FURTHER CASES

Prophylactic topical eye treatments given at birth will not reliably prevent development of ophthalmia neonatorum due to *C. trachomatis*. There is a strong case for screening for *Chlamydia* among all women having terminations of pregnancy or receiving antenatal care. Since 1998 it has been policy in England and Wales to undertake opportunistic screening in general practice (i.e. offering screening to all those attending for other reasons) for genital chlamydia among sexually active adolescent girls and young women (under age 25 years) and older women with recent new partners. All those testing positive (and their sexual partners) should receive treatment.

CHLAMYDIA PNEUMONIAE

ORGANISM

C. pneumoniae is an obligate intracellular parasite. This was referred to as the TWAR strain and has distinct morphological and serological differences from *C. psittaci* and *C. trachomatis*.

EPIDEMIOLOGY

This organism is found worldwide, with man as the only host. Antibodies are uncommon in preschool children, rising among teenagers so that 50% of the 20–30-year-old group are positive. Prospective studies in young adults have suggested that up to 20% of lower respiratory tract infections are caused by this organism. It has been suggested that infection with *C. pneumoniae* increases the risk of arterial disease in later life.

Transmission

By aerosol from person to person.

Incubation period

More than 10 days, considered to be around 3 weeks.

NATURAL HISTORY AND CLINICAL FEATURES

The infection is thought to be spread by droplets and the incubation period is more than 10 days. Most infections resemble those caused by *Mycoplasma pneumoniae* with fever, cough, malaise, headache, sore throat and pharyngitis. Children may be asymptomatic or only moderately ill. However, a small number of infections result in severe disease, respiratory failure and pleural effusion. Auscultation of the chest may identify crackles, and chest X-ray may show a patchy infiltrate restricted to only part of the lungs.

Diagnosis

Culture is difficult and diagnosis is usually made on serology. Criteria for diagnosis of infection have been defined and are as follows: a fourfold rise of IgG titre, or a single IgM titre of 1 in 16 or greater, or a single IgG titre of 1:512 or higher. PCR detection is increasingly available.

MANAGEMENT

Because studies have shown that the organism is slow to clear with antibiotics, long courses are recommended: for the older child, doxycycline 21 days or erythromycin for the same period for younger children.

PREVENTION OF FURTHER CASES

No action is needed.

CHLAMYDIA PSITTACI

ORGANISM

C. psittaci, a bacterium that is an obligate intracellular pathogen. It differs from *C. trachomatis* by lacking glycogen in the inclusions. There are several serovars, with preferences for different hosts.

EPIDEMIOLOGY

This infection occurs worldwide. Although most cases occur in adults, children may be affected. Disease occurs among individuals or in families exposed to infected psittacine birds (parrot family – parrots, cockatiels and budgerigars), turkeys, pigeons and ducks. Cats, sheep, goats and cattle can also be infected. Birds with this infection usually appear unwell, with anorexia, ruffled feathers and green droppings. Outbreaks have been reported in workers from duck and turkey processing plants. Infection in sheep during lambing can be transmitted to pregnant women and result in spontaneous abortion or a neonate with severe infection (sepsis neonatorum).

Transmission

Person-to-person spread by aerosol is rare. Birds can excrete this organism intermittently and do not necessarily appear unwell.

Incubation period

From 5 to 21 days.

NATURAL HISTORY AND CLINICAL FEATURES

The onset of illness is abrupt, with fever, cough and often severe headache. Examination of the chest reveals crackles. Chest X-ray usually shows signs of patchy infiltrates and sometimes pleural effusions. The white blood cell count is of little diagnostic help but liver function may be abnormal.

Diagnosis

A history of contact with psittacine or other birds at risk of infection is invariably a feature. Culture of *C. psittaci* is not available but the diagnosis can be confirmed by serology. A fourfold rise in complement fixation antibodies is considered diagnostic, although the test is genus-specific so that infection with *C. pneumoniae* may produce high titres.

MANAGEMENT

Treatment is with oral erythromycin, or doxycycline in the older child. Treatment for 7–10 days is recommended.

PREVENTION OF FURTHER CASES

When pet birds die with suggestive symptoms they should be examined by a veterinary pathologist. If suspected birds cannot be killed then the droppings may be examined, but discuss first with microbiologists. If infection is confirmed, exposed individuals should be made aware of the most likely signs of infection (fever and respiratory symptoms). The cage of the dead bird should be thoroughly disinfected and surveillance maintained over other exposed birds.

44 Cholera

Notifiable disease

ORGANISM

Widespread epidemic disease is associated with *Vibrio cholerae* serogroup O1, a Gram-negative motile rod-like bacteria. There are two biotypes, classical and El Tor; the latter has mostly dominated the seventh pandemic. El Tor is further subdivided into three subtypes: Ogawa, Inaba and Hikojima. In 1992 a new and distinct strain causing epidemic cholera appeared, *V. cholerae* O139. Other species may cause diarrhoea but not epidemics.

EPIDEMIOLOGY

Humans are a reservoir of infection, along with algae and plankton in salt water and estuaries. After 1961 what is known as the 'seventh pandemic' of cholera spread from south Asia to south-east Asia, Africa, the Middle East, some parts of southern Europe and finally (in 1991) South America, from which it had been absent for 100 years. In 1992 an outbreak of cholera due to *V. cholerae* serogroup O139 appeared in South Asia and has since spread rapidly in Asia. Some authorities are characterising this as the start of the eighth pandemic. In 1999 approximately 254 300 cases were reported to the World Health Organization, including 9175 deaths. Attack rates can be 10% or more in nonimmune populations. Worldwide case fatality rates of 2–3% are cited.

Refugees and other displaced persons are especially liable to experience epidemics, which also occur frequently after natural disasters as where health and hygiene infrastructures are prejudiced cholera can be catastrophic. For example, in an El Tor outbreak of cholera in Rwandan refugees in camps in western Zaire in 1994 there were over 10 000 deaths, with case fatality rates of 20% overall, but approaching 50% in some places. When much of the adult population is immune, infection becomes endemic and occurs mostly among the very young and women looking after children (who are exposed to large inocula). Those occurring in western Europe are almost all imported following infection elsewhere. Sixty-three isolations of *Vibrio cholerae* were reported from laboratories in England and Wales. Under ordinary circumstances and where there are reasonable health facilities care fatality rates are under 1%. Disease tends to be milder in children and is most severe in young adult males.

Transmission

V. cholerae is often acquired through intrafamilial spread by direct contact. However the O1 and especially O139 organisms are suited to survival in aquatic environments and transmission from infected person is also through contaminated water and food. Shellfish are important vehicles of transmission and a particular hazard arises from the use of waste water or sewage to irrigate vegetables. With modern sanitation, widespread transmission is uncommon in industrialised countries and areas of low-income countries with reasonable sanitation. Epidemics typically follow natural disasters where there is contamination of food and water and a breakdown of hygiene and sanitation.

Incubation period

This is usually 1–3 days with a range of a few hours to 5 days. The greater the infective dose ingested, the shorter the incubation period and the more severe the disease. Ingestion with food protects the vibrio from stomach acids. The period of infectivity is highly variable, and a carrier state may last several months or longer. Antibiotics such as co-trimoxazole can shorten this period.

NATURAL HISTORY AND CLINICAL FEATURES

Asymptomatic infection is more common than disease but cholera is unique among diarrhoeal diseases in its rapidity of onset and in potentially having a very high mortality rate. Illness is caused by an enterotoxin consisting of two subunits – A, the toxin itself, and B, a carrier. It acts on cyclic-AMP-dependent secretion and absorption. Its action is characterised by a rapid onset of severe diarrhoea followed by vomiting. Profuse, frequent and sometimes painless bowel evacuations accelerate severe dehydration. Stool output can reach a litre an hour and hence shock and collapse may occur. Hypoglycaemia and convulsions are particularly common in children. 'Ricewater diarrhoea' describes the stools, which are typically colourless and contain flecks of mucus.

Complications of delayed treatment are hypovolaemic shock, uncompensated metabolic acidosis and renal failure. Proper management will reduce case fatality from a potential 50% to less than 1%.

Diagnosis

In endemic areas, especially during epidemics, there is no difficulty in diagnosis but sporadic cases will require differentiation from other forms of severe diarrhoea. Diagnosis can be made by microscopic examination of the stool. Culture on bile-salt agar will produce characteristic colonies in 24 hours. The organism can be typed from culture colonies by agglutination with specific antisera. This is rarely performed routinely on diarrhoea specimens. Specific antibody titres can also be measured and a rise in titre may be used for diagnosis.

MANAGEMENT

The most important aspect of treatment is the restoration of plasma volume and electrolyte balance. In many cases this can be achieved using oral rehydration therapy (ORT), which promotes absorption via cyclic-AMP-independent mechanisms. The introduction of ORT has resulted in a dramatic decrease in mortality in many countries. However, if dehydration is severe intravenous rehydration may also be necessary. Antibiotics are used for eradication of *V. cholerae* from the gastrointestinal tract. Co-trimoxazole or erythromycin should be given to children under 12 years of age and doxycycline to older children and adults. The infected child needs to be barrier-nursed during the acute phase and special care should be taken when handling stools (enteric precautions) until demonstrated to be noninfectious. Stools of close contacts should be cultured and carriers should be given antibiotics (treatment dose). Attempts must be made to identify the source of infection and appropriate control measures taken.

PREVENTION OF FURTHER CASES

Cases in Europe require prompt notification of public health officials to ensure that further spread does not occur. Prevention is achieved by good standards of hygiene, education to promote this and good sanitation, especially the establishment and maintenance of sewage disposal systems. Where safe water cannot be provided through a mains water supply, point-of-use-water disinfection should be used. Parental-inactivated vaccines have been in use for many years against Cholera O1, but they confer only limited protection (estimated at 50%) for a few months and have no role in disease control. No country officially requires certification for visitors; however it may occasionally be demanded by officials at some border crossing points in low-income countries. Oral inactivated vaccines have been developed. They are based on the nontoxic B subunit of the toxin and have been shown to be safe and efficacious, at least in the short term, in clinical trials. They are starting to become available; however, no cholera vaccine is currently available in the UK. There is no vaccine against cholera O139 and the vaccine against O1 seems to give limited cross-immunity.

ORGANISM

Causative organisms are: *Chlamydia trachomatis*, serotypes D to K; *Neisseria gonorrhoeae*; other bacteria such as *Haemophilus influenzae* and *Streptococcus pneumoniae* (*Staphylococcus aureus* and *Pseudomonas aeruginosa* in neonates); adenoviruses, especially types 3, 4 and 7; picornaviruses, especially enterovirus 70 and Coxsackie virus A24; and herpes simplex virus.

EPIDEMIOLOGY

All these organisms are found worldwide. About 35–50% of neonates will acquire chlamydial eye infection when delivered through an infected cervix. One in 300 people with a genital infection develops eye disease. Chlamydial conjunctivitis can also occur in the sexually inactive. Gonococcal conjunctivitis is also acquired at birth. Other bacterial conjunctivitis most often affects preschool children. It is common, especially in warmer climates, and may be epidemic. Viral conjunctivitis may be sporadic or occur in epidemics. Enteroviral acute haemorrhagic conjunctivitis (AHC) occurs mainly in the tropics but also in some European countries and in people coming from areas with AHC outbreaks. Adenoviral conjunctivitis often occurs as summer epidemics.

Transmission

The spread of nongonococcal bacterial conjunctivitis is by infected material, either directly or on objects such as make-up, clothing and multiple-dose dispensers of eye-drops or ointment. Viral conjunctivitis is spread by direct or indirect contact with infected material from a discharging eye. Transmission within a household is common. Adenoviral disease has been associated with the use of poorly chlorinated swimming pools.

Incubation period

Chlamydia trachomatis, 5–12 days; *Neisseria gonorrhoeae*, 1–5 days; other bacterial infections, usually 1–3 days; adenovirus, 3–29 days; picornavirus, 12 hours to 3 days.

NATURAL HISTORY AND CLINICAL FEATURES

For chlamydial and gonococcal conjunctivitis, see Chapters 43 and 55. Nongonococcal bacterial conjunctivitis presents with irritation and redness of the conjunctiva, followed by oedema of the lids, photophobia and mucopurulent discharge. The severity varies from minor hyperaemia and a slight discharge to ecchymoses and infiltration of the cornea. Adenoviral conjunctivitis usually presents with lymphoid follicles and often small subconjunctival haemorrhages. It usually lasts 7–15 days and may be accompanied by upper respiratory illness (pharyngoconjunctival fever). The onset of AHC is sudden, with redness, pain and swelling, frequently in both eyes. The inflammation subsides over the next few days, but petechiae appear on the conjunctivae. These enlarge and coalesce to produce subconjunctival haemorrhages, which resolve over the next week or two. Some outbreaks have been associated with polio-like paralysis, starting anything from a few days to a month after the conjunctivitis. Often there is some residual paralysis.

Diagnosis

It is important to exclude chlamydial and gonococcal conjunctivitis (see Chapters 43 and 55). Bacterial cultures should be taken before antibiotics are started.

MANAGEMENT

For chlamydial and gonococcal conjunctivitis, see Chapters 43 and 55. If a bacterial aetiology is suspected, topical neomycin or chloramphenicol is first-line treatment. Neomycin is to be preferred in the neonatal period because, unlike chloramphenicol, it will not mask a chlamydial infection. Ointment is often better than drops, especially in young children, as it can be difficult to administer drops reliably. Both eyes should be treated, as the infection, even if initially unilateral, often spreads from one eye to the other. Different dispensers should be used for each eye to prevent cross-infection.

PREVENTION OF FURTHER CASES

Strict attention to hygiene may prevent the transmission of nongonococcal bacterial conjunctivitis and viral conjunctivitis. Swimming pools should be properly chlorinated. The value of excluding children from school because they have conjunctivitis is not clear. In younger children, it is probably wise to exclude them until treatment has been initiated, as there is more likelihood of transmission in this group.

46 Cryptosporidiosis

ORGANISM

Cryptosporidium parvum is a protozoan parasite. Infected individuals excrete large numbers of thick-walled oocysts which can persist in the environment.

EPIDEMIOLOGY

Cryptosporidia can be found worldwide in a variety of hosts including humans, domestic animals (especially sheep and cattle), birds and pets. Prevalence of infection in humans is higher in low-income countries, where infection in children is associated with higher risk of mortality. Both children and adults are affected, although cases under 1 year are unusual.

Outbreaks occur in child-care centres and major outbreaks through contamination and poor maintenance of water supplies have recently been increasingly recognised.

Transmission

Faecal–oral, person- or animal-to-person and through contamination of water supplies, milk. The infective dose can be as low as one oocyst.

Incubation period

Not clearly known – a likely range is 1–14 days with an average of 7 days.

NATURAL HISTORY AND CLINICAL FEATURES

The parasite invades epithelial cells in the intestine and then produces oocysts, which are infectious and excreted. In children the commonest signs are watery diarrhoea, low-grade fever, abdominal pain, anorexia and mild weight loss. Severe illness is rare in immunocompetent children and adults. Asymptomatic infections occur. Symptoms frequently wax and wane. The infection is usually self-limiting to 10 days on average (maximum 3–6 weeks). Persistent infection leading to failure to thrive may occur in those with severe T-cell immunosuppression such as severe HIV disease and AIDS, and children with SCID (severe combined immunodeficiency).

Diagnosis

This can be difficult. Diagnosis relies on microscopic examination of stained stool smears for oocysts. These are small bodies and false-positive and -negative results occur such that repeated specimens and specialist assistance is usually required. Yeasts typically cause false positives. This is especially so when examining water supplies for evidence of contamination.

MANAGEMENT

Treatment in the immunocompetent child is usually symptomatic, with rehydration therapy as required. If an immunocompromised child (e.g. a child with HIV infection) is infected, a specialist opinion should be sought from the physician providing care. There is no wholly effective anticryptosporidial agent. Although spiramycin, paromomycin or paromomycin/azithromycin combination have been shown to suppress the symptoms, they are not curative.

PREVENTION OF FURTHER CASES

When cases occur, enteric precautions should be applied. However the main method of prevention in industrialised counties is the delivery of safe domestic drinking water. This is the responsibility of the suppliers. Domestic water supplies must be well maintained. The cysts are resistant to chlorination and therefore filtration is needed to deliver safe water supplies. Immunocompromised patients with T-cell-based conditions should only take water-based drinks if the water has been boiled. See page 126 for prevention in immunocompromised individuals.

47 Cytomegalovirus

ORGANISM

Cytomegalovirus (CMV), also known as human herpesvirus 5 (HHV-5), is an enveloped DNA virus.

EPIDEMIOLOGY

Serological studies show that approximately 50% of women of childbearing age are seropositive. Congenital infection occurs in about 3/1000 newborn infants in the UK. Most cases result from primary rather than reactivated or secondary infection during pregnancy. Infection in the infant may be acquired later, either at delivery or after birth. CMV is one of the commonest causes of congenital hearing loss in the UK, with an estimated 200 cases per year.

Transmission

CMV can be cultured or identified in a number of body fluids. Congenital infections are thought to occur via transplacental blood-stream spread at any stage of pregnancy, with acquired infection in the newborn resulting from contamination by cervical secretions. CMV is present in the white blood cells of seropositive individuals and transfusion of CMV-infected blood to preterm infants results in a systemic illness with pneumonia and hepatitis. Transmission may also occur in breast milk. Most transmission in children is thought to be through saliva, but urinary spread may be a factor, although it is less important, even in a nursery setting. The agent is transmitted sexually and can be identified in semen and cervical secretions. Organ transplantation is also a source of infection. Immunosuppressed individuals may experience a reactivation of latent CMV infection.

Incubation period

This is unknown for person-to-person spread. The incubation period for transmission during blood transfusion or transplantation is 1–4 months.

NATURAL HISTORY AND CLINICAL FEATURES

Congenital and acquired infection in the newborn

Some 3–5% of infants with congenital infection develop cytomegalic inclusion disease (CID), with features that include petechiae from thrombocytopenia, hepatitis, chorioretinitis, intracranial calcification and microcephaly. Survivors may develop cerebral palsy. Sensorineural deafness alone may occur in up to 10% of infants with congenital infection. Excretion of virus may persist for several years.

Acquired infection in the child

Children at risk are those immunosuppressed with symptomatic HIV infection or following bone marrow and organ transplantation. They develop disseminated disease, with pneumonia, hepatitis and retinitis. Mortality rates of up to 10% have been reported following CMV infection in this group.

Diagnosis

Diagnosis is difficult. To make a diagnosis of congenital infection, specimens have to be taken for culture within 3 weeks of birth. Such evidence of infection is supported by a positive IgM anti-CMV antibody. Virus can be isolated in tissue culture from a number of sources, including throat swabs, urine, breast milk, semen, cervical secretion and peripheral blood leukocytes. Although routine tissue culture is slow to produce results, more rapid identification is obtained by a short period of culture following a specific immunofluorescence test, of which there are several available. PCR diagnosis is possible using commercially available kits

MANAGEMENT

There is no conclusive evidence as yet that any antiviral agents alter the course of the disease in congenital infection. Ganciclovir, an acyclic nucleoside related to aciclovir has been shown to eradicate CMV excretion for a short period following treatment of an infant with congenital infection. Case reports describe the successful use of ganciclovir in acquired neonatal infection when used in a dose of 5 mg/kg twice daily for 14 days, although the long-term results of such treatment are unclear.

Ganciclovir has been used with success in both the prevention and treatment of CMV infection following bone marrow and organ transplantation (see Chapter 22). The main side-effect of ganciclovir is neutropenia. Foscarnet is effective in the treatment of CMV retinitis in the immunosuppressed and is also used.

PREVENTION OF FURTHER CASES

Children with congenital CMV infection excrete virus. The importance of hand-washing for staff looking after such children should be reinforced. As yet a vaccine has not been developed. There is insufficient evidence to exclude pregnant nurses from contact with infants and children with CMV infection. Prophylactic high dose oral aciclovir has been shown to reduce the incidence of CMV disease after solid organ transplantation and is also increasingly used for this purpose after marrow transplantation.

48 Dermatophytoses: tinea capitis, corporis, pedis and unguium

TINEA CAPITIS (SCALP RINGWORM)

ORGANISM

Fungi from the genera *Trichophyton* and *Microsporum* are responsible.

EPIDEMIOLOGY

The disease is found worldwide. It can affect some animal species as well as humans. All ages can be infected. Zoophilic fungi (those spread from infected animals) used to be most important, in particular *Microsporum canis* from dogs and cats and, less commonly, *Trichophyton verrucosum* from cattle. Recently, increasing numbers of cases due to anthropophilic fungi (those spread from humans) have been seen, especially *Trichophyton tonsurans*. This has resulted in increased rates of transmission within families and schools.

Transmission

Direct contact with infected humans, animals or fomites. Spread may occur via combs, hairbrushes, hats, etc., on which the organism may remain viable for long periods.

Incubation period

10–14 days.

NATURAL HISTORY AND CLINICAL FEATURES

The lesions often start as small papules, which spread outwards leaving scaly areas of hair loss. The remaining hairs are brittle, leaving short stubs when broken. Other presentations are possible – pustules with little scaling or hair loss, or areas of scaling like dandruff with varying degrees of hair loss. The lesions may progress to form a raised, boggy area known as a kerion. Infections with anthropophilic, rather than zoophilic, fungi are often less severe. Confusion can arise with other conditions such as impetigo, dandruff, seborrhoeic dermatitis, psoriasis, trichotillomania, folliculitis, alopecia areata and, rarely, lupus erythematosus. Reinfection is uncommon.

Diagnosis

Microsporum spp. will fluoresce under ultraviolet light (Wood's lamp). This is not true for *Trichophyton* spp. and so lack of fluorescence cannot be used to exclude the diagnosis. Scrapings taken from the outer margin of a lesion should be sent to the laboratory on dark paper. They will be treated with 10% potassium hydroxide and examined for fungal filaments. Culture on Sabouraud's medium provides the definitive diagnosis and can be important.

MANAGEMENT

Oral griseofulvin (10 mg/kg daily) should be given for 8–10 weeks; this treatment may occasionally fail. An alternative if this occurs is terbinafine

125 mg daily for 2–4 weeks, although specialist opinion should be sought as this drug is not licensed for use in children. Topical antifungal agents have only a secondary role. They should not be used as a substitute for systemic treatment.

PREVENTION OF FURTHER CASES

All members of the household, including pets such as cats and dogs, should be examined and treated if infected. Combs, brushes, pillows and hats should not be shared. Selenium sulphide shampoo, if applied twice weekly for 2 weeks, has been shown to kill fungal spores and may be an aid to the prevention of the spread of infection. All infected members of the family, and any infected pets, must be treated at the same time. Exclusion from school is not indicated.

TINEA CORPORIS (RINGWORM OF THE BODY)

ORGANISM

Fungi from the genera *Trichophyton* (in particular *T. rubrum* and *T. mentagrophytes*), *Microsporum* (in particular *M. canis*) and *Epidermophyton floccosum*.

EPIDEMIOLOGY

The disease is found worldwide. It can affect some animal species as well as humans. All ages can be infected.

Transmission

By direct contact with infected humans, animals or fomites.

Incubation period

Not known for certain but thought to be 4–10 days.

NATURAL HISTORY AND CLINICAL FEATURES

The typical lesion is found on the hairless parts of the face, trunk and limbs (see Plate 3). The groins, hands and feet are spared. The typical lesion is round with a red, scaly border. The border tends to expand slowly outwards, leaving a pale centre, often of normal skin. Topical corticosteroid treatment can alter this characteristic appearance. The lesions are usually pruritic.

Diagnosis

Diagnosis can often be made clinically but should usually be confirmed microbiologically. Scrapings should be collected for microscopy (see Tinea capitis, above)

MANAGEMENT

Topical preparations alone are often ineffective in the long term. Griseofulvin for 6 weeks should be combined with a topical antifungal agent such as clotrimazole, ketoconazole or miconazole for 2 weeks. When the fungus is resistant to griseofulvin, oral itraconazole should be used instead.

PREVENTION OF FURTHER CASES

The lesions should be covered. All infected members of the family, and any infected pets, must be treated at the same time.

TINEA PEDIS (ATHLETE'S FOOT)

ORGANISM

Fungi from the genus *Trichophyton* (in particular *T. rubrum* and *T. mentagrophytes*) and *Epidermophyton floccosum*.

EPIDEMIOLOGY

Tinea pedis occurs worldwide, affecting adults more frequently than children and men more commonly than women. It is more common in summer.

Transmission

From infected skin scales, by direct contact with an infected person or from places on which an infected person has shed scales, e.g. changing rooms, swimming pools and bath mats.

Incubation period

Unknown.

NATURAL HISTORY AND CLINICAL FEATURES

The typical appearance is of scaling and cracking of the skin of the feet, especially between the toes. It is usually pruritic. Occasionally there may be a hypersensitivity reaction with vesicular lesions on the palms of the hands and sides of the fingers.

Diagnosis

Diagnosis is usually made on the basis of the appearance of the lesions. The diagnosis can be confirmed by taking skin scrapings (see Tinea capitis, above).

MANAGEMENT

Topical treatment with an antifungal such as clotrimazole, ketoconazole or miconazole for 2 weeks.

PREVENTION OF FURTHER CASES

Good hygiene is necessary in communal places where feet may be uncovered. Exclusion from swimming is not necessary.

TINEA UNGUIUM (NAIL RINGWORM)

ORGANISM

Fungi from the genus *Trichophyton*, *Epidermophyton floccosum* and, rarely, *Microsporum* spp.

EPIDEMIOLOGY

The fungi are found worldwide, but the only important reservoir is in humans.

Transmission

Thought to be predominantly by direct contact with infected skin or nails. It is not very contagious and spread within families is low.

Incubation period

Unknown.

NATURAL HISTORY AND CLINICAL FEATURES

The nail becomes thickened, brittle and discoloured. White caseous material may collect under the nail, which in turn may disintegrate.

Diagnosis

By examination of scrapings (see Tinea capitis, above).

MANAGEMENT

Oral terbinafine has been shown to be more effective than griseofulvin. Although it is more expensive, it has a lower relapse rate and a shorter course is needed, so it is more cost-effective. However it is not licensed for use in children. The first-line treatment is therefore oral griseofulvin, which should be given until the nail has grown out. Where it fails, treatment with terbinafine may be considered. Topical antifungal agents have no role.

PREVENTION OF FURTHER CASES

No special measures are necessary as the condition is not very contagious.

FURTHER READING

Leyden JJ (ed) (1999) Update on Tinea capitis and new antifungal therapies. Paediatr Infect Dis J 18(suppl.): 179–215.

49 Diphtheria

Notifiable disease

ORGANISM

Corynebacterium diphtheriae – a Gram-positive bacterium. There are three biotypes (colony types): gravis, mitis and intermedius. Strains may be toxigenic or nontoxigenic depending on the presence of the tox+ gene, which is thought to be transmitted by a bacteriophage. Toxigenic strains are considered to have some selective advantage in nonimmune populations. A diphtheria-like illness is also occasionally caused by toxin-producing C. ulcerans.

EPIDEMIOLOGY

Humans are the only source of infection of C. diphtheriae. C. ulcerans is a zoonosis associated with cattle and goats and infections in humans are usually, but not always, associated with the consumption of unpasteurised milk. There are two major sites of infection, the upper respiratory tract and the skin – 'cutaneous diphtheria'. Diphtheria is now rare in most industrialised countries because of routine immunisation. It still causes considerable morbidity and mortality in the low-income countries, where much of the circulating infection is through cutaneous diphtheria, and an important source of strains in the UK, toxigenic or otherwise, is from the Indian subcontinent. There has recently been a massive resurgence in the newly independent states of the former USSR and adjoining parts of eastern Europe, because of a breakdown in immunisation programmes, loss of confidence in vaccination in the population and lack of familiarity of the disease among clinicians. In 1993 there were 15 211 cases in the Russian Federation; numbers have decreased since. Imported cases in western Europe are uncommon but include both throat and cutaneous diphtheria.

Transmission

C. diphtheriae is spread by droplet infection from nose and throat secretions. Cutaneous diphtheria spreads from direct contact through fomites. Untreated patients with pharyngeal diphtheria are considered infectious for 2–3 weeks. Correct antibiotic treatment usually makes the patient noninfectious in 24 hours.

Incubation period

This is usually 2–5 days but can be longer.

NATURAL HISTORY AND CLINICAL FEATURES

The disease is clinically classified according to the anatomical site of infection: pharyngeal, laryngeal, nasal and cutaneous. In pharyngeal, laryngeal and nasal diphtheria, disease usually involves cervical lymphadenopathy and the development of a membraneous nasopharyngitis or laryngotracheitis. Onset is often insidious with a low-grade fever for 1–2 days and perhaps a sore throat. The membrane may be classical, grey/white, thick and spreading and firmly adherent to the throat, where it may cause respiratory obstruction (diphtheritic croup). However it may be more focal on one tonsil or deeper in the larynx causing stridor while nasal diphtheria will manifest itself as a serous and then serosanguinous nasal discharge. **Because of these atypical presentations and the severity of the illness, a high degree of suspicion should be maintained if a patient with any such symptoms has travelled to an endemic area or has been in close contact with a case**. The bacterium releases a powerful exotoxin that causes local tissue necrosis and attacks the myocardium of the heart and motor nerves, notably of the soft palate, eyes and diaphragm. The course of the illness depends on the severity of the toxaemia and the degree of immunity conferred by previous immunisation. Milder infections in the partially immune may lead to uneventful recovery, with the membrane sloughing off in 6–7 days. Severe infections occur in the unimmunised and untreated and are characterised by increasing toxaemia. Cardiac symptoms appear in the second week and neurological features after 2–6 weeks. These may progress to cardiovascular collapse, stupor, coma and death. Case fatality rates are 5–10%.

Diagnosis

Although diphtheria is a rare condition in the UK, cases still occur and the diagnosis must be considered in any membraneous condition of the throat, especially in children recently arrived from abroad or their unimmunised contacts, and in those of doubtful immune status. Cases of infection with toxigenic strains occur even in persons who have not had any recent contact with abroad. Cultures should be taken from the nose and throat or from any site that may be contaminated (e.g. weeping skin ulcers). If possible, the swab should be taken from under the membrane. The laboratory should be consulted in advance as special media will be used to accelerate growth and thus identification of the organism. Most isolates of *C. diphtheriae* from the upper respiratory tract or skin in the UK are nontoxigenic, including those associated with time spent abroad, and it is often the case that the organism is isolated but it is unclear whether a toxigenic strain is involved and whether control measures should be employed. The **rapid** identification of toxigenic strains is possible and essential by the use of methods such as polymerase chain reaction (PCR).* A serum sample should also be obtained before antitoxin treatment is administered for measurement of antibodies to toxin.

MANAGEMENT

Individual management consists of counteracting the effects of toxin and treating the infection to eliminate the infection and prevent transmission. When the diagnosis of diphtheria is suspected, expert advice should be sought from a specialist with relevant clinical infectious disease experience before administering antitoxin. However, the patient should be isolated and the antitoxin administered without unnecessary delay. The dose is calculated according to the size of the membrane, the degree of toxicity and the duration of illness. A diluted test dose must first be given intradermally. If the test is negative, antitoxin may be given intramuscularly or intravenously depending on the volume required and the severity of illness. If the patient is hypersensitive then expert advice must be sought to discuss the possibility of attempting desensitisation. If acute anaphylaxis develops, intravenous adrenaline (0.2–0.5 mL of 1:1000 solution) should be administered immediately.

Dosages of antitoxin that have been recommended are listed in Table 49.1.

---

* **In England and Wales isolates can be rapidly tested by the Diphtheria Reference Unit at the Central Public Health Laboratory, which maintains a 24-hour on-call service (020 8200 4400).**

Table 49.1 Recommended dosages of diphtheria antitoxin

Type of diphtheria	Dosage (units)	Route of administration
Nasal	10 000–20 000	i.m.
Tonsillar	15 000–25 000	i.m. or i.v.
Pharyngeal or laryngeal	20 000–40 000	i.m. or i.v.
Combined or delayed diagnosis	40 000–60 000	i.v.
Severe diphtheria (by either extensive membrane and/or severe oedema)	40 000–100 000	i.v.

Other dosage regimens are also suggested. In England and Wales diphtheria antitoxin is available from the Immunisation Division at the Communicable Disease Surveillance Centre and in Scotland a small stock is held at Glasgow Royal Infirmary.
i. m. = intramuscular; i.v. = intravenous.

Antitoxin is not generally considered useful for cutaneous diphtheria, although wounds should be cleaned with soap and water and antibiotic treatment given.

Penicillin should also be given to treat the infection. Benzylpenicillin (penicillin G) for 14 days is the treatment of choice and should be given intravenously or intramuscularly. An alternative is parenteral erythromycin for 14 days. This should be continued until the child can swallow again, at which point treatment can switch to oral medication. The patient should also be given a booster dose of vaccine.

PREVENTION OF FURTHER CASES

Once it is clear that a toxigenic strain is involved (see Diagnosis, above) or is very likely, specialist advice is essential and public health measures must be instituted with urgency. The Consultant in Communicable Disease Control (or Director of Public Health) and CDSC or the Scottish Centre for Infection and Environmental Health must be contacted urgently. Close contacts (defined as household members, regular household visitors, kissing contacts, classroom contacts and health-care staff exposed to oropharyngeal secretions), whether immunised or not, must have throat swabs (carriage may be up to 25%) and be given a 7-day course of penicillin or oral erythromycin irrespective of the swab result or vaccine history. Carriers should have a second swab to ensure clearance. Patients with cutaneous diphtheria should have the lesion covered and be isolated. Contacts previously immunised should receive a booster dose of monovalent diphtheria vaccine or tetanus/diphtheria (Td) as appropriate if not boosted with a diphtheria-containing vaccine in the previous 12 months.

Immunisation

Diphtheria immunisation, a toxoid, has been routinely available in the UK for about 60 years. In the UK it is given at 2, 3 and 4 months of age with tetanus and pertussis (the 'triple vaccine') and before starting school with tetanus (the 'preschool booster'). Since the end of 1994 it has also been given with tetanus (Td) before leaving secondary school and may also be given as part of antitetanus prophylaxis for wounds or burns. The strength of this dose of diphtheria toxoid is 4 IU, compared to 30 IU in the preparation given to children below 10 years old. A monovalent vaccine is available for children up to age 9 years. Low-dose single-antigen diphtheria vaccine for children of 10 years and older and adults is not always available but if a patient has had recent tetanus vaccine it is possible to give one-fifth (30 IU) of the monovalent diphtheria vaccine for children on a named patient basis to adults and children 10 years or older. Contraindications to the vaccine are few and adverse events rare.

FURTHER READING

Begg NT (1994) Diphtheria: manual for the management and control of diphtheria in the European Region. World Health Organization (Europe), Geneva. (Available from the PHLS Communicable Disease Surveillance Centre with companion *Manual on Laboratory Diagnosis* by A. Efstratiou.)

Begg N, Balraj V (1995) Diphtheria: are we ready for it? Arch Dis Child 73; 568–572.

Bonnet JM, Begg NT (1999) Control of diphtheria: guidelines for Consultants in Communicable Disease control. Comm Dis Public Health 2:242–249.

50 Ehrlichioses

ORGANISM

The genus *Ehrlichia*, named in honour of Paul Ehrlich in 1945, comprises some 18 species of obligate intracellular Gram-negative bacteria. Most are of veterinary importance but three, *E. chaffeensis*, *E. sennetsu* and the agent of human granulocytic ehrlichiosis (HGE) are pathogenic to man. HGE infects and grows in neutrophils whereas the other two predominantly infect monocytes and macrophages.

EPIDEMIOLOGY AND CLINICAL FEATURES

E. chaffeensis infection was first described in North America in 1986 and is predominantly confined to south and south-eastern USA. Its distribution reflects the distribution of its vector, *Amblyomma americanum* (the lone star tick), although it has also been detected in *Dermacentor variabilis* (the American dog tick). Ticks are a biological vector (i.e. the bacterium replicates in the tick). Deer and dogs are the major reservoir hosts, although small rodents may also be infected. Human infection is rural (60% of cases) and seasonal (66% of cases occur from May to July) and most infections occur in adults, although 37 infections in children (aged 7 months to 14 years) have been described. The most frequent clinical manifestations in children are fever, rash (macular, maculopapular, petechial or a mixture of these), hepatosplenomegaly and a systolic murmur. Over 80% of the children gave a history of tick bite. In most cases the infection is not fatal and recovery is complete. However at least one child has died and two have had long-term neurological sequelae.

E. sennetsu causes an infectious mononucleosis-like illness and was first described in 1945 in Japan, where most cases are reported. It is thought to be transmitted by ingestion of raw fish.

The agent of HGE was first described in 1994 in the USA. It is very closely related (at the genomic level, antigenically and by cross-species infectivity) to *E. phagocytophila*, *E. equi* and the agent of llama granulocytic ehrlichiosis, which infect sheep and cows, horses and llamas respectively. It is transmitted by the bite of ixodid ticks (*Ixodes pacificus*, *I. scapularis* and *I. ricinus* in Europe). The reservoir hosts are thought to be small rodents, wild deer and some domestic animals. Although most infections are reported from the USA there is evidence of HGE in Sweden and Slovenia. In a UK serosurvey, 1.5% of farm-workers had antibody to the agent of HGE. It has been transmitted perinatally but whether this was transplacentally (which occurs in other species), during delivery or via breast milk is not known. The incubation period is 1–60 days (median 8 days) following a tick bite, followed by pyrexia (mean 39.3°C), myalgia, headache, nausea, rigors and arthralgia. Most often disease is short-lived and self-limiting. Up to 25% of patients require hospitalisation but a minority develop opportunistic infections and die. Co-infection with Lyme borreliosis should also be considered.

Diagnosis

Monocytic ehrlichiosis or HGE should be considered in patients presenting with a 'flu-like' illness following outdoor activity where they may have been exposed to tick bites. Morulae (inclusions containing the bacteria) may be seen in monocytes or neutrophils in stained buffy coat smears. *E. chaffeensis* and HGE can be cultured (2–3 days) in human-monocyte-derived cell lines. Serological diagnosis can be made using either *E chaffeensis* or *E. equi* as antigens. Polymerase chain reaction (PCR) detection is possible using primers directed to regions of the 16S rRNA operon.

MANAGEMENT

Tetracycline or doxycycline are the treatments of choice and prolonged administration (up to 2 weeks) may be needed to avoid relapses. In children the risk of tooth and bone damage must be balanced against the risk of damage if left untreated.

PREVENTION

Prevention is by avoidance of tick bites, by not visiting their habitat or by using insect repellent.

51 Enteroviruses

Excluding polioviruses – see Chapter 87

ORGANISM

Genera within the family Picornaviridae, which are small nonenveloped RNA viruses, fall into four major groups:

- Coxsackieviruses: two families – A and B
- Echoviruses
- Enteroviruses
- Hepatoviruses (includes Hepatitis A virus, see Chapter 63).

Humans are the only hosts.

EPIDEMIOLOGY

Enteroviruses are found worldwide, with infection rates highest in younger children. The USA, with a population of 260 million, has an estimated 30 million nonpolio enterovirus infections per annum. Epidemics of particular virus types occur most notably in the autumn in the northern hemisphere. These are more frequent in institutional settings such as day care for the under-5s and primary schools. There are occasionally severe outbreaks of infection and severe disease; for example, an epidemic of enterovirus 71 probably caused over 40 deaths among children in Taiwan in 1998. Enteroviruses can persist in the watery environment if the temperature remains low, pH is neutral and there is sufficient organic material. Recreational or occupational exposure to contaminated water may result in infection.

Transmission

Person-to-person spread predominates through faecal–oral and respiratory routes. Infectivity is high in the acute phase of illness and may be prolonged since presence of virus in the faeces may be prolonged (for up to 2 months).

Incubation period

Variable – considered to be usually between 2 hours and 6 days, although it may be shorter for haemorrhagic conjunctivitis.

NATURAL HISTORY AND CLINICAL FEATURES

Infection is usually asymptomatic (60–70% of echovirus and 40–50% of Coxsackie virus infections). However, a considerable range of clinical conditions can result from infection with these viruses. Although certain viruses tend to be associated with particular syndromes there is considerable overlap and the listing below should only be seen as approximate:

- Viral (aseptic) meningitis and encephalitis (echo 3–7, Coxsackie A9, B1–5, enterovirus 71)
- Haemorrhagic conjunctivitis (Coxsackie A25, enterovirus 70)
- Hand, foot and mouth disease (see Chapter 59) (Coxsackie A5, A16; enterovirus 71)
- Myo/pericarditis (Coxsackie B1–5)
- Exanthems (echo 7, 9, 16; Coxsackie A4)
- Enanthems (echo 3, 6, 9, 16, 17; Coxsackie A1, 3; B1–5)
- Pleurodynia (Bornholm disease) (Coxsackie B1–6)
- Upper respiratory disease (echo 1, 3, 4, 20, 22; Coxsackie B)
- Lower respiratory disease (echo 9, Coxsackie B1, 4)
- Neonatal infections (echo 9, 11, 14; Coxsackie B1–5)
- Hepatic failure (neonatal infection) (echovirus 20)
- Polio-like syndrome (echovirus type 11, enterovirus 71)
- Diarrhoea (echoviruses, enteroviruses but unproven)
- Intrauterine death (echovirus 11).

Each condition can be caused by a number of viruses, including others outside this group; for example, respiratory conditions are more commonly caused by rhinoviruses and mumps; polio, herpes, varicella and arbovirus also cause aseptic meningitis – hence the clinical range of signs and symptoms that can result from these viruses. While most infections are self-limiting, some can be lethal and substantial supportive therapy may be needed.

Neonatal enterovirus infection can result in severe disease. Infection is usually acquired from family members. Infection manifests as irritability, fever, anorexia, lethargy, jaundice and respiratory signs. Severe multisystem disease may develop. The latter is more likely with early-onset disease (especially day 1), an ill mother and viraemia.

Diagnosis

Specimens for viral culture should be taken using throat swabs and stools, which are placed in viral culture medium – although it must be borne in mind that, particularly during epidemics, viral isolation may represent asymptomatic infection. If illness is severe CSF and blood specimens should also be taken. It is worthwhile setting serum aside and taking a convalescent specimen later to check for a rising antibody titre.

MANAGEMENT

This is usually supportive. Intravenous immunoglobulin may be of benefit in neonatal outbreaks of echovirus infection and when infection occurs in an immunocompromised child. A new antiviral drug, pleconasil, has been used with good results in the latter.

PREVENTION OF FURTHER CASES

Enteric precautions are obligatory during hospitalisation and in institutional outbreaks.

52 Epstein–Barr virus infections: infectious mononucleosis (glandular fever)

ORGANISM

Epstein–Barr virus (EBV) is one of the herpes viruses and is also known as human herpes virus 4 (HHV-4 – see Table 68.1 for list of all herpes viruses). A similar clinical illness can occasionally be caused by cytomegalovirus (see Chapter 47), *Toxoplasma gondii* (see Chapter 104) and newly acquired HIV infection in adolescents.

EPIDEMIOLOGY

EBV only infects the human host. Most people are infected in childhood or adolescence so that serological evidence of past infection is present in up to 90% of individuals by early adulthood. Many infections occur asymptomatically, particularly in early childhood. Symptomatic infection – infectious mononucleosis ('glandular fever') – is commonest in adolescence. Like other herpes viruses, EBV exhibits latency and has been shown to rekindle in immunocompromised individuals such as those undergoing renal transplantation. It is associated (in such patients) with lymphoproliferative disease (of B-cell lineage), which is either polyclonal or true malignant lymphoma. The virus has been more generally implicated in the oncogenesis of nasopharyngeal carcinoma and Burkitt's lymphoma and may also be involved in the development of other B-cell lymphomas. In X-linked lymphoproliferative disorder (Duncan's syndrome), affected boys develop severe illness with EBV, most often resulting in a fatal outcome.

Transmission

This is directly via saliva, by kissing or other close contact, or by droplet transmission. The infectious period lasts for at least 2 months after acute infection.

Incubation period

33–49 days. Reactivation disease occurs in the immunocompromised.

NATURAL HISTORY AND CLINICAL FEATURES

The clinical features vary from asymptomatic infection through typical glandular fever to (rarely) severe, prolonged and sometimes fatal illness. Glandular fever is characterised by fever, malaise, pharyngitis (often exudative) and cervical lymphadenopathy. Hepatosplenomegaly and/or hepatitis (usually anicteric) are relatively common features. Oedema in the throat may occur, leading to 'nasal' voice and difficulty swallowing. A sparse maculopapular rash is present in 10–15% of cases. Petechiae may be seen on the palate. Most cases develop a florid rash if given ampicillin or amoxycillin (see Plate 4). In severe cases, central nervous system involvement with meningoencephalitis, transverse myelitis or Guillain–Barré syndrome may develop. Myocarditis, orchitis and blood dyscrasias can also occur.

Severe and, usually, fatal disease in X-linked lymphoproliferative syndrome is associated with one or more of prolonged and severe infectious mononucleosis, aplastic anaemia, hypogammaglobulinaemia or lymphoma.

Diagnosis

This is usually based on the typical clinical features. The blood picture shows a lymphocytosis with atypical lymphocytes. A heterophile antibody (agglutinating sheep red blood cells) is produced and is the basis of the slide agglutination tests – monospot and Paul–Bunnell test. This antibody doesn't usually appear until the second week of illness or even later and in young children may not be produced at all. Specific EBV serology is more reliable. A positive IgM to viral capsid antigen (VCA) is diagnostic early in the disease. IgG anti-VCA indicates past infection, but a positive titre with a negative anti-EBNA (antibody to Epstein–Barr nuclei antigen – an antibody produced very late in the illness) is suggestive of recent infection. Antibody response to an early antigen (EA) can also be used in diagnosis.

Differential diagnosis includes other causes of infectious-mononucleosis-like illness such as cytomegalovirus and acquired toxoplasmosis, as well as other causes of pharyngitis (streptococcus, diphtheria, respiratory viruses) and other hepatitides. The blood picture may be confused with acute leukaemia, necessitating bone marrow examination.

MANAGEMENT

This is generally symptomatic with analgesics and antipyretics. Corticosteroids may help when massive pharyngeal swelling threatens airway obstruction or there is other severe disease. If infection with EBV is suspected, ampicillin and amoxycillin use should be avoided because of the rash they induce.

PREVENTION OF FURTHER CASES

Isolation is not required and there is no quarantine period. Vaccines against Epstein–Barr virus are not available. Recent infection with EBV is considered a contraindication to blood donation.

53 *Escherichia coli* diarrhoea

This section deals only with those *Escherichia coli* that cause diarrhoea. Details of meningitis and septicaemia in neonates and of urinary tract infection due to *E. coli* are to be found in Chapters 10 and 19 respectively. There is a separate chapter (Chapter 56) on the haemolytic uraemic syndrome (HUS) usually associated with verotoxin-producing *E. coli*.

ORGANISM

Escherichia coli is a Gram-negative motile bacillus. Strains can be differentiated for epidemiological purposes on the basis of O-antigens (on lipopolysaccharide on the bacterial surface), H-antigens (on the flagella used to propel the bacterium) or K-antigens (on the capsule). Although these antigens were used originally to define *E. coli* that caused diarrhoea (all were termed enteropathogenic *E. coli*), serogrouping is not a useful method except when an epidemic occurs. Currently, five different mechanisms of pathogenicity have been described. The strains are thus described as enteropathogenic (EPEC), enterotoxigenic (ETEC), enteroinvasive (EIEC), enterohaemorrhagic (EHEC) and enteroaggregative (EAggEC) *E. coli* (Table 51.1).

EPIDEMIOLOGY AND CLINICAL FEATURES

Enterotoxigenic *E. coli*

Enterotoxigenic *E. coli* produce a noninflammatory (secretory) small-bowel diarrhoea. They produce either or both heat-labile toxin (LT; similar to cholera toxin) and heat-stable toxin (ST). These have secretory and antiabsorptive effects on the enterocytes and are a major cause of infantile diarrhoea in low-income countries (up to three episodes per child per year) and of travellers' diarrhoea (60–70% of cases). The incubation period is 3 hours–7 days (median 4 days) followed by anorexia, vomiting and abdominal cramps and voluminous watery diarrhoea with a frequency of up to 10 times per day. The infection is self-limiting and usually resolves in 1–5 days. In malnourished children it may be prolonged (up to 3 weeks). Dehydration occurs in up to 46% of adults and 16% of children.

Enteroinvasive *E. coli*

Enteroinvasive *E. coli* produce an inflammatory large-bowel diarrhoea. Their pathogenesis is identical to that of shigellas. They invade and kill colonic enterocytes. They are responsible for up to 4% of cases of diarrhoeal disease in children in low-income countries but are rarely found in those under 1 year. They may also be a cause of travellers' diarrhoea. After an incubation period of 1 hour to 6 days (mean 3 days), patients develop fever, abdominal pain and dysentery characterised by frequent but scanty stools with blood and mucus. The illness is less severe than that caused by *Shigella*.

Enteropathogenic *E. coli*

Enteropathogenic *E. coli* produce a noninflammatory (osmotic) small-bowel diarrhoea. They adhere intimately to the enterocyte brush border and cause loss of the microvilli (attaching–effacement). This results in a loss of absorptive area and of the brush border disaccharidase enzymes. EPEC are rarely encountered in developed countries but are a major cause of infantile and neonatal gastroenteritis in low-income countries. The incubation period varies from 2–48 hours (median 8 hours), after which there is a profuse watery diarrhoea, fever and dehydration. Infection can be very prolonged, with relapses over a period of weeks.

Table 51.1 Strains of E. coli

Type of E. coli	Epidemiology	Mechanism of action	Clinical features	Transmission	Incubation period	Period of infectivity
Enteropathogenic (EPEC)	Acute and chronic endemic and epidemic diarrhoea in infants and neonates	Adherence, effacement	Watery diarrhoea	Contaminated infant formula and weaning foods. Nosocomial infection	2–48 h (median 18 h)	While organism being excreted; may be prolonged
Enterotoxigenic (ETEC)	Infantile diarrhoea in low-income countries and travellers' diarrhoea	Adherence, enterotoxin production	Watery diarrhoea and abdominal pain	Contaminated food, especially weaning foods, and less commonly water	3 h–7 d (median 4 d)	While organism being excreted; may be prolonged
Enteroinvasive (EIEC)	Diarrhoea with fever at all ages	Adherence, invasion of mucosa. Similar to Shigella	Fever, often bloody diarrhoea, vomiting, abdominal pain and tenesmus	?Contaminated food	1 h–7 d (median 4 d)	While organism being excreted
Enterohaemorrhagic (EHEC)	Haemorrhagic colitis and HUS in all ages and thrombocytopenic purpura in adults	Cytotoxin production, adherence, effacement	Nonbloody diarrhoea progressing to bloody diarrhoea and abdominal pain. Fever in 1/3	Contaminated food, including hamburgers and milk	12–60 h	While organism being excreted; up to 2–3 weeks
Enteroaggregative (EAggEC)	Diarrhoea in adults and children worldwide; travellers' diarrhoea	Adherence, ?toxin	Bloody, chronic diarrhoea	Food and water	Not known	While organism being excreted; long period

HUS = haemolytic uraemic syndrome.

Enterohaemorrhagic *E. coli*

Enterohaemorrhagic *E. coli* produce an inflammatory large-bowel diarrhoea (haemorrhagic colitis). They produce attaching effacement on the distal ileum and colon and release either or both verocytotoxins 1 and 2. These toxins inhibit protein synthesis and kill the enterocytes. In some cases the toxins enter the bloodstream and result in HUS (see Chapter 56). EHECs (also called verotoxin-producing *E. coli*, VTEC) can be part of the normal intestinal flora of cattle and pigs and are transmitted via undercooked meat or unpasteurised milk. Outbreaks of infection due to serotypes O157:H7, O26:H11 and O111:H8 have been described, often linked to undercooked beefburgers. Contamination of meat products occurs through poor hygiene (e.g. carrying out production of cooked and uncooked meats in the same area in a butcher's) and can result in fatal outbreaks. One involving elderly patients in Lanark, Scotland in 1996 killed 19 people. There is also evidence of person-to-person transmission of *E. coli* O157. After an incubation period of 1–10 days (median 4 days), the patient experiences abdominal cramps and a watery diarrhoea, followed rapidly by haemorrhagic diarrhoea containing frank blood. The patient is rarely febrile and diarrhoea lasts for 5–7 days. *E. coli* O157 is an emerging infection that appeared in the early 1980s. Because it is the most important cause of HUS it is probably the most important common gut pathogen in the UK (see Chapter 56).

Enteroaggregative *E. coli*

Enteroaggregative *E. coli* produce a chronic inflammatory diarrhoea. They adhere well to colonic mucosa and produce haemorrhagic necrosis of villi. They were or are responsible for 13% of cases of acute diarrhoea and 30% of cases of chronic diarrhoea in rural Indian children. They are also responsible for diarrhoea in industrialised countries, where they can cause acute watery diarrhoea, chronic diarrhoea and abdominal colic. They are a cause of travellers' diarrhoea. The incubation period is unknown but they produce fever, vomiting and diarrhoea with frank blood in the stool. The mean duration of diarrhoea in one study was 17 days.

Infectivity

This is for as long as the bacteria are excreted; however, the infective doses for EPEC and EIEC are quite high (c. 10^6 bacteria) but for *E. coli* O157 much lower (c. 10^1–10^2 bacteria).

Diagnosis

Diagnosis is by culture of stool; however, *E. coli* is part of the normal intestinal flora (see Chapter 30) and commensal *E. coli* must be differentiated from pathogenic strains. Therefore in symptomatic cases isolates should be sent to reference laboratories. The majority of enterohaemorrhagic *E. coli* are serogroup O157 and are sorbitol-nonfermenting.

MANAGEMENT

Dehydration and electrolyte imbalance should be corrected (see Chapter 18). Antibiotics should not be used unless diarrhoea is severe, chronic, dysenteric or systemic spread has occurred, and should be based on antimicrobial susceptibility testing. Antimicrobial therapy of *E. coli* O157 diarrhoea may actually predispose to the development of HUS.

PREVENTION OF FURTHER CASES

In babies one of the most potent preventive measures is the promotion of breastfeeding and good household hygiene. In hospitalised cases enteric precautions are obligatory. In outbreaks it is important that Consultants in Communicable Disease Control are informed. *E. coli* isolates in England and Wales should be forwarded for typing by microbiologists to the Laboratory of Enteric Pathogens at the Central Public Health Laboratory and in Scotland to the Scottish Centre of Infection and Environmental Health. This is particularly important for VTEC and where a food source is suspected. If VTEC are isolated or one or more cases of HUS occur the possibility of an outbreak must be considered (see Chapter 33).

FURTHER READING

PHLS/SCIEH (2000) Guidelines for the control of infection with VTEC. Comm Dis Public Health 3: 14–23.

54 Giardiasis

ORGANISM

Giardia lamblia, a primitive binucleate flagellate protozoan also called *G. intestinalis* and *G. duodenalis*.

EPIDEMIOLOGY

The life-cycle of *Giardia lamblia* is one of the simplest of those seen in parasites. There are only two stages: the trophozoite, which exists freely in the human small intestine, and the cyst, which passes down the intestine into the environment. The cycle is completed when the cyst is reingested orally and excysts in the stomach and duodenum, releasing the trophozoite. The parasite is found worldwide and in animal species including sheep, cattle, cats and dogs, although epidemiological studies have failed to confirm them as an important source. Cysts from human sources may be more infectious to man than those from animal sources; hence giardiasis is probably best not considered to be a zoonosis. Under favourable conditions the cysts may remain viable for several months. Boiling destroys the cysts but not freezing. As few as 10 cysts can be infective.

Children are infected more frequently than adults, although breastfed infants may receive protection from breast milk. Prevalence is higher in areas with poor sanitation and in facilities with young children such as day-care centres. The prevalence of stool positivity in different areas ranges between 1% and 30%, depending on the community and age surveyed. Water-borne outbreaks occur most often in communities that derive drinking water from streams or rivers without a water filtration system. Giardiasis is prevalent in certain temperate as well as tropical countries, with frequent infection of tourists related to drinking inadequately treated water or eating contaminated food.

Transmission

Person-to-person transmission occurs by hand-to-mouth transfer of cysts from the faeces of an infected individual, especially in institutions and day-care centres. Asymptomatic infected individuals (being commoner) are probably more responsible for transmission than those with diarrhoea. Localised outbreaks may occur from ingestion of cysts in faecally contaminated water and less often from faecally contaminated food. The cysts are hardy and partially resistant to chlorination. Concentrations of chlorine used in routine water treatment do not kill *Giardia* cysts, especially when the water is cold; unfiltered stream and lake waters that are open to contamination by human and animal faeces are a frequent source of infection.

Incubation period

This depends on the inoculum and can be as extreme as 5–20 days, but the median is 7 days. Infectivity lasts for the entire period of infection.

NATURAL HISTORY AND CLINICAL FEATURES

Giardiasis is an infection principally of the upper small intestine; while usually asymptomatic (the asymptomatic carrier rate is high and infection is frequently self-limiting), it may occasionally be associated with a variety of intestinal symptoms, such as chronic diarrhoea; steatorrhoea; abdominal cramps; bloating; frequent loose, pale, greasy stools; fatigue and weight loss. Malabsorption of fats and of fat-soluble vitamins may occur, especially when there is damage to duodenal and jejunal mucosal cells in severe giardiasis.. There is usually no extraintestinal invasion, but occasionally trophozoites may migrate into the bile or pancreatic ducts, producing inflammatory processes. Chronic or recurrent infection is a particular problem in immunocompromised individuals.

Diagnosis

Made by the identification of cysts or trophozoites in faeces. Specimens need to be repeated at least three times over a number of days (because of intermittent release) before being considered negative. An alternative is searching for trophozoites in duodenal fluid (by aspiration or string test) or in mucosa obtained by small-intestine biopsy. The latter may be tried when results of stool examination are questionable but only rarely provides additive information to well-conducted stool testing. Because *Giardia* infection is usually asymptomatic, the presence of *G. lamblia* (either in stools or duodenum) does not necessarily indicate that *Giardia* is the cause of an illness. Faecal specimens are examined by microscopy looking at a fresh specimen for active trophozoites (in liquid stools) or for cysts in preserved specimens and formed stools. Tests for *G. lamblia* antigen in the stool are becoming available. However since the clinician frequently wishes for a search for multiple parasites, e.g. in a child returning from a low-income country, such specific tests cannot replace a search for ova and parasites.

MANAGEMENT

Metronidazole is the drug of choice. Quinacrine and tinidazole are alternatives; furazolidone is available in paediatric suspension for young children and infants but relapses may occur with any medication. When *G. lamblia* is found in well-nourished, asymptomatic children it is not always necessary to apply treatment. Considerations should include an assessment of whether other children are being put at risk, e.g. if the child attends a day-care centre. In children with persistent symptoms, even in the absence of microbiological proof of diagnosis, 'blind' treatment may be justified.

PREVENTION OF FURTHER CASES

When a case is found it is worth testing other close household members, whether symptomatic or not, supplemented by a search for environmental contamination.

If a child is hospitalised enteric precautions should be taken and soiled articles disinfected. In communities with a modern and adequate sewage disposal system, faeces can be discharged directly into sewers without preliminary disinfection.

In the epidemiological investigation of clustered cases in an area or institution to determine source of infection and mode of transmission, a common vehicle, such as water or association with a day-care centre, should be sought. If found, appropriate preventive or control measures should be applied. Control of person-to-person transmission requires special emphasis on personal cleanliness and sanitary disposal of faeces.

Education of families, personnel and inmates of institutions, and especially adult personnel of day-care centres, in personal hygiene and the need for hand-washing before eating and after toilet use is of use. As for other enteric pathogens, public water supplies need to be protected against contamination with human and animal faeces.

FURTHER READING

Ortega YR, Adam RD (1997) Giardia: overview and update. Clin Inf Dis 25: 545–50.

55 Gonococcal infection

Notifiable as eye infection in the newborn – ophthalmia neonatorum

ORGANISM
Neisseria gonorrhoeae – a Gram-negative diplococcal bacterium.

EPIDEMIOLOGY
Humans are the only reservoir of infection. There are two clinical entities in children.

Newborn infants
Infection usually involves the eye (ophthalmia neonatorum*), although systemic infection can also occur.

Children and adolescents
Infection involves the genital tract and extragenital sites. Infection in pre-pubertal children is commonly the result of child sexual abuse (see Chapter 20) and in adolescents through sexual activity. In most countries the levels of infection are highest in young adolescent females in the age-group 16–19 years. In England and Wales numbers of cases of gonorrhoea have been rising recently, the largest rises being in adolescents. Between 1995 and 1997 numbers of new gonorrhoea cases diagnosed at STD clinics rose among all age groups but the rise was highest (over 50%) for 16–19-year-old males and females. The incidence of infection in younger adolescents is not well known because of asymptomatic infection (especially common in females) and the reluctance of young persons to use clinics or family doctors. In both adolescents and adults it is common to find gonococcal and chlamydial infections coexisting. Unlike some other commoner infections (genital chlamydia and warts), but like HIV and syphilis, there are some clear risk factors for gonorrhoeal infections. In England and Wales these risk factors are having previously had other sexually transmitted infections and being of black ethnic group. However it remains the case that the majority of gonorrhoeal infections are among persons of white ethnic group.

Transmission
Transmission occurs through close intimate contact – in the newborn from an infected mother during the passage through the birth canal. Infection at later ages occurs from sexual contact. Casual transmission does not occur. Infectivity continues as long as no treatment is given and discharges continues, though infectivity may occur with no or minimal symptoms in females. In adults without treatment infectivity can continue for 3–6 months.

---

* **Ophthalmia neonatorum is also caused by other organisms, notably *Chlamydia trachomatis* – see Chapter 43.**

36–48 hours for neonatal infection; 2–7 days for infection in older children.

NATURAL HISTORY AND CLINICAL FEATURES

Newborn infants

Acute inflammation and exudate of the conjunctiva of one or both eyes develops within 5 (usually 2) days of birth. Without treatment corneal ulceration, perforation and blindness can occur. In contrast, chlamydial ophthalmia usually presents after 48 hours.

Children and adolescents

Sites involved are any mucosal membrane that is exposed to sexual contact, i.e. the genital tract, urethra, pharynx and rectum. The genital tract of prepubertal and adolescent girls is considered to be more susceptible to damage than that of older women. The clinical spectrum runs from asymptomatic infection through a simple discharge to pelvic inflammatory disease, epididymitis and perihepatitis. Systemic spread is uncommon, although septicaemia and meningitis have been described.

Diagnosis

Microscopic examination and culture of exudate. Culture media that inhibit other organisms (such as chocolate agar with appropriate antibiotics) should be used when sampling from mucosal surfaces, which will be colonised by nonpathogenic organisms. Hence it is important that laboratory staff realise that they may be culturing for gonorrhoea. Once *N. gonorrhoeae* is isolated it is obligatory to test for antibiotic resistance. Adolescents will require further investigation by taking a history for risk factors and screening for other infections including *Chlamydia*, syphilis and HIV. It is important to consider the possibility of same-sex sexual orientation and drug use. This often requires specialist expertise undertaken in a genitourinary (STD) clinic, or at least with advice from their specialist services.

MANAGEMENT

Newborn infants

Treatment of uncomplicated gonococcal ophthalmia neonatorum is with parenteral penicillin with or without chloramphenicol eye drops. Eye drops alone are inadequate, although irrigation of the eyes assists in clearing infection. The possibility of chlamydial infection should also be considered (see Chapter 43). Investigation and treatment of the mother is obligatory and should involve a specialist in genitourinary medicine.

Children and adolescents

Treatment is with penicillin or ampicillin and probenecid, which can be given at all ages. Many specialists also give treatment for chlamydial infection because of the likelihood of dual infection and because of difficulties in reliably detecting *C. trachomatis*. In the prepubertal child treatment is with erythromycin while in those over age 12 doxycycline is the drug of choice. Where complications have occurred, such as pelvic inflammatory disease, advice should be sought from specialists in genitourinary medicine who, with their staff, can also assist in tracing and treating sexual contacts of adolescents through partner notification. The possibility of child sexual abuse should be considered for children at all ages but is obligatory for the prepubertal child (see Chapter 20).

PREVENTION OF FURTHER CASES

Newborn infants

Where incidence of gonorrhoea is high antimicrobial eye drops are used routinely after birth.

Children and adolescents

Children require protection from adults who seek underage sex and sex without consent in older children. Prevention of all sexually transmitted infections should not be considered in isolation but should be integrated with other aspects of sexual and reproductive care in a comprehensive sexual health policy with adolescents as a prime group for targeting. Sex education and accessible sexual health services (involvement of specialists in genitourinary medicine) are necessary for adolescents. Partner notification (contact tracing) by genitourinary medicine services is essential for gonorrhoea to prevent further spread of infection.

56 Haemolytic uraemic syndrome

Haemolytic uraemic syndrome (HUS) is a clinical syndrome defined by the presence of microangiopathic haemolytic anaemia, thrombocytopenia and acute renal dysfunction. It is closely related to thrombocytopenic purpura. It comprises a set of heterogeneous conditions but more than 90% of cases are caused by toxin-producing diarrhoeal organisms. There are other rare aetiologies (atypical HUS) that have a worse prognosis; for example, some are inherited disorders and tend to relapse. The condition has also been reported in association with some drugs (such as antineoplastic agents and cyclosporin A) and some other diseases such as systemic lupus erythematosus. The features of HUS also occur in thrombotic thrombocytopenic purpura (TTP).

ORGANISM

In 95% of cases HUS occurs following an episode of diarrhoea, usually bloody, caused by enterohaemorrhagic *Escherichia coli* infection. These organisms produce verotoxin also known as Shiga-like toxins, and are therefore referred to as verotoxin-producing *E. coli* (VTEC or STEC). Among *E. coli* serotypes the most commonly associated with HUS in the

UK is *E. coli* O157 and the most prevalent exotoxin is VT-2. In other countries O111 and O26 are more important. Because VT production is encoded on a promiscuous bacteriophage, which can be transferred between serotypes or even between species, this pattern of serotype prevalence may change. *Shigella dysenteriae* type 1 produces a homologous toxin and can also cause HUS as a complication of classical dysentery.

EPIDEMIOLOGY

E. coli O157 is an emerging infection that appeared in the early 1980s. Because it is the most important cause of HUS it is probably the most important common gut pathogen in the UK. Around 90% of cases of HUS occur in early childhood and most cases are in children between the ages of 6 months and 5 years of age. A survey in the UK between 1986 and 1989 through the British Paediatric Surveillance Unit found an incidence of 0.82 per 100 000 child population per annum. This survey resumed in 1997 and in combination with laboratory reporting has detected many cases. Numbers of cases of O157 VTEC in England and Wales have increased dramatically from under 100 a year in the 1980s to 600–700 a year in the period 1995–97. Outbreaks of VTEC have been reported in association with nurseries, improperly chlorinated swimming pools and among tourists. The main reservoir of VTEC is considered to be cattle, although the organism is also found in other species such as sheep, pigs and goats. Levels of VTEC are high in UK herds (around 60% of herds are carrying the organism) and contact with animals, e.g. on farm visits, is a risk factor for infection with VTEC and HUS in children. The organisms persist in faecally contaminated soil so that children do not have to touch animals on farm visits to become infected.. Contamination of meat products occurs through poor hygiene (e.g. carrying out production of cooked and uncooked meats in the same area in a butcher's) or food production (e.g. undercooking beefburgers). The organisms can also enter ground water supplies. *E. coli* O157 infections occur both sporadically and as outbreaks.

Transmission

Substantial outbreaks of HUS due to VTEC in the UK, North America, Australia and Japan have been associated with consumption of undercooked hamburgers, unpasteurised milk, contaminated water and other food products (such as vegetables) and contaminated water (including swimming in untreated water and paddling pools). Sporadic cases and outbreaks also occur through contact with farms and farm animals. Because the organism persists in the environment children do not have to have direct contact with animals. Person-to-person spread, presumed faecal–oral, of VTEC is also important.

Incubation period

E. coli O157 has a usual incubation period of 3–4 days, although both shorter and longer periods have been observed, the outside limit being 10 days. When HUS follows there is usually a period of about a week between the onset of diarrhoea and the first signs of HUS.

NATURAL HISTORY AND CLINICAL FEATURES

VTEC can cause asymptomatic infection, diarrhoea, abdominal cramps, haemorrhagic colitis or complete or partial HUS. The pathogenesis is complex (see Further reading), the key being production of verocytotoxin in the gut. Its entry into the mucosa causes microvascular injury and then cytotoxic and inflammatory events, particularly affecting the glomerular microvascular endothelial cells of the kidney but also causing haemolysis and neutrophil activation. The chance of a child with VTEC-induced diarrhoea progressing to HUS is considered to be about 10%. In those who proceed to HUS the diarrhoea is often initially nonbloody but becomes grossly bloody in 75% of cases and is often associated with severe abdominal pain. Patients may present with surgical emergencies such as intussusception, rectal prolapse, toxic dilatation of the colon, bowel ischaemia and perforation. The acute oliguric renal failure develops abruptly and usually coincides with the onset of anaemia. The abruptness of oliguria is such that it may rapidly lead to extracellular fluid overload, hyperkalaemia, acidosis and hypertension. Fever occurs in less than 20% of affected children. Broadly speaking those with the worse colitis have the worse renal damage but this is not always the case. An adverse prognostic feature is an elevated peripheral blood neutrophil count at presentation. Counts in excess of 20×10^9/L predict poor outcome. Central nervous system involvement usually occurs early in the course of HUS and presents with irritability, seizures, drowsiness, coma and hemiplegia. Neurological damage is the principal cause of death. Insulin-dependent diabetes mellitus can also appear during the acute illness. Cardiomyopathy can occur up to 4 months after onset.

Diagnosis

The clinical diagnosis of HUS is based on the clinical triad: microangiopathic haemolytic anaemia, thrombocytopenia and acute renal dysfunction, remembering that the thrombocytopenia is often transient. Children whose HUS does not follow a diarrhoeal prodrome may still have VTEC infection and should be appropriately investigated. Other atypical, usually nondiarrhoeal forms of HUS are rare and include red cell polyagglutination syndrome, which usually follows pneumococcal infection, familial forms including those associated with hypocomplementaemia, thrombotic thrombocytopenic purpura, systemic lupus erythematosus, the antiphospholipid antibody syndrome and renal venous thrombosis for whatever cause.

Diagnosis of infection with VTEC can be on the basis of detection of either the expected VTEC or the toxin (VT) itself. The organism may be isolated from stool specimens, although it can be undetectable by the time that HUS develops. Specialist and reference laboratories will be able to detect the toxin from organism-negative stools and antibody tests for anti-E.-coli-O157 (IgG and IgM) are becoming available and will be useful in establishing whether a single-source outbreak is occurring. It is vital that isolates are sent on from primary to central laboratories for typing so that common source outbreaks can be detected promptly.

MANAGEMENT

The child with diarrhoea only (see also Chapter 18)

Electrolyte and fluid balance should be corrected and maintained in all children with diarrhoea irrespective of whether HUS develops (see Chapter 18, pp. 95–95). Stool specimens for culture should be obtained from all children with diarrhoea and when the diarrhoea has been bloody the culture should specifically be for VTEC and the laboratory should be appraised of the likelihood of this diagnosis. It is recommended that all diarrhoeal specimens should be tested by laboratories for VTEC. If the diarrhoea is severe, or VTEC is detected, it will also be wise to establish baseline blood count and metabolic status.

Children with haemorrhagic colitis require close follow-up to detect early signs of surgical complications as well as pallor, oliguria or hypotension, which may suggest HUS. In VTEC infection, antibiotic therapy is not thought to reduce the likelihood of HUS developing. Indeed some antibiotics (e.g. fluoroquinolones) increase toxin release. Antidiarrhoeal agents may also be positively harmful and should not be given.

The child with haemolytic uraemic syndrome

Specialist advise should be sought early. Fluid balance must be monitored with great care. In the first instance vascular volume must be corrected with isonatraemic fluids. Thereafter fluid prescription should be restricted to the estimated insensible losses plus urine output. Particular attention must be given to the restriction of potassium and the correction of acidosis. Transfusion of packed red blood cells should be undertaken for symptomatic anaemia if the haemoglobin falls below 6 g/100 mL, although transfusion should be slow and cautious taking care to avoid fluid overload. Dialysis is needed in about 50% of cases to support homeostasis and nutrition.

With meticulous attention to care the acute mortality from HUS has declined to less than 5%. Atypical forms of HUS (see above) have a much higher morbidity and mortality and should always be managed in paediatric nephrology centres. Chronic renal failure follows HUS in about 10% of cases, but one-third of survivors exhibit renal impairment, proteinuria or hypertension. Some of these abnormalities appear after many years and therefore long-term follow-up of these children is mandatory.

PREVENTION OF FURTHER CASES

General considerations for prevention of gastrointestinal infections apply (see Chapter 33). In any single case of infection-associated HUS it is important that Consultants in Communicable Disease Control or other public health specialists are informed at an early stage. It is recommended that all laboratories should test all diarrhoeal specimens routinely for VTEC and that this should particularly apply for bloody diarrhoea. *E. coli* isolates in England and Wales should be forwarded for typing by the Laboratory of Enteric Pathogens at the Central Public Health Laboratory and in Scotland by the Scottish Centre of Infection and Environmental Health. This is particularly important for VTEC and where an outbreak is suspected. Serum samples should be retained from affected children to identify serotypes retrospectively where there are outbreaks.

FURTHER READING

PHLS/SCIEH (2000) Guidelines for the control of infection with VTEC. Comm Dis Public Health 3: 14–23.

Taylor CM, Monnens LAH (1998) Advances in haemolytic uraemic syndrome. Arch Dis Child 78: 190–193.

57 *Haemophilus influenzae* infection

Notifiable disease if resulting in meningitis. Paediatricians also notify **all invasive *H. influenzae* whether type b or not** to the BPSU.

ORGANISM

Haemophilus influenzae is a Gram-negative bacterium. Six serotypes (a–f) are defined by polysaccharide antigens in the capsule. Other isolates are nonencapsulated and hence are classified as nontypable.

EPIDEMIOLOGY

Humans are the only hosts. *Haemophilus influenzae* type b (Hib) is the most virulent serotype. Before routine vaccination, it accounted for more than 90% of invasive *H. influenzae* disease (such as meningitis) in children. The disease rate is maximal in the second half of the first year of life. Day care attendance, lower socioeconomic status and overcrowding are risk factors. Before routine vaccination, Hib was a principal cause of bacterial meningitis, the predominant cause of epiglottitis and also the most common bacterial pathogen in septic arthritis and cellulitis among children aged less than 2 years. Most serious *Haemophilus* disease in neonates is caused by nontypable organisms. Later in life, these mainly cause less serious mucosal infections, e.g. otitis media and bronchitis. However, they are becoming relatively more important as causes of invasive disease with the decline in Hib.

Until recent times, the rate of Hib disease below 5 years of age varied between 1:200 and 1:600 in the developed world and was even higher in low-income countries and in aboriginal populations of Australia, Canada and the USA. The introduction of efficacious vaccines against Hib produced dramatic declines in the overall rate of invasive *H. influenzae* disease (see Fig. I.4, p. 447). The few cases of invasive disease in fully immunised infants now seen are more likely to be caused by another serotype or nontypable *H. influenzae* organisms than by Hib.

Because the organism only infects humans, hope has arisen that the disease can be eliminated and perhaps even the organism eradicated. This is supported by studies of the effect of vaccination on Hib throat carriage, which have shown a reduced rate of acquisition and transmission within families in which an infant is immunised.

Transmission

The respiratory route is most common. Shared handkerchiefs in day care have been implicated.

Incubation period

This is uncertain. Although it is suspected that most invasive disease occurs within days of nasopharyngeal acquisition, this has not been proved.

NATURAL HISTORY AND CLINICAL FEATURES

Asymptomatic nasopharyngeal carriage with nontypable organisms is common. Prior to the introduction of routine vaccination the carriage rate was about 5% for encapsulated strains and peaked at pre-school age. Carriage of Hib is now very uncommon in countries where vaccine is used. Only a small minority of carriers develop bacteraemia and invasive disease. Meningitis accounts for 70% of invasive Hib disease, epiglottitis about 10%, with cellulitis and bone or joint infections around 5% each. Hib pneumonia is more common than diagnoses based on blood culture isolates would suggest, and before vaccination Hib was probably the second most common cause of bacterial pneumonia after pneumococcus in children. Cardinal signs of meningitis in the older child include stiff neck and photophobia but in infants less specific features such as fever, irritability and vomiting may be all that is seen (see Chapter 10).

Diagnosis

Accurate diagnosis requires the collection, ideally before antibiotic administration, of samples such as blood, joint fluid or cerebrospinal fluid (CSF) for Gram stain and culture from which serotyping and genotyping can take place. Careful characterisation of *H. influenzae* isolates is important for epidemiological purposes. Antigen detection by latex agglutination or countercurrent immunoelectrophoresis, where available, are especially useful when antibiotics have been given before samples are obtained. It should, however, be recognised that these tests have a false-positive rate that, although low, is especially relevant in the case of a recent recipient of Hib vaccine in whom CSF and urine Hib antigen (polyribosylribitol phosphate – PRP) may be detectable for weeks and perhaps even months. Collection of acute and convalescent sera for antibody to PRP may be helpful if cultures are negative, but do not rule out Hib infection if no rise is seen in an infant younger than 2 years because the immature immune system may not respond to polysaccharide antigens such as PRP.

Lumbar puncture should be delayed if signs suggesting dangerously raised intracranial pressure are present such as coma, pupillary abnormalities, papilloedema or abnormal posturing. Molecular techniques such as polymerase chain reaction are available in some reference laboratories for typing in cases of diagnostic difficulty.

MANAGEMENT

The treatment of choice for invasive disease such as meningitis is a third-generation cephalosporin such as cefotaxime or ceftriaxone. About 15% of Hib isolates are ampicillin-resistant as are a similar percentage of noncapsulate isolates. Chloramphenicol resistance in Hib, although rare, is increasing, so its combination with ampicillin is now less justifiable as a first-line treatment. A minimum of 7 days treatment is required for uncomplicated meningitis. If response to treatment is slow, such as when fever is prolonged, a second lumbar puncture may be helpful. It is reassuring if the CSF is returning to normal (negative), although another source of infection should be sought by the methods described above and could direct a change in antibiotic treatment if viable organisms, whether resistant or not, are found. To reduce the incidence of neurological sequelae in Hib meningitis, dexamethasone 0.6 mg/kg per day in four divided doses should be started (concurrent with the first dose of antibiotics) and be continued for 2 days. Hearing tests for sensorineural deafness should be performed in convalescence.

Young children, especially those under 2 years, will often not produce a protective antibody response after invasive Hib disease, whether previously immunised or not, so Hib vaccine should be offered in convalescence if it is not possible to check the serum antibody response. If Hib infection is proved in an adequately immunised child, immunodeficiency is a strong possibility and must be investigated (Chapter 21). Children with non-type-b invasive H. influenzae disease also merit investigation.

In the UK, mucosal infections such as otitis media are usually managed without obtaining an isolate. About 15% of H. influenzae (usually nontypable) and all isolates of Moraxella catarrhalis (two of the three commonest causes) often produce the enzyme β-lactamase, rendering amoxycillin ineffective. To maximise successful treatment, antibiotics like co-amoxiclav, cefaclor, clarithromycin or azithromycin should be used.

PREVENTION OF FURTHER CASES

When a case of Hib disease occurs in a child or an adult the immunisation records of all children under 4 years in the household should be checked and any unimmunised children should be offered vaccine as soon as possible. Elimination of carriage with antibiotic (usually rifampicin) is no longer indicated if all contacts aged under 4 years have been fully immunised (three doses for children aged less than 12 months and one dose for those aged 12–48 months). In households where there is one or more children aged under 4 who is unvaccinated or incompletely vaccinated, rifampicin should be offered to all home contacts irrespective of age and Hib immunisation history. Similar treatment should be offered to all room contacts (teachers and children) when two or more cases of Hib disease have occurred in a playgroup, nursery or creche within 120 days. Unimmunised children under 4 should also receive vaccine. Cases of Hib disease should be offered both vaccine and antibiotic treatment to eliminate carriage before discharge from hospital as Hib disease occasionally fails to generate immunity, especially in the very young. Rifampicin is the drug of choice for elimination of carriage. The recommended dose is 20 mg/kg/day (up to a maximum of 600 mg daily) once daily for 4 days. This is longer than the 2-day regimen used for meningococcal infection, which will not always clear Hib. Recipients need to be advised of possible adverse reactions, which include interference with the oral contraceptive and red coloration of urine and other body fluids.

Immunisation

In the UK routine vaccination against Hib in the form of a PRP conjugate is given at 2, 3 and 4 months of age. A booster is not currently offered in the second year of life (unlike in most other western countries). This policy appears to have been successful, with the national coverage for three doses approaching 95% (see Fig. I.8, p. 450), estimated effectiveness in those under 4 years old in excess of 95% and a minimal fall-off in protection thereafter. The UK's early accelerated schedule ensures that virtually all infants can be protected before reaching the age of susceptibility.

Although all children under 4 years old should be immunised, those at increased risk of invasive infection by encapsulated bacteria like Hib should be especially targeted for vaccination. These include premature babies, children with asplenia and functional asplenia (as in sickle cell disease) and children infected with HIV. There is evidence for adequate, though reduced, immunogenicity in these groups. The widespread use of Hib conjugate vaccines in many western countries has been highly effective in diminishing the incidence of invasive *Haemophilus influenzae* disease. There is no evidence that Hib is being replaced by similarly virulent organisms and neither has the possibility of vaccine escape mutants arisen. However, vigilance will need to be maintained to ensure the continued success of the vaccine programme and this should include characterisation of invasive *H. influenzae* isolates from all children with this infection.

58 Viral haemorrhagic fevers

Notifiable conditions

Viral haemorrhagic fevers (VHFs) are severe viral infections in which haemorrhage is an important clinical feature. Several different VHFs exist and the pathogenesis of the bleeding differs between them. The importance of managing potential VHFs lies in the differential diagnosis from other, more treatable, life-threatening haemorrhagic diseases such as malignant malaria or meningococcal disease.

ORGANISM

Several groups of viruses are responsible for viral haemorrhagic fevers. Most have an animal reservoir and several are transmitted by an insect vector (Table 58.1).

EPIDEMIOLOGY AND TRANSMISSION

'Arboviruses'

The Flaviviridae and Alphaviridae were previously grouped as arboviruses (arthropod-borne). All are able to replicate both in the insect vector and their vertebrate host.

Yellow fever is an important endemic and epidemic disease of tropical and subtropical Africa and South America. Its insect vector is the mosquito *Aedes aegypti*, which is no longer found in Europe. Jungle or sylvatic yellow fever is transmitted from nonhuman primates. Urban yellow fever is transmitted from infected humans. Both types occur in all age groups with equal frequency and, where further transmission is possible through mosquitoes, cases must be isolated (see Chapter 32).

Dengue is present in the tropics and subtropics worldwide. Its insect vector is also *A. aegypti* and in epidemics can have a very high attack rate. Dengue haemorrhagic fever (DHF) is usually confined to children. It occurs when a child is re-infected with a heterologous dengue serotype (there are four serotypes) and is thought to be caused by pre-existing antibody binding to virus and facilitating infection of monocytes or macrophages via Fc receptors. DHF occurs more frequently in south-east Asia.

The other arboviral haemorrhagic fevers may have a reservoir in chimpanzees or monkeys. They have a similar course to dengue but without a rash.

Arenaviruses

Lassa fever occurs in West Africa, notably in parts of Sierra Leone. It persistently infects the multimammate rat (*Mastomys natalensis*) and humans become infected by inhaling or ingesting infected urine. Other haemorrhagic fevers caused by arenaviruses Machupo, Junin and Sabia are transmitted from persistently infected *Calomys* species in South America.

Bunyaviruses

The nairovirus causing Crimean–Congo haemorrhagic fever (CCHF) is transmitted to man from many vertebrate species, including hares, hedgehogs and domestic animals via the tick (*Hyalomma* spp.). CCHF has been described in Russia, Bulgaria, former Yugoslavia, Pakistan, Iraq, Tanzania, Zaire, Uganda, Burkina Faso and South Africa. Infection can spread from person to person by aerosol to hospital staff or to other family members, often with increased severity of disease in the recipient.

Hantaviruses

Hantaviruses cause haemorrhagic fever with renal syndrome (HFRS). Hantaan virus, which is found in Korea, Japan, far-eastern Russia and China, persistently and silently infects fieldmice (*Apodemus agrarius*).

Table 58.1 Viruses and haemorrhagic fevers

Virus group	Virology	Reservoir	Direct person-to-person spread	Vector	Incubation period (days)	Geographical distribution
Flaviviridae	Enveloped RNA					
Yellow fever		Monkeys, man	No	Mosquito (Aedes aegypti)	3–6	Tropics and subtropics
Dengue		Man	No	Mosquito (Aedes aegypti)	2–7	Tropics and subtropics
Omsk haemorrhagic fever		Musk rat	No	Ticks (Dermatocentor)	3–7	Russia, Rumania
West Nile fever	–	Birds	No	Mosquito	3–10	Middle East, Africa, France, USA
Togaviridae	Enveloped RNA					
Chikungunya*		Man (?monkeys)	No	Mosquito (Aedes aegypti)	1–6	Sub-Saharan Africa, India, SE Asia
Arenaviridae	Unenveloped RNA					
Lassa fever		Multimammate rat	Yes	Aerosol (urine)	10–11	Sub-Saharan Africa
Junin (Argentinian fever)		Calomys musculinus	Yes	Aerosol (urine)	10–11	South America
Machupo (Bolivian haemorrhagic fever)		Calomys callosus	Yes	Aerosol (urine)	10–11	South America
Sabia (Venezuelan haemorrhagic fever)		?	Yes	Aerosol (urine)	10–11	South America

Bunyaviridae	Enveloped RNA				
Phlebovirus: Rift Valley fever	Sheep, cattle, goats	Mosquito, sandfly	No	3–12	Sub-Saharan Africa
Nairovirus: Crimean–Congo haemorrhagic fever	Many vertebrates	Ticks (Hyalomma, etc.)	Yes†	3–12	Russia, sub-Saharan Africa
Hantavirus: Hantaan	Fieldmice (Apodemus)	Aerosol (excreta)	No	7–42	Far East
Seoul	Rattus norvegicus	Aerosol (excreta)	No	7–42	Worldwide
Puumala	Bank vole (Clethrionymus)	Aerosol (excreta)	No	7–42	Northern Europe
Filoviridae	Enveloped RNA				
Ebola	Possibly bats‡	Aerosol	Yes	7–9	West and central Africa
Marburg	Bats‡	Aerosol	Yes	7–9	West and central Africa

* Usually causes arthritis and fever but in children produces a bleeding diathesis. † Nosocomial infection via blood and interfamilial aerosol spread. ‡ Isolated from monkeys but these are thought not to be the definitive host.

Infection occurs when man enters the fieldmouse's ecological niche or vice versa, and virus is usually transmitted via inhalation of excreta or saliva. Seoul virus is present throughout the world and persistently infects the brown rat (*Rattus norvegicus*). For example, in Baltimore, USA, 50% of rats have been found to be excreting virus. Puumala virus persistently infects the bank vole (*Clethrionymys glareolus*) and is found in Scandinavia and other parts of northern Europe. Hantaviruses have been found in man and animal reservoirs in the UK. In most surveys 5–10% of cases are reported in children. Person-to-person spread (apart from two cases of transplacental spread) has not been described. These and related viruses (Sinnombre, Black Creek Canyon, Bayou, etc.) can cause a severe inhalation pneumonitis, hantavirus pulmonary syndrome (HPS), which rarely spreads from person to person.

Filoviruses

The filoviruses Marburg and Ebola are transmitted via blood and other bodily fluids and occasionally by the respiratory route. Ebola outbreaks have occurred in Zaire, Sudan, Uganda, Gabon and Côte d'Ivoire with high mortality. Health-care facilities have acted as foci for transmission, e.g. through emergency surgery on Ebola cases. Marburg fever occurred initially in monkey handlers in a laboratory in Germany but subsequent sporadic cases have occurred in travellers in Kenya and Uganda and there have been outbreaks in Zaire. Although monkeys have been found to be infected, it is thought that they are not the definitive host. Persistent asymptomatic infection of bats has been induced experimentally and there are some epidemiological links between bats and human Ebola fever.

Incubation period

This varies from 1 day to 6 weeks (Table 58.1).

NATURAL HISTORY AND CLINICAL FEATURES

Arboviruses

Dengue may be an undifferentiated febrile illness. Nausea and vomiting occur in 60% of cases, being more common in children and the elderly. Over 50% of patients will have cough. Older children and adults display the more classical disease. This begins with a sudden onset of fever (which may be biphasic), severe muscle aches, bone and joint pains, severe headache and altered taste (a metallic taste is described). Lymphadenopathy and rash appear 2–3 days after onset of fever. The rash is preceded by skin flushing and can be maculopapular, petechial or purpuric. There is a spectrum of disease from mild dengue fever (DF) to dengue haemorrhagic fever and dengue shock syndrome (DSS) but DHF and DSS should not be diagnosed unless the criteria in Table 58.2 are met. DHF usually occurs in two stages. The first resembles classical dengue with fever, malaise, headache, anorexia and vomiting. Some 2–5 days later the condition worsens with the onset of shock. There is restlessness, irritability, cold extremities, narrowed pulse pressure and petechiae on the face and extremities. Frank ecchymoses

Table 58.2 Diagnosis and staging of DHF and DSS (Adapted from Belshe RB (ed.) (1990) *A textbook of Human Virology*. Mosby, St Louis, MO)

Clinical

Acute high fever	> 2–7 days
Haemorrhage	Tourniquet test positive (> 20 petechiae/inch)
	Plus one or more of epistaxis, gum bleeding, melaena, haematemesis, ecchymoses
Hepatomegaly	
Shock	Hypotension, narrow pulse pressure, cold clammy skin

Laboratory

Thrombocytopenia (< 100 000/µL)
Haemoconcentration (haematocrit increase by 20% or more)

Staging

Grade I	Fever, nonspecific symptoms, positive tourniquet test
Grade II	As above plus spontaneous bleeding
Grade III	Circulatory failure, rapid weak pulse, hypotension, narrowing pulse pressure
Grade IV	Profound shock with blood pressure not measurable

(10% of cases), bleeding from gums and venepuncture sites can occur and the tourniquet test will produce petechiae.

Children will also have thrombocytopenia and haemoconcentration, which helps to differentiate early or low-grade DHF from dengue. If there is circulatory failure (hypotension or narrowed pulse pressure) this is diagnostic of DSS. Approximately 30% of children with DHF progress to DSS. The mortality rate of DHF is 5–10%.

Arenaviruses

It is estimated that Lassa fever virus (LFV) affects up to 50 000 persons each year in west Africa. In a study in Sierra Leone it was estimated that 12% of 3849 hospital admissions were for Lassa fever and that LFV was responsible for 30% of the deaths in hospital. Nevertheless, not all cases are severe. Infection begins insidiously with generalised myalgia, chills, sore throat, fever and dry cough. This can progress with manifestations of increased capillary permeability such as pulmonary oedema and subconjunctival oedema. Subsequently haemorrhagic complications such as epistaxis, haemoptysis, haematemesis, petechiae at pressure points and oozing from venepuncture sites develop. This terminates with abrupt shock and death. The overall mortality is 7–10% but rises to 30% in the first trimester of pregnancy. Viraemia is heavier in pregnant women.

Bunyaviruses

Crimean–Congo haemorrhagic fever begins abruptly with fever, myalgia, malaise and headache. This lasts 2–3 days when the patient then has full development of haemorrhagic features. Petechiae develop over the chest and abdomen and epistaxis is common. Spreading cutaneous ecchymoses and bleeding from every orifice, together with neurological signs, indicate very severe disease. Death occurs following circulatory collapse. There may be hepatomegaly and occasionally splenomegaly.

Haemorrhagic fever with renal syndrome varies in severity. That due to Hantaan virus (sometimes termed Korean haemorrhagic fever) is the most severe. Classically it evolves through five phases (febrile, hypotensive, oliguric, diuretic and convalescent). Mild haemorrhagic signs occur first in the hypotensive phase, which lasts from 2 hours to 3 days. Major haemorrhages and most of the deaths occur in the oliguric phase (3–7 days). The diuretic phase lasts from days to weeks with polyuria (3–6 L/day) and convalescence takes weeks to months. A mortality rate of 15% is not uncommon. Balkan HFRS is due to a similar virus, has a similar clinical pattern but is acquired from the yellow-necked fieldmouse (*Apodemus flavicollis*). Nephropathia epidemica (NE) occurs in northern Europe and is due to Puumala virus. It is far milder than Hantaan infection; indeed, only one in 15–20 cases of infection is symptomatic and the mortality is less than 1%. Seoul virus infection occurs worldwide and is intermediate in severity between Hantaan and Puumala. It usually does not show phase progression but patients do show hepatomegaly. There is some evidence that hantavirus infection might predispose to development of chronic renal failure.

Filoviruses

Illness due to filoviruses usually begins with fever, myalgia and headache. Some 2–3 days later diarrhoea and a morbilliform rash appear. This is followed by widespread haemorrhagic manifestations. Mortality is high (Marburg 50%; Ebola 80%).

Diagnosis

Travel history and history of contact with arthropods and animals will help to reach a diagnosis. Malaria, meningococcal septicaemia and rickettsioses are part of the differential diagnosis. The specific diagnosis depends upon detection of virus or a serological response to it. Great care must be exercised in handling specimens from patients with VHF. Samples will need to be examined under category 4 containment at specialist centres such as the PHLS Virus Reference Laboratory, Colindale.*

MANAGEMENT AND PREVENTION

All viral haemorrhagic fevers require immediate specialist care and advice. Infections with arenaviruses, filoviruses and CCHF are transmissible from person to person and cases (suspected or proven) should be managed in a high-security infectious disease unit. Supportive therapy includes fluid management and administration of fresh frozen plasma and platelets. Ribavirin (intravenous) may be of benefit in arenavirus, bunyavirus and filovirus infections. Immune plasma may also be of benefit in some cases of VHF.

---

* **Contact PHLS Virus Reference Division – tel. 020 8200 4400. Out of working hours contact the on-call doctor for the Communicable Disease Surveillance Centre – tel. 020 8200 6868.**

If VHF is considered possible or likely the Consultant in Communicable Disease Control must be informed immediately by telephone. The names and addresses of family and health-care contacts should be noted in case the VHF is one that is transmissible from person to person.

A vaccine is available to prevent yellow fever.

FURTHER READING

Advisory Committee on Dangerous Pathogens (1996) Management and control of viral haemorrhagic fevers. HMSO, London.

59 Hand, foot and mouth disease

See also Chapter 51

ORGANISM

Causative organisms are Coxsackie viruses of a number of types, especially A16 and A5, and less often A10 and enterovirus 71. They are small, nonenveloped RNA viruses of the picornavirus family. Coxsackie A16 and enterovirus 71 are those most commonly associated with epidemics.

EPIDEMIOLOGY

Children between 1 and 4 years are most commonly affected, with those between 5 and 14 years less so. The disease is uncommon in older and younger people. Infection has not been reported in neonates or adults older than 65 years. The disease occurs worldwide, both sporadically and in epidemics, especially in preschool child-care establishments. It shows a bimodal seasonal pattern, being more common in summer and late autumn/early winter. The interepidemic period in the UK is 2–3 years.

Transmission

By droplets, direct contact with nasal secretions and the rash, and the faecal–oral route. The risk of interfamilial spread is low (three examples from 26 cases in one study).

Incubation period

3–5 days.

NATURAL HISTORY AND CLINICAL FEATURES

The illness usually begins with a mild pyrexia followed 3–5 days later by a rash. In the mouth a vesicular rash 4–8 mm across is present on the tongue and buccal mucosa. Similar lesions occur on the hands and less commonly the feet. They are more common on the dorsal surfaces than on the palms and soles. The typical distribution of the rash is on the hands, feet and mouth (60%) and less commonly on only the hands and feet or hands and mouth only (c. 20% each). Lesions may occasionally be present on the buttocks, trunk, genitalia, face and limbs. The rash lasts about a week and the disease is typically mild and self-limiting. It is usually the severity of the buccal lesions that determines how ill a child is.

Recently there have been outbreaks of severe (epidemic) hand, foot and mouth disease (HFMD), which is not seen in the UK. The outbreaks were in Malaysia (1997 and 2000), Taiwan (1998), Hong Kong (1999) and Singapore (2000). These have been atypical in that the initial presentation was as classical HFMD but subsequently a significant number of children developed rapid clinical deterioration as a result of cardiopulmonary failure. There was also central nervous system involvement (meningitis, encephalitis or acute flaccid paralysis) in a high proportion. The hospital mortality for the epidemic in Taiwan was about 15% (55 deaths), most deaths occurring within 24 hours of admission. Enterovirus 71 has been associated with some cases in the Malaysian and Taiwan epidemics though the aetiology in some outbreaks has not yet been fully elucidated.

Diagnosis

Virus can be isolated from the lesions and stools but this is not usually necessary as the diagnosis can be made clinically.

MANAGEMENT

Management is symptomatic only except for the very rare severe case with cardiac involvement (see Chapter 17).

PREVENTION OF FURTHER CASES

Isolation is of little value as the virus may persist in the stools for several weeks. Sharing of cups, cutlery, etc. should be prohibited. Strict attention to personal hygiene may have some effect.

60 Hantavirus pulmonary syndrome

ORGANISM

Hantavirus is an enveloped virus with a segmented RNA genome in the family Bunyaviridae and, unlike the other family members, is not spread by insect vectors. In general the hantaviruses found solely in the Americas cause hantavirus pulmonary syndrome (HPS) and those with a worldwide distribution cause haemorrhagic fever with renal syndrome (HFRS), see Chapter 58. At least six different hantaviruses (Sin nombre, New York, Andes, Bayou, Black Creek Canal and Laguna Negra) can cause HPS.

EPIDEMIOLOGY

Sin nombre virus ('without a name' – nobody wished to have such a rapidly fatal virus infection named after where they lived) was the first HPS-associated hantavirus to be described in 1993. Since then large numbers of 'new' hantaviruses have been discovered, some of which infect man. However, it is unlikely that it is an entirely new virus; indeed, examination of post-mortem material from a case of unexplained adult respiratory distress syndrome in 1978 has demonstrated that it was HPS. The epidemiology involves a rodent host (e.g. the deermouse, *Peromyscus maniculatus*, for Sin nombre) which is persistently and asymptomatically infected. The virus is persistently excreted and man becomes infected, usually by inhalation of dried excreta, when the rodent enters man's ecological niche or vice versa. Infection is more common in males (M:F, 2:1 to 3:1) and occurs most often in those aged 20–30 years with little evidence of person-to-person spread. The exception to this is Andes virus (reservoir *Oligoryzomys longicaudatus*), which has been associated with person-to-person spread and high attack rates in children in Argentina.

Incubation period

Not known.

NATURAL HISTORY AND CLINICAL FEATURES

Unlike some hantaviral HFRS, most infections are clinically apparent and severe. One 4-year-old child whose mother had died of HPS had a mild respiratory hantavirus infection. A prodromal phase in which patients complain of fever, myalgia, gastrointestinal problems and headache lasts for up to 7 days. This is followed by a nonproductive cough and rapidly progressing tachypnoea and tachycardia as a result of noncardiac pulmonary oedema. The mortality rate is high (c. 50%) and predictors of mortality include increases in haematocrit and prolonged prothrombin and partial thromboplastin times. Features distinguishing HPS from pneumococcal and influenzal pneumonia are dizziness, nausea and vomiting, absence of cough and, in the laboratory, thrombocytopenia, high haematocrit and low serum bicarbonate. The pulmonary disease is caused by increased permeability pulmonary oedema. The oedema fluid has a protein content equivalent to serum, indicating the severity of the capillary leak. Death occurs as a result of myocardial depression unresponsive to therapeutic interventions.

Diagnosis

Viral RNA is detectable in peripheral blood mononuclear cells by reverse transcription–polymerase chain reaction (RT-PCR) at presentation. Detection of IgM antihantavirus can also aid specific diagnosis.

MANAGEMENT

Early admission to intensive care and ventilatory support are essential. Ribavirin, although effective in vitro, has been disappointing in open trials. Extracorporeal membrane oxygenation has proved a useful adjunct to therapy.

PREVENTION OF FURTHER CASES

Prevention is by avoiding exposure to rodent excreta. Rodent-proofing houses has been shown to be effective in excluding *P. maniculatus* and should prevent transmission of hantaviruses. There is no vaccine currently available.

61 Helicobacter pylori

ORGANISM

Helicobacter pylori is a Gram-negative, spiral organism that grows under microaerophilic conditions.

EPIDEMIOLOGY

In developed countries the prevalence of *H. pylori* colonisation of the gastric mucosa increases with age. Serological studies have shown the prevalence of infection is approximately 10% at 15 years of age and rises to 60% at 60 years of age. However, in low-income countries the prevalence of infection is between 80% and 100% by 10 years. Recent studies suggest that the marked difference in infection rates between children in different countries is related to living standards. Children from families with low incomes in developed countries are much more likely to be infected than children from higher income families. The increase in prevalence of *H. pylori* infection with increasing age noted in developed countries is probably due to a cohort effect. *H. pylori* is acquired in childhood and the high prevalence of infection in older age groups in developed countries probably relates to poorer living conditions in those countries 40 years ago.

There is marked clustering of infection within families. In one study, more than 80% of the siblings of *H.-pylori*-colonised children had serological evidence of infection in comparison to 13% of age-matched controls. Clustering of *H. pylori* infection has also been identified within institutions for the mentally handicapped.

Transmission

No environmental source of infection has been identified. The human stomach remains the only site from which *H. pylori* is consistently isolated. In two studies *H. pylori* has been cultured from the faeces of some infected individuals. The method of transmission of *H. pylori* is still unknown. Oral–oral or faecal–oral transmission between humans is most likely. The lack of a serotyping system for the organism is a major problem in conducting studies of transmission.

Incubation period

Unknown

NATURAL HISTORY AND CLINICAL FEATURES

H. pylori colonisation of the gastric mucosa is always associated with histological evidence of chronic gastritis in children. *H. pylori* is present in most cases of primary or unexplained gastritis. There is a strong correlation between duodenal ulceration and *H. pylori* gastritis in children and adults. Almost 100% of primary duodenal ulcers are associated with *H. pylori* gastritis. In adults, duodenal ulcers do not recur if *H. pylori* is cleared from the gastric mucosa. Studies in children have produced similar findings. *H. pylori* colonisation of the gastric mucosa and the associated chronic gastritis may be important factors in the development of gastric cancer. *H. pylori* has recently been classified as a group 1 carcinogen by the World Health Organization. However, only about 1% of infected individuals will develop gastric cancer.

There is little evidence that *H. pylori* gastritis in the absence of duodenal ulcer disease is a cause of abdominal pain in children. Children with *H.-pylori*-associated gastritis are often asymptomatic. Large serological studies of healthy children have found *H. pylori* infection in up to 30% of asymptomatic children. Furthermore, it is not possible to differentiate children who are infected with *H. pylori* from uninfected children on the basis of their symptoms. Following eradication of *H. pylori*, symptoms appear to improve consistently only in those children who have an associated duodenal ulcer and not in those who have *H. pylori* gastritis alone.

Diagnosis

In adults the presence of *H. pylori* gastritis has usually not been associated with any morphological evidence of inflammation. However, the presence of a nodular appearance of the antral mucosa has been noted in over 50% of children with chronic *H.-pylori*-associated antral gastritis.

Culture

The ultimate test to confirm the presence of *H. pylori* on the gastric mucosa is to culture the organism from a mucosal biopsy. However, culturing *H. pylori* is slow and expensive and many laboratories have difficulty in consistently culturing the organism. Incubation under microaerophilic conditions for a period of between 5 and 7 days is usually required.

Staining techniques

Silver stains are almost 100% sensitive in identifying the presence of *H. pylori* in children. A modified Giemsa stain is also sensitive in identifying the organism and is easier to perform. Gram's staining of gastric mucosal material is a practical way of identifying this organism but it has a low sensitivity.

Urease test

H. pylori produces large amounts of urease, which can be detected by various tests. When a full biopsy specimen is placed in urea medium the sensitivity of this test is close to 100%. It is important to note that using only half a biopsy specimen in such tests significantly lowers the sensitivity in children. This is probably because there are fewer organisms present in children.

Urea breath test

The production of urease by *H. pylori* has also resulted in the development of urea breath tests. The patient ingests ^{13}C-labelled urea. The presence of urease in the stomach results in the release of ^{13}C-labelled CO_2 in the expired air. These tests are very sensitive in detecting *H. pylori* colonisation of the gastric mucosa. In children, the test can be carried out after a 2-hour fast without any test meal being required. Under such circumstances it was recently reported to be 100% sensitive and 97% specific in children.

Serology

The sensitivity and specificity of commercially available ELISAs to detect the *H.-pylori*-specific IgG response can be very variable. This is especially true in children. It is important that ELISAs used to diagnose *H. pylori* colonisation in children are standardised by use of children's sera. If the assay is based on adult antibody cut-off levels a significant number of children colonised by *H. pylori* are not detected.

MANAGEMENT

In children, as in adults, eradication of *H. pylori* from the gastric antrum is associated with healing of antral gastritis. In children, triple therapy combining two antibiotics and a bismuth preparation for 1 week appears to be successful in eradicating *H. pylori*. Colloidal bismuth subcitrate is the bismuth preparation most extensively studied for use in children. Bismuth subcitrate prescribed at a dose of 480 mg BiO_3/1.73 m^2 of body surface area per day resulted in bismuth concentrations that varied between 5 mg/L and 28 mg/L with the toxic range being above 50 mg/L. Bismuth should be prescribed on a four times per day basis. Recently, triple therapy for 1 week incorporating colloidal bismuth subcitrate 480 mg/1.73m^2/day (maximum 120 mg four times a day) combined with metronidazole 20 mg/kg/day (maximum 200 mg three times a day) and clarithromycin 15 mg/kg/day (maximum 250 mg twice a day) was successful in clearing *H. pylori* infection in 95% of treated children. Compliance was very closely monitored in the study. This high success rate may not be achievable in routine clinical practice when compliance may not be so closely monitored.

Concern has been expressed about the use of bismuth in the treatment of *H. pylori* gastritis in children. In studies to date using bismuth preparations to treat *H. pylori* gastritis in children no case of bismuth toxicity or adverse side-effect has been reported. Toxic effects of bismuth have been reported in adults and include encephalopathy which is reversible after withdrawal of the drug and acute renal impairment after ingestion of a large overdose.

In adults, 1 week of triple therapy using a combination of a proton pump inhibitor and two antibiotics (metronidazole and clarithromycin, amoxycillin or tetracycline) is very effective. Recently, a number of studies have been published on the use of omeprazole rather than bismuth, combined with two antibiotics (clarithromycin and metronidazole or amoxycillin) to treat *H.-pylori*-infected children. Preliminary reports from across Europe suggest that clarithromycin-resistant strains are much more prevalent in children than in adults, possibly because of the widespread use of clarithromycin for childhood infections. If clarithromycin resistance is present, the success rate of triple therapy that includes this antibiotic appears to be markedly reduced.

Children with duodenal ulcer disease who have confirmed *H. pylori* infection of the gastric mucosa should all be treated to eradicate this infection. Eradication of *H. pylori* from the gastric mucosa will result in long-term healing of duodenal ulcers in children as in adults. The question as to whether or not children with chronic *H.-pylori*-associated gastritis who do not have duodenal ulcer disease should be treated remains debatable. As noted above, the evidence suggests that the majority of these children do not have symptoms as a result of the chronic gastritis. There is therefore at this point no definite indication to treat the infection in such children. However, this situation may change in the next few years if evidence supporting an association between early infection with *H. pylori* and chronic gastritis with the subsequent development of gastric cancer continues to increase.

FURTHER READING

Rowland M, Drumm B (1998) Clinical significance of *Helicobacter* infection in children. Br Med Bull 54; 95–105.

62 Invasive helminths causing multisystem disease

Ascariasis cysticercosis, gnathostomiasis, hydatid disease, schistosomiasis, strongyloidiasis, toxocariasis, trichinosis. See also Chapter 103.

ORGANISM

This chapter describes conditions caused by a number of organisms: *Ascaris lumbricoides*, *Clonorchis sinensis*, *Echinococcus granulosus*, *E. multilocularis* and *E. vogeli* (causing hydatid disease), *Fasciola hepatica* (fascicoliasis or liver fluke disease), *Gnathostoma spinigerum*, *Schistosoma japonicum*, *S. mansoni*, *S. haematobium* (schistosomiasis and Katayama fever), *Strongyloides stercoralis* (strongyloidiasis and *Strongyloides* hyperinfection syndrome), *Taenia solium* (cysticercosis) *Toxocara canis*, *T. cati* and *Trichinella spiralis* (trichinosis).

EPIDEMIOLOGY

Worldwide the invasive helminths are a major source of childhood ill-health. Apart from sometimes causing severe invasive disease, the commoner varieties, hookworm and *Schistosoma haematobium*, cause major morbidity through anaemia and chronic ill-health. *A. lumbricoides* is an intestinal roundworm found in temperate and tropical regions but is uncommon in the UK. The adult ranges from 20–35 cm long and is as thick as a pencil, although the male tends to be smaller. They are particularly prevalent in conditions of poor sanitation, with an individual patient harbouring up to 1000 worms and mature females producing up to 200 000 eggs daily. In 1947 it was estimated that 18 000 tons of *Ascaris* eggs were produced annually in China alone. *A. suum*, the pig ascarid, can also infect man and cause intestinal obstruction. The eggs need to mature for 2–3 weeks in the soil. The spread is faecal–oral with an incubation period of 4–8 weeks.

G. spinigerum is mainly confined to south-east Asia and is a parasite of dogs and cats, being accidentally transmitted to man by the ingestion of undercooked fish or poultry.

F. hepatica, the liver fluke, is a parasite of sheep, cattle and other large animals and occurs worldwide, including the UK. Cysts are ingested in contaminated water plants such as watercress.

S. stercoralis is a human gut parasite but can also exist as a free-living form in damp soil and occurs throughout the tropics. Infection arises when larvae from stool (including autoinfection) or contaminated soil penetrate the skin or gut wall.

Schistosomiasis (bilharzia) is caused by parasites that are predominantly of human origin and is found in parts of sub-Saharan and northern Africa, the Middle East, south-east Asia, Central and South America and some Caribbean islands. The larvae (cercariae), which have developed in snails, penetrate the skin of anyone swimming or wading in contaminated water.

Cysticercosis occurs following ingestion of food or water contaminated with *T. solium* eggs (cf. tapeworm, which is acquired by eating improperly cooked pork containing *T. solium* larvae). The eggs remain viable in soil for many weeks after excretion in human faeces. It is also possible for a patient harbouring an adult worm to autoinfect from anus to mouth via the hands. Cysticercosis is endemic in South and Central America, south-east Asia and parts of Africa. It affects both sexes equally and may become apparent in infancy. The adult tapeworms of *Echinococcus granulosus*, *E. multilocularis* and *E. vogeli* are found in dogs (and other Canidae), foxes (but now also spread to domestic dogs and cats) and Latin American bush dogs respectively. The larval forms (hydatid cysts) are found normally in herbivores (sheep and cattle) and small rodents (voles, rats and mice) but occur in man following ingestion of eggs excreted in canine faeces. *E. granulosus* is the commonest cause of human hydatid disease and is found worldwide, particularly in association with sheep-raising areas. *E. multilocularis* is enzootic in subarctic areas, China and continental Europe and *E. vogeli* in Central America.

T. canis and *T. cati*, dog and cat ascarids respectively, can undergo limited growth in man. They are similar to *A. lumbricoides* but only one-quarter of their size. In their natural host (and especially in young animals) they undergo a full developmental cycle and become mature worms in the intestine. The adult worms produce eggs, which are excreted in the puppies' or kittens' faeces. The eggs require a period of maturation (1–3 weeks) in the soil, after which they are infective for dog, cat or man. Soil from parks in London has been shown to contain eggs in up to 25% of samples. In older dogs and cats the worms do not undergo full development and encyst in tissues; however, in pregnant dogs and cats the worms excyst and cross the placenta. Thus even very young puppies and kittens can be parasitised and infective. Children become infected by ingestion of contaminated soil (pica). Other potential sources of infection include play-pit sand and unwashed faecally contaminated vegetables. Infections are more common with *T. canis* and the incubation period can be weeks to months for development of visceral larva migrans or years for ocular granulomas.

Trichinella spiralis has a worldwide distribution in man and carnivorous animals. The major (but decreasing) reservoir for human infection is the pig. Man becomes infected by ingestion of improperly or incompletely cooked pork containing encysted larvae. In industrialised countries the incidence of infection is decreasing; for example, in the USA, autopsy surveys in 1941 and 1970 showed that the prevalence had dropped from 16% to 4.7%. This has largely been achieved by banning raw pork scraps from pig-feed, by deep freezing meat (which kills cysts) and by education on cooking meat.

Incubation period

These primary systemic illnesses usually present within 3 months of infection, although *Strongyloides* can be harboured as a symptomless infection for many years until systemic invasion occurs following an event that lowers immunity. For both cysticercosis and hydatid disease the incubation varies according to the site of infection and rate of growth of cysts. For example, in cysticercosis, full maturation of cysts takes 3–4 months when they achieve diameters of 2 mm to 2 cm. Hydatid cysts reach a diameter of 1 cm in 5 months but continue to grow as large as 35 cm containing litres and 'hydatid sand'. The incubation of trichinosis is 5–15 days (average 10 days).

NATURAL HISTORY AND CLINICAL FEATURES

Ingested embryonated eggs of *A. lumbricoides* hatch in the duodenum and the larvae penetrate through the wall into blood or lymphatics. They are carried to the liver, heart and thence to the pulmonary circulation. Here they penetrate through the capillaries into the alveoli. They then ascend the bronchial tree, enter the oesophagus and pass down to the small intestine. Here they mature, mate and produce eggs 45–60 days after initial ingestion. In the majority of cases (80%) the only manifestation is excretion of worms or eggs in stool. In a small proportion of cases gastrointestinal or pulmonary symptoms may arise, probably related to the numbers of eggs ingested. Löffler's syndrome (larval pneumonitis) occurs as the larvae migrate through the lungs. Cough, wheezing and breathlessness are the most common presenting features. An urticarial rash may be present and crepitations and ronchi may be detected on chest auscultation. Heavy bowel infestation may cause obstruction. Children with very heavy worm loads may show failure to thrive.

Gnathostomiasis may present with recurrent cutaneous swellings and pulmonary and peritoneal effusions. *Strongyloides* hyperinfection syndrome may rarely present with the primary infection, although it is more commonly seen in children who have carried the organism in the gut for many years and then become immunocompromised, for instance following renal transplantation, the onset of leukaemia or HIV infection. This leads to massive tissue invasion by *Strongyloides* larvae. Clinical features include severe, acute onset of fever, diarrhoea, pneumonitis and sometimes eosinophilic meningoencephalitis. The blood eosinophil count may not be raised. Gram-negative septicaemia is also a common complication. The mortality is high in the immunocompromised.

Katayama fever is seen 2–6 weeks after infection with schistosome cercariae; the child develops high fever, hepatosplenomegaly and a very high blood eosinophilia. There is always a history of contact with fresh water in an area endemic for schistosomiasis.

Cysticercosis can develop in any organ but the common sites are brain, subcutaneous tissues, muscle and eye. There are usually multiple cysts. The chance of clinical infection is less if infection is light. In muscle, cysts frequently calcify and do not initiate disease but subcutaneous infection, painless lumps varying in size from that of a rice grain to a pigeon's egg, may become apparent, predominately over the abdomen. Neurocysticercosis usually appears 5–7 years after infection. The most common presentation is epilepsy but single cysts may present as for a space-occupying lesion with raised intracranial pressure and focal neurological features. Spinal cord involvement is rare but may present as compression or arachnoiditis. Ocular cysts (often subretinal) may lead to blindness. Death of cysticerci may be accompanied by increased disease manifestation as an intense inflammatory response occurs.

In hydatid disease there is usually a single cyst but in up to 30% multiple cysts, usually in a single organ, can occur. Cysts have been described in every organ system but favoured sites are liver, lungs, spleen, brain, eye, heart, bone and genitourinary system. Brain hydatid disease is commoner in children than adults and bone cysts are seen in infants. Infection become manifest either because of expansion of the cysts or because of rupture and release of cyst contents. The signs and symptoms will depend on the site of the cyst. For example, bone cysts give bone pain and pathological fractures; pulmonary cysts cause fever, cough, chest pain and haemoptysis (in adults, if the cysts rupture into a bronchus the patient may complain about coughing up 'grape-skins') and brain cysts present with raised intracranial pressure and fits but few localising signs.

In toxocariasis there are two distinct disease presentations and it is rare for children to progress from one to the other.

Visceral larva migrans is a syndrome of fever, hepatomegaly, pulmonary symptoms (especially wheezing) and signs and eosinophilia. The latter is often very high and occurs as the larvae move through the tissues, eliciting an immune response. A minority may also develop splenomegaly and lymphadenopathy. This form occurs most often in children aged 1–3 years and symptoms can persist for up to a year.

Eye involvement (**ocular larva migrans**) is detected in older children (6–8 years old), when the optic fundus is examined for strabismus or poor visual acuity. The dead larva causes a granulomatous reaction (which has been mistaken for retinoblastoma), which is most damaging when close to the macula. It is, fortunately, rare for this to be bilateral.

Most infections with *T. spiralis* are asymptomatic. When clinically expressed, disease occurs in three phases. The intestinal phase occurs as diarrhoea with abdominal pain due to penetration of the intestinal wall by larvae that have been born to the mature encysted worms. Larvae leave the intestine via the lymphatics, enter the blood stream and are distributed to striated muscle throughout the body. In the muscle fibres, they initiate the phase of muscle invasion with fever, eosinophilia, myositis and the classical sign of periorbital oedema. Dyspnoea occurs because of invasion of the respiratory muscles. In moderate infection the convalescent phase begins in the fifth week of disease. Fatalities occur 4–6 weeks after infection as a result of cardiac or central nervous system involvement.

Diagnosis

The initial diagnosis of each of the individual syndromes is often made on clinical features alone initially as specific antibody tests are usually negative at this stage, except in strongyloidiasis. *Strongyloides* larvae can be found in stool or sputum during hyperinfection if examined immediately by an experienced observer.

Microscopy of stool or urine may reveal eggs in schistosomiasis. In long-standing cases, the bladder may be calcified. Serology is often difficult to interpret.

There is usually eosinophilia with ascariasis and in pneumonitis the chest X-ray may show diffuse mottled opacities. Larvae may be found in sputum and adult worms and eggs may be seen in the stool. Care must be taken not to confuse earthworms that a child has eaten with *A. lumbricoides*.

The specific diagnosis of cysticercosis generally follows radiological demonstration of calcified cysts in brain or muscle, histological examination of surgically removed subcutaneous nodes or visualisation of the cysticercus in the eye. Serological tests (indirect haemagglutination or ELISA) are available but false negatives occur regularly in central nervous system disease.

Asymptomatic or symptomatic hydatid cysts are often picked up on radiography where the disease is prevalent. Outlined cysts with fluid levels may be seen. Nonsurgical aspiration of cysts is dangerous and should be avoided. Serological tests such as indirect haemagglutination or ELISA can be of value but false negatives occur, particularly in pulmonary disease and in children. The Casoni skin test is less reliable than serological tests.

Visceral larva migrans due to *Toxocara* is diagnosed on the basis of multisystem disease accompanied by eosinophilia in a child who has not been out of northern Europe. After foreign travel *F. hepatica*, *G. spinigerum*, *A. lumbricoides* and *C. sinensis* should be considered. Serum *Toxocara* antibodies may be raised, although not reliably, in acute disease. Tissue biopsies might demonstrate larvae. Ocular toxocariasis is diagnosed by its appearance on fundoscopy but serum antibodies might not be raised.

The diagnosis of trichinosis is primarily clinical. Muscle biopsy to demonstrate encysted larvae can be of benefit.

Other diagnoses to be considered in a child with acute illness and eosinophilia include haematological malignancies and an acute vasculitic illness.

MANAGEMENT

Piperazine (75 mg/kg up to a maximum of 4 g on two successive evenings) is effective in eliminating *A. lumbricoides* from the intestine. In children sensitive to piperazine, mebendazole (100 mg twice daily for 3 days) is equally effective but should not be given to those under 2 years. There is no specific treatment for Löffler's syndrome.

Strongyloides hyperinfection syndrome requires urgent therapy with thiabendazole 25 mg/kg twice daily for at least 3 days, albendazole 400 mg daily for at least 5 days (by nasogastric tube if necessary) or ivermectin (200 µg/kg as a single dose) and the latter is becoming the drug of choice. Intravenous antibiotics are also required for the septicaemia. This condition carries a high mortality.

The other acute syndromes, especially Katayama fever, may be worsened by antihelminthic therapy in the acute phase but steroids can be of benefit by dampening the vigorous immune response. Specific antihelminthic therapy, such as praziquantel 20 mg/kg twice daily for 2 days in the case of schistosomiasis, would be introduced after the acute symptoms have resolved and an aetiology has been confirmed.

In cysticercosis many cases are asymptomatic and require no treatment. In some cases surgical removal is needed but therapy has been revolutionised by praziquantel. For neurocysticercosis, dosage is 50 mg/kg/day in three divided doses daily for 15 days. Concurrent administration of dexamethasone may be of benefit to suppress inflammation around moribund cysts. Praziquantel should not be used for ocular cysticercosis.

Hydatid disease is often treated by surgical removal (with a 3–5% morality rate). Albendazole and praziquantel should also be given over the perioperative period. Albendazole can be useful in inoperable or recurrent disease but is of less value in bone disease. *E. multilocularis* is much more difficult to treat.

Toxocaral visceral larva migrans is most often self-limited and watchful waiting is advised. In severely affected children corticosteroids might be beneficial as might treatment with thiabendazole (25 mg/kg twice daily until symptoms resolve) or diethylcarbamazine (2 mg/kg thrice daily for 30 days). Ocular infections do not respond to antihelminthics.

In severe trichinosis corticosteroids should be administered; they can be life-saving.

PREVENTION

Simple hygiene measures prevent the acquisition of ascariasis.

F. hepatica is usually acquired after eating wild watercress or other water plants. Cultivated watercress is safe.

S. stercoralis is initially caught by walking barefoot on damp soil in the tropics and prevented by the use of footwear. It is important to screen children from the tropics for this infection prior to the use of immunosuppressives.

Schistosomiasis may be avoided by keeping out of rivers, streams and lakes in endemic areas. Prevention of cysticercosis and hydatid disease is by preventing ingestion of pig and dog tapeworm eggs. Toxocariasis could be largely prevented if pet owners regularly dewormed their cats and dogs and prevented them from defecating in public places (or at least cleaned up after them). Sand-pits should be covered to prevent cats defecating in them. There is no benefit in giving antihelminthics prophylactically. Prevention of trichinosis can be achieved by good pig husbandry, storing pork deep-frozen and ensuring that pork (including sausages and 'beefburgers') is cooked well prior to ingestion.

63 Hepatitis A

Hepatitis A infection is a notifiable disease*

ORGANISM

An RNA enterovirus, a hepatovirus of the picornavirus family. Humans are the only host. The virus can survive for some time outside the body so that water and food contaminated by sewage or faeces constitute environmental reservoirs.

EPIDEMIOLOGY

Hepatitis A is the commonest cause of infectious hepatitis in most countries. In low-income countries most individuals are infected in childhood and acquire lifelong immunity. In industrialised countries rates of infection in the population are highly variable but lower than in the developing world

---

* In the UK the reporting doctor is currently asked to report viral hepatitis but to categorise it as type A, B, non-A non-B (includes hepatitis C and E) or type not known.

and many children and adults remain nonimmune. In 1998 1515 cases were notified and 1104 cases reported by laboratories in England and Wales to the PHLS Communicable Disease Surveillance Centre; most occurred in children and young adults. Cases occur either sporadically or as outbreaks. In industrialised countries such as the UK, outbreaks occur within families and in settings where there is close physical contact and the potential for faecal–oral spread is high. Examples include day-care centres, nurseries and primary schools. In addition, common source outbreaks occur through consumption of food or water contaminated by sewage, consumption of contaminated shellfish (shellfish concentrate the sewage content of seawater) and food contaminated by infectious foodhandlers. Particular risk groups are drug injectors, gay men and the homeless, while individuals with pre-existing liver disease are at highest risk of severe disease. Travel to low-income countries places individuals at higher risk of infection, especially if they fail to take precautions against enteric infections and are unimmunised (see Prevention of further cases, below).

Transmission

The virus replicates primarily in the intestines and liver and is shed through the biliary tree and bile duct into faeces. Most transmission is via the faecal–oral route. Food or water contaminated by sewage are important vehicles. Among adults faecal–oral transmission can take place through sexual activity. Transmission from blood transfusion can occur but is very rare, and the potential for transmission is far less than for hepatitis B and C virus because of the short duration and low level of viraemia. Vertical (mother to fetus) transmission has been recorded but is exceptionally rare. Sexual transmission also occurs, especially between men having sex with other men involving oral–anal contact.

Incubation period

There is a range of 15–50 days with a median of 33 days.

Infectivity

Infectivity increased during the latter half of the incubation period and is maximal just before the onset of dark urine and jaundice when the virus is replicating and being shed into the faeces. Infectivity of faeces decreases quickly in the week following the darkening of the urine and the appearance of jaundice. There is little risk of transmission in a school setting after the onset of jaundice unless there are concerns over the child's personal hygiene. There is no chronic infection (carrier) state.

NATURAL HISTORY AND CLINICAL FEATURES

Severity of disease is closely related to age. In childhood many infections are asymptomatic or without jaundice (anicteric), especially in younger children. The most specific sign is the onset of dark urine (due to the presence of urobilinogen) which precedes jaundice. In symptomatic cases common symptoms and signs include fever, headache, anorexia, nausea, vomiting and abdominal pain from a tender, enlarged liver. Splenomegaly occurs in a minority of cases. Once the urine darkens the child often feels better, although return of appetite and full vigour may be delayed for 1–2 weeks. However, convalescence is generally brief in children and full recovery is usual. The return of normal stool colour can be taken as indicative of the end of the disease process. In adolescents and adults symptoms are more often severe and prolonged. The development of fulminant hepatitis due to hepatitis A is rare in children, but does occur.

Diagnosis

Diagnosis is often made on the basis of the clinical features and a history of likely exposure to hepatitis A. Urobilinogen can be detected in the urine shortly before the onset of jaundice. Laboratory testing will show a transient rise in serum transaminase (ALT and AST) levels for 1–3 weeks with a rise in bilirubin around the peak of transaminase disturbance. Serological tests for recent hepatitis A infection, IgM anti-HAV (antibody to hepatitis A virus), as well as tests for anti-HBV and anti-HCV, are in common use. Hepatitis B, C and E infection should also be considered and appropriate tests undertaken when the course of the illness appears to be more severe or prolonged than expected, e.g. measuring coagulation indices (prothrombin and partial thromboplastin times), or there has been a probable exposure to these other infections (see Chapters 64–66). Other infections to exclude are infectious mononucleosis and infection with cytomegalovirus. Salivary and urine tests for anti-HAV are becoming available for use in outbreaks where it is impractical or undesirable to take blood.

MANAGEMENT

There is no specific treatment. Hospital admission is undesirable and rarely necessary. However, if admission is unavoidable, the patient should be nursed in a cubicle and enteric precautions taken. Should the hepatitis be severe and hepatic failure seem imminent it is important to contact a specialist liver unit immediately. Important signs include persisting anorexia, progressively deepening jaundice, reappearance of the initial symptoms or the development of ascites. A late sign is behavioural change prior to encephalopathy. Worrying laboratory signs are rising bilirubin, prolongation of the prothrombin time, a falling serum albumin or hypoglycaemia. Enteric precautions also apply in the community and it may be desirable or necessary to exclude children with hepatitis A from nurseries while infectious (see Chapters 32 and 33). If jaundice appears, these precautions can be discontinued 3 days after its appearance.

PREVENTION OF FURTHER CASES

UK cases

The importance of personal hygiene in preventing spread of this and other enteric pathogens must be emphasised to parents and other carers (see Chapter 33). Particular care must be taken within day care, nurseries and primary schools, centres where the potential for spread is higher. Children with clinical hepatitis should be excluded and managed with precautions applicable to hepatitis A, B and C until a specific diagnosis is made. Blood, faeces and other body fluids/products should be the subject of universal precautions (see Chapter 33). All cases of hepatitis A should be notified by the attending doctor. When two or more cases of hepatitis A occur in association the Consultant in Communicable Disease Control or Director of Public Health should be contacted immediately, as well as notification made. This is especially important where food or water contamination is possible or where a number of adults and children may have been exposed, such as in a day nursery. When adults or adolescents have been recently exposed they should be advised to have the active vaccine intramuscular human normal immunoglobulin (HNIG; there is no specific immunoglobulin). HNIG is considered to prevent infection or at least attenuate disease if given within 2 weeks of exposure (HNIG is being used less now). It is not needed for those with a history of two or more doses of hepatitis A vaccine. Dosage is 250 mg for children up to the age of 9; 500 mg for children of 10 and over and adults.*

Adults who are likely to be exposed to infection are those working in a day-care centre where a case has occurred, household contacts, kissing contacts and those sharing meals with an index case. Testing of exposed individuals for anti-HAV IgG (evidence of preceding infection or active immunisation) is not recommended because of the low prevalence of prior infection and the delay and expense that this will cause. Most hepatitis A cases occurring in schools with children over age 5 will be the result of household transmission and so HNIG for school contacts in this age-group rarely has any use in preventing further cases.†

Travel abroad

Travellers to endemic countries (most low-income countries) should be advised to take precautions to avoid infection with hepatitis A and other enteric pathogens (see Chapter 26). Active immunisation is recommended to frequent and long-stay travellers. Inactivated vaccines are available for adults and children but are mostly used in adults at risk of exposure from frequent travel. The vaccine is given in two doses separated by 2 weeks to 1 month and a booster given 6–12 months following the initial dose. It is not licensed for use in children under 1 year old. A combined Hepatitis A and B vaccine is now available.

---

* **An alternative dosage is 0.06–0.12 mL/kg, which applies at all ages. Note that these regimens contain dosages higher than that recommended for short-duration travel abroad – see Chapter 26.**
† **Exceptions would be when cases occur within a limited time (6 weeks or less) in the same class in children who do not come from the same family, or in children attending a boarding school.**

Acute hepatitis B infection is a notifiable disease*

ORGANISM

An enveloped DNA virus of the genus *Hepadnavirus*. The hepatitis B virus (HBV) is a double-shelled particle with an outer lipoprotein envelope containing the surface component hepatitis B surface antigen (HBsAg) and a core containing the core antigen (HBcAg), the e antigen (HBeAg) and viral DNA (HBV DNA). Humans are the main host. HBV infects other higher primates but they are not a source of human infection and there are no important environmental reservoirs.

EPIDEMIOLOGY

The prevalence of hepatitis B infection in the general population varies between global regions and between groups inside countries. In 1998 there were 886 notifications and 843 laboratory reports of acute hepatitis B in England and Wales, however, in parts of Africa, east and south-east Asia, infection is common, with up to 70% of children being infected by adolescence. In a number of these the infection fails to resolve and a persistent infectious state of carriage develops.[†] The proportion of acute infections that progress to become carriers varies according to the age at infection and therefore the prevalence of carriage reaches 7% is Africa and Asia. In these areas most transmission occurs perinatally as vertical transmission from 'carrier' mothers. Some is also thought to occur horizontally from child to child and perhaps also from adult to child.

The Middle East, the Amazon basin in South America, the Pacific islands and parts of south-eastern (Turkey, Greece) and eastern Europe have intermediate prevalence of 2–7% HBsAg positivity). Population prevalence is generally low (under 2% HBsAg positivity) in indigenous populations in other countries including western and northern Europe and the UK and most new transmissions occur between adults in these countries. Exceptions are aboriginal groups in Australia, New Zealand and Canada/Alaska, which have high prevalences. Groups migrating from high- to low-prevalence areas retain their prior prevalence rates for some time and consequently substantial variations in prevalence, and rates of perinatal exposure, are found between ethnic groups in low-prevalence countries according to their group country of origin. Mothers at particular risk of being carriers are those originating in higher-prevalence countries (including second- and subsequent-generation immigrants) and to a lesser extent those who have injected

---

* **In the UK the reporting doctor is currently asked to report viral hepatitis but to categorise it as type A, B, non-A non-B (includes hepatitis C and E) or type not known.**

† **Defined as being HBsAg-positive and anti-HBc-IgM-negative or HBsAg-positive on two occasions more than 6 months apart.**

drugs or with other behavioural risks. Children at risk of postnatal acquisition in the UK are those who receive frequent transfusions of blood and blood products such as children on haemodialysis and with severe haemoglobinopathies, all of whom should be protected by active immunisation (see Prevention of further cases, below).

Incubation period

This is usually 60–90 days (from exposure to initial disease), but may be as long as 6 months.

Infectivity

Infectivity is greatest in individuals who are both HBsAg- and HBeAg-positive (Table 64.1). Carriers who are HBsAg-positive but have antibody to e antigen (anti-HBe-positive) are of lower infectivity. Transmission efficiency for perinatal infection from HBeAg-positive (anti-HBe-negative) mothers is approximately 80% if vaccine and immunoglobulin are not given. Efficiency of transmission after the perinatal period is much lower.

Transmission

HBV may be transmitted through exposure to the following body fluids (in descending order of viral concentration): blood, tissue fluid, semen and cervical secretions, and saliva. Perinatal transmission occurs to infants born to infectious mothers (see Infectivity, above). The virus does not usually cross the placenta and most vertical (mother-to-child) transmission is thought to occur during or just after birth by infant exposure to maternal blood. Mother-to-child transmission is thought also to take place postnatally but it is unclear whether HBV is transmitted through breastfeeding; however, it is prevented by immunising all children born to HBsAg-positive mothers. In countries where prevalence is high and immunisation unavailable, child-to-child and late mother-to-child transmission probably takes place through accidental sharing of blood and wound fluids, particularly within families. In day-care facilities and schools in the UK the risk of child-to-child transmission is very low and can be minimised by normal infection control procedures (see Chapter 33). In adults, parenteral exposure to blood and sexual intercourse are the predominant modes of transmission, with sharing of equipment by injecting drug users, unprotected sex and frequent partner change having the highest associated risk. Health-care workers who are exposed to blood are at risk of infection, which has occurred from and to surgeons, theatre staff and dentists undertaking 'exposure-prone' procedures. The risk can be minimised by ensuring that all such staff are immunised and have serological evidence of immunity.

NATURAL HISTORY AND CLINICAL FEATURES

In most perinatally exposed children infection is asymptomatic or symptoms are minimal and there is no apparent jaundice. Fulminant neonatal hepatitis has been described but is unusual. It has been seen at around 3 months of age in infants born to low-risk mothers (i.e. HBsAg-positive but HBeAg-negative). The risk of perinatally infected babies becoming carriers is higher (approximately 90%) than for any other group of infected individuals, and those who acquire persistent infection as babies are also more at risk of developing chronic liver disease and hepatocellular carcinoma in later life. Children infected after the birth period are quite likely to experience either no symptoms (90%) or a mild illness with anorexia, nausea and general malaise. A prodrome with arthralgia and a rash may occur but is unusual. Although the serum bilirubin is usually elevated and serum transaminases are disturbed for a number of weeks, obvious jaundice is unusual and less common than in adolescents and adults. In most children the infection resolves. The probability of a child becoming a carrier is estimated to be 30%. Older adolescents are similar to adults in showing symptoms in up to 30% but a risk of developing carrier status of only 10%. The most serious sequelae of infection are developing fulminant hepatitis as part of acute hepatitis or becoming a carrier, following which severe chronic hepatitis, cirrhosis and primary hepatocellular carcinoma can develop. Fulminant hepatitis occasionally occurs, with onset of hepatic failure within a few weeks after the onset of acute hepatitis. Hepatocellular carcinoma is commoner among individuals infected in Africa or Asia and is seen in adults with coexisting liver cirrhosis three or more decades after initial infection.

Diagnosis

Clinical signs and symptoms and a history of exposure can give rise to a suspicion of hepatitis B but diagnosis is dependent on serology. Serological testing for antibodies and antigens relating to hepatitis B make the diagnosis and indicate whether an individual is infectious, has natural immunity or immunity relating to vaccination (Table 64.1) Other infections (and noninfectious aetiologies) should be considered, including hepatitis A, hepatitis C, infectious mononucleosis and infection with

Table 64.1 Interpretation of serological markers of hepatitis B virus infection

HBsAg	Anti-HBc IgG	IgM	Anti-HBs	HBeAg	Anti-HBe	Interpretation
+	+	+ or –*	–	+	–	Hepatitis B carrier of high infectivity (chronic hepatitis B)
+	+	+ or –*	–	–	+	Hepatitis B carrier of low infectivity
+	–	–	–	+ or –	–	Very early infection/ late incubation period
+	+	+	–	+ or –	+ or –	Acute hepatitis B
–	+	–	+ or –	–	+ or –	Immune as a result of previous infection
–	–	–	+	–	–	Immune as a result of immunisation

* Usually negative or low ressure.

cytomegalovirus. Clinical hepatitis developing in a child who is HBsAg-positive may represent hepatitis A infection and IgM tests should be used for distinguishing between acute and chronic infections.

MANAGEMENT

There is no specific treatment for acute hepatitis B infection at any age. The majority of cases can be cared for at home. Where hospitalisation is required, infected children should be nursed with standard universal precautions taken in handling blood and other body fluids (see Chapter 22). Patients with undiagnosed jaundice should be managed with universal precautions applicable to both hepatitis A and B until the aetiology is established. If a child is seeming to progress to fulminant hepatitis, referral to a specialist liver unit is urgently required (guidance on the signs of this are given in Chapter 63, p. 305). Infants born to HBsAg-positive mothers do not need to be isolated but will require immunisation within 24 hours of birth. If the mother is e antigen-positive or not known to be anti-HBe-positive, or suffered acute hepatitis B in pregnancy, hepatitis B specific immunoglobulin is also given (see Prevention of further cases, below). Some specialists are now using recombinant interferon-alpha to clear infection in adults with chronic hepatitis and trials are under way in children, where it seems more or less effective depending on the time of infection, therapy being less effective for children with perinatally acquired infection. Oral lamivudine is also being evaluated in children. However, the course of some of these treatments is long, there are troublesome, though reversible, side-effects and treatment is not always successful.

PREVENTION OF FURTHER CASES

Immunisation

Perinatal exposure

In the UK, since April 2000, it has officially been required that all pregnant women should be screened serologically for their hepatitis B status (presence of HBsAg). This is a change from a previous practice of screening only those considered to be at higher risk. Mothers found to be HBsAg-positive are then tested for other HBV markers (Table 64.1). All babies born to women known to be HBsAg-positive should commence a course of hepatitis B vaccine within 24 hours of birth. Three doses are given as an accelerated course at 0 (birth), 1 and 2 months, with a booster at about 12 months of age when the infant's infection status is checked. An acceptable alternative is to boost and check serological status at the time of giving the measles, mumps and rubella (MMR) vaccine. Breastfeeding is permissible and should be encouraged as long as immunisation is given. If the mother is HBsAg-positive but also HBeAg-positive or not known to be anti-HBe-positive, or if she has had acute hepatitis B in pregnancy, then the baby should also receive 200 IU of hepatitis B specific immunoglobulin (HBIG) intramuscularly within 24 hours of birth and at a contralateral site from the vaccine. Because of the importance of early immunisation, preparations to provide immunisations should be made during the pregnancy of the carrier mother. These regimens have an efficacy of over 90% in preventing infection in the infant. There is no clear evidence that giving HBIG to babies of mothers known to be anti-HBe-positive has any additional value to giving vaccine alone. Immunised infants should be tested for HBsAg at 1 year of age when the vaccine booster is given. In most cases the child will be anti-HBs-positive and HBsAg-negative, indicating that immunisation was successful and that no further follow-up is needed. In a few cases the child will be HBsAg-positive, indicating that infection has occurred and follow-up is required.

Mothers found to be chronic carriers will also need to be assessed and referred for their care. The majority will have themselves been infected perinatally. However, household contacts should also be screened.

Routine immunisation

The World Health Organization (WHO) recommendations are that where population prevalence of HBsAg is 2% or over all infants should be immunised, starting at birth. Where prevalence is low (under 2%), WHO recommends universal childhood or adolescent vaccinations. In a number of low-prevalence countries (e.g. the USA, France and New Zealand) it is now policy to incorporate hepatitis B immunisation in primary immunisation courses for children. This is not yet the case in the UK, which is following a policy of attempting selective immunisation of those at risk combined with universal antenatal screening. It is important to appreciate that, even if there was universal childhood or adolescent vaccination, it would still be necessary to have universal antenatal screening.

Immunisation of individuals at risk

Immunisation is recommended for those who might have been exposed (see Postexposure prophylaxis, below) and those more likely to be exposed to hepatitis B, including injecting drug users and homosexual and bisexual men. Those at higher risk in relation to care of children are: household contacts of carriers of hepatitis B; health-care workers who have direct contact with blood, blood-stained body fluids or patients' tissues; staff and clients of residential accommodation for the mentally handicapped (including handicapped children); foster parents; children of parents who inject drugs; children with chronic renal failure* and haemodialysis patients; haemophiliacs and other children likely to be receiving repeat blood transfusions; and relatives responsible for the administration of such products. The routine immunisation course is three doses at 0, 1 and 6 months. An alternative accelerated schedule is four doses at 0, 1, 2 and 12 months; this is used when there has been exposure to infection, e.g. at birth from an infectious mother. Immunisation is given intramuscularly (not intradermally and not in the buttock). The dose varies according to the manufacturer but is lower in children and when the vaccine is given

---

* **Response to vaccination is poor in those with advanced disease and HBV vaccine should be given early in the course of the disease.**

Table 64.2 Hepatitis B virus prophylaxis for reported exposure incidents (Source: Communicable Disease Review (1992) 2: R97–101)

	Significant exposure*			Nonsignificant exposure	
HBV status of person exposed	HBsAg-positive source	Unknown source	HBsAg-negative source	Continued risk	No further risk
Received one dose HB vaccine or none	Accelerated course of HB vaccine† HBIG × 1	Accelerated course of HB vaccine†	Initiate course of HB vaccine	Initiate course of HB vaccine	No HBV prophylaxis; reassure
Two or more doses HB vaccine pre-exposure (anti-HBs not known)	One dose of HB vaccine followed by second dose 1 month later	One dose of HB vaccine	Finish course of HB vaccine	Finish course of HB vaccine	No HBV prophylaxis; reassure
Known responder to HB vaccine (anti-HBs ≥ 10 mIU/mL 2–4 months postvaccination)	Booster dose of HB vaccine	Consider booster dose of HB vaccine	Consider booster dose of HB vaccine	Consider booster dose of HB vaccine	No HBV prophylaxis; reassure
Known nonresponder to HB vaccine (anti-HBs < 10 mIU/mL 2–4 months postvaccination)	HBIG × 1 Consider booster dose of HB vaccine	HBIG × 1 Consider booster dose of HB vaccine	No HBIG Consider booster dose of HB vaccine	No HBIG Consider booster dose of HB vaccine	No HBV prophylaxis; reassure

* A significant exposure is one from which HBV transmission may result. It may be: (1) percutaneous exposure (needlestick or other contaminated sharp object injury, a bite that causes bleeding or other visible skin puncture), (2) mucocutaneous exposure to blood (contamination of nonintact skin, conjunctiva or mucous membrane); or (3) sexual exposure (unprotected sexual intercourse). Percutaneous exposure carries a higher risk than mucocutaneous exposure and exposure to blood is more serious than exposure to other body fluids. Hepatitis B virus does not cross intact skin. Exposure to vomit, faeces and sterile or uncontaminated sharp objects poses no risk.

† An accelerated course of vaccine consists of doses spaced at 0, 1 and 2 months. A booster dose is given at 12 months to those at continuing risk of exposure to HBV.

intradermally. Health-care workers receiving vaccination require serological checking (anti-HBs titres) 2–4 months after completing the course. The aim is to achieve antibody levels of over 100 mIU/mL. Persons with levels of under 10 mIU/mL are given further doses but if they still show these low titres they are classified as nonresponders and will require hepatitis B specific immunoglobulin if exposed to infection (Table 64.2). A combined hepatitis A and B vaccine is now available but it should not be used for postexposure prophylaxis.

Postexposure prophylaxis

A common occurrence is a child receiving an injury from a needle found on the ground. In these circumstances an immunisation course is started but immunoglobulin is not given. It is considered that immunisation has to commence within 7 days if it is going to give protection against infection from the needlestick injury (see Chapter 33, p. 222). This and indications for use of HBV vaccine and HBIG following other types of exposure are shown in Table 64.2. When exposure has occurred a history must be taken, which allows an assessment of risk. In the case of a bite from another child, unless the biting child is known to be HBsAg-positive the hepatitis status of the biting child is assumed to be unknown and immunisation is given (Table 64.2). For further guidance see the article listed in Further reading.

FURTHER READING

Public Health Laboratory Service Hepatitis subcommittee (1992) Exposure to Hepatitis B virus: guidance on post-exposure prophylaxis. CDR Review 2: R97–101.

65 Hepatitis C

Acute hepatitis C infection is a notifiable disease*

Information specifically relating to hepatitis C infection in children remains limited. Much of what is written here is derived from what is known about the infection in adults. The field is rapidly evolving and the information should be regarded as provisional. The reader is therefore advised to consult a recent review.

* In the UK the reporting doctor is currently asked to report viral hepatitis but to categorise it as type A, B, non-A non-B (includes hepatitis C and E) or type not known. It is likely that in the future the doctor will be asked also to categorise acute hepatitis C.

ORGANISM

An enveloped RNA virus classified as a flavivirus. The major cause of parenterally acquired 'non-A non-B' hepatitis.

EPIDEMIOLOGY

As tests for antibody to hepatitis C (anti-HCV) have become available and more specific, it is becoming clear that hepatitis C infection is present worldwide. Prevalence is higher in Japan, the southern USA, Africa, the Middle East and European countries bordering on the Mediterranean. Prevalence is especially high in Egypt. In the UK, prevalence of anti-HCV among new blood donors is thought to be around 1 in 2000. Most HCV-infected adults in the UK are persons who have injected drugs, were born in higher-prevalence countries or have received blood transfusions before screening was introduced (in the UK blood donations have been screened for anti-HCV since September 1991). Many persons with haemophilia are infected if they received plasma products before inactivation with heat or detergent/solvent became standard in 1985.

Transmission

Parenteral exposure (including blood transfusion) is the most important mode of transmission for children. Surveillance has indicated that most current paediatric infections in UK and Ireland have been acquired from contaminated blood products. Transmission through pre- and perinatal vertical exposure (mother-to-child) does occur but the risk of transmission is low (probably under 7%) unless there is coexisting HIV infection in the mother, which considerably increases infection risk. If transmission also takes place through breastfeeding it is a rare event. Risk of mother-to-child transmission seems to be negligible if the mother is not viraemic. Transmission from an infected blood transfusion is thought to be almost 100% efficient. In adults, parenteral transmission predominates, such as through injecting drug use and in association with use of unscreened blood products. Transmission can occur following needlestick injury, with a risk of transmission of around 3%. Transmission through sexual intercourse is uncommon and it is generally not required that HCV-infected men and women use condoms routinely, although this is appropriate for people having multiple partners.

NATURAL HISTORY AND CLINICAL FEATURES

The natural history of infection acquired at or before birth or in childhood has yet to be properly described. Around 20% of children have seemingly cleared their infections, while hepatitis C infection persists in others and a few have developed active hepatitis. In adult transfusion-associated cases the incubation period from infection to appearance of altered transaminases is usually 6–8 weeks (range 2–29 weeks). Infection persists in 80% of cases but initial disease is usually mild or asymptomatic. It may lead to chronic 'active' or 'persistent' hepatitis but cohort studies of individuals with known dates of infection have found that at 10 years over 80% still remain symptom free. It is estimated that about 20% of infected individuals develop cirrhosis. Some may advance to hepatocellular carcinoma. However, it may be that children suffer less disease than adults, as acquiring infection at older ages is associated with more severe disease. Infection with particular HCV genotypes (type 1 and especially type 1b) seems to be associated with a worse prognosis in adult cohorts. Use of alcohol increases the risk of progression to disease in adults but to date there is no evidence that knowledge of being HCV-infected results in less risk-taking behaviour.

Diagnosis

Serological screening enzyme-linked immunosorbent assays (ELISAs) for antibodies to hepatitis C (anti-HCV) are in their third generation. Their sensitivity and specificity approach 100%. However false positives occur and can contribute a substantial proportion of positives in low-prevalence populations. Seroconversion may not occur in adults for up to 6 months after exposure (the mean period is 12 weeks) so that early tests relying on antibodies may show false-negative results following exposure and infection and repeat testing is often required. Anti-HCV seropositivity detected by ELISA has to be followed by supplementary testing with recombinant immunoblot (RIBA) synthetic peptide assays or genome detection (usually by polymerase chain reaction – PCR) One recommended algorithm is to follow ELISA reactivity directly with PCR for subjects at higher risk (e.g. patients reporting a risk factor) but to apply RIBA as an intermediary step in low-risk (general population) patients. If clinical evidence is strong, seronegative results should not deter repeat antibody testing and use of antigen (or genome) tests. However these may also show false negatives because of intermittent expression of viral RNA.

Screening

Because of the lack of knowledge about the natural history of the disease, the relatively low effectiveness of anti-HCV therapy (and its significant side-effects), the high cost per case for routine screening and the lack of interventions that have been shown to prevent transmission, the case for routine screening of the general population is currently weak. However, in adults with known risk factors (e.g. injecting drug use in the past, coming from a high-prevalence country or receipt of blood products prior to 1991) the case for and against testing should be discussed on an individual basis.

MANAGEMENT

In adults, interferon-alpha is considered to be of value in treating chronic hepatitis C infection and experience is growing in children. It seems to be around 20% effective in clearing infection in both adults and children. Combinations of interferon and ribavirin achieve clearance in around 40% of adults. However the therapy has significant side-effects and is expensive. Children should be referred to a specialist centre for assessment and decisions on treatment. No vaccine is available.

PREVENTION OF FURTHER CASES

In a number of countries, including the UK and most of Europe, blood donations are screened for anti-HCV and donation by those who have ever injected drugs is actively discouraged. It remains to be determined whether HCV-infected mothers in industrialised countries should be advised to breastfeed. Until the role of breastfeeding in HCV transmission is clarified, some have argued that it would seem wise to advise against breastfeeding by known HCV-infected women in situations where the risks associated with use of artificial feeds can be minimised. However the case is much less clear cut than for HIV (see Chapter 23). Antenatal screening for HCV is not advised.

FURTHER READING

Anonymous (1998) Recommendations for prevention and control of hepatitis C virus (HCV) infection and HCV-related chronic disease. Centers for Disease Control and Prevention. MMWR Morb Mortal Wkly Rep 47: 1–39.

66 Hepatitis E

Acute hepatitis E infection is a notifiable disease*

ORGANISM

Hepatitis E virus (HEV) is a small nonenveloped RNA virus similar in morphology to the Caliciviridae.

EPIDEMIOLOGY

Hepatitis E infection was originally described as enterically transmitted non-A non-B hepatitis (ET-NANBH). It produces explosive outbreaks of hepatitis in low-income countries, on a background of sporadic endemicity. Large epidemics have occurred in Asia (India, Nepal, Kyrgyzstan, Myanmar, Indonesia, Pakistan, China), Africa and the Middle Eastern crescent (Ethiopia, Sudan, Algeria, Saudi Arabia), North America (Mexico) and eastern Europe (west Ukraine). During epidemics the attack rate is highest in adolescents and young adults. In one survey in Egypt of endemic NANBH in children, 40% of cases were due to HEV. Recent surveys of HEV suggest that is responsible for 50% of cases of non-A, non-B, non-C hepatitis.

---

* In the UK the reporting doctor is currently asked to report viral hepatitis but to categorise it as type A, B, non-A non-B (includes hepatitis C and E) or type not known.

Infection has been described from the UK but usually in travellers returning from endemic regions. Blood donor surveys have demonstrated HEV seropositivity rates of 1.7%, 1.1%, 3.4% and 14% from the UK, the Netherlands, California and France respectively. However, in most cases those who were seropositive could have acquired the infection outside Europe.

Transmission
Direct person-to-person spread via the faecal–oral route can occur but is rare. In most epidemics transmission occurs indirectly via consuming food or, more commonly, water contaminated by human faeces.

Incubation period
2–9 weeks (mean 6 weeks).

NATURAL HISTORY AND CLINICAL FEATURES
The disease is similar clinically to hepatitis A virus (HAV) infection. It has a preicteric phase of 1–10 days with abdominal pain, nausea and vomiting. The icteric phase lasts 12–15 days with complete recovery within 1 month. Chronic infection has not been described. As with HAV, the disease tends to be milder in children.

Mortality rates are higher than for HAV. For example, in the Rangoon, Nepal and Azamgarh epidemics mortality rates were 1%, 6.6% and 11% respectively. Pregnant women are at particularly high risk, especially in the third trimester, with mortality rates ranging from 11–39%.

Diagnosis
The mainstay of diagnosis is detection of IgM or IgG antibodies by enzyme-linked immunosorbent assay (ELISA) using HEV recombinant antigens. The sensitivity and specificity of the currently available tests are poor (80–85% and 90% respectively). Virus is present in faeces and serum in largest amounts prior to jaundice. Electron microscopy and reverse transcription–polymerase chain reaction have been used for diagnosis.

MANAGEMENT
There is no specific antiviral chemotherapy; thus, treatment is supportive. In pregnancy both mother and baby are at high risk and there are suggestions that caesarean section under epidural anaesthesia may save some mothers. No vaccine is available.

67 Other hepatitis viruses

From virological studies of hepatitis it is apparent that hepatitis viruses A–E do not account for all cases. For this reason it is likely that the alphabet of hepatitis viruses will continue to expand.

HEPATITIS D (HDV)

This small, defective RNA virus was described in 1977 and called the delta agent. It cannot replicate except in the presence of hepatitis B virus. In infected blood, HDV is found as a nucleocapsid core surrounded by a hepatitis B surface antigen envelope. It is present worldwide. In the Mediterranean basin, parts of Africa, the Middle East and the Amazon basin infection is endemic. Elsewhere it is sporadic. Spread is blood-to-blood. In endemic areas the virus is spread by direct contact, with family members and intimate contacts at greatest risk. In nonendemic areas those at risk of percutaneous exposure, e.g. in intravenous drug abuse or haemophilia, are most often affected.

There are two patterns of infection. Patients may be infected with HBV and HDV simultaneously (coinfection) or have HDV superimposed on existing chronic HBV (superinfection). Coinfection usually produces mild self-limiting disease whereas superinfection is more often associated with fulminant life-threatening hepatitis and has a greater risk of rapidly progressive chronic hepatitis.

There is no specific therapy but HBV vaccination will prevent both HBV and HDV infections.

HEPATITIS F (HFV)

For obvious reasons the designation hepatitis F was kept for a faecal–orally transmitted virus. An unenveloped DNA virus was described in India and provisionally called HFV but this has not yet been confirmed.

HEPATITIS G (HGV)

HGV was originally called GB agent (the initials of the surgeon in whom it was first detected). The surgeon's blood was used to infect tamarin monkeys, which subsequently developed acute hepatitis. Infection could then be passed by blood to other monkeys. Two viruses, GB-A and GB-B, were detected in the monkey plasma, using reverse transcription-polymerase chain reaction (RT-PCR); these viruses were also detected in west African patients' sera, as well as a third virus called GB-C. Unfortunately, GB-A and GB-B appear to be endogenous simian viruses. However GB-C appears identical to a virus detected independently in patients with hepatitis. This is now termed hepatitis G virus. It is also a flavivirus (enveloped RNA virus) but is different from HCV. It is transmitted blood-to-blood and there is some evidence for mother-to-baby transmission. Although HGV has been detected in acute hepatitis, fulminant hepatitis, cirrhosis and hepatocellular carcinoma, its disease associations are not entirely clear. Some 5–10% of blood donors have evidence of these viruses, detected by RT-PCR. HGV is detected more frequently in the blood of those frequently receiving blood or blood products and in intravenous drug abusers. It is possible that there is some interaction between HCV and HGV in hepatitis.

TT VIRUS (TTV)

In 1998 Japanese workers using representation difference analysis detected a novel single-stranded DNA virus (TTV) in the plasma of a patient (named TT) with post-transfusion non-A, non-B, non-C hepatitis. TTV is most closely related to the parvoviruses. It has been detected in the blood of 1.9% of blood donors but was more prevalent in older age groups. It was frequently (44–56%) detected in factor VII and IX concentrates. As with HGV the role of TTV in hepatitis remains to be clarified. For example, TTV was detectable in 25% of patients with chronic liver disease but also in 10% of 'normal' controls.

68 Herpes infections

See also Chapters 42 (varicella-zoster virus, HHV-3), 47 (cytomegalovirus, HHV-5) and 54 (Epstein–Barr virus, HHV-4)

ORGANISM

Human herpes simplex type 1 (HHV-1, HSV-1) and human herpes simplex type 2 (HHV-2, HSV-2) are enveloped DNA viruses. They grow readily in tissue culture and can be distinguished by differences in cytopathic effect and immunologically (Table 68.1). Epstein–Barr virus (Chapter 52) and cytomegalovirus (Chapter 47) are covered elsewhere.

NEONATAL INFECTION

EPIDEMIOLOGY

Most neonatal HSV infection results from type 2 (genital herpes). Data from the British Paediatric Surveillance Unit (BPSU) suggest that 1 in 50 000 newborn infants is infected. The incidence in the USA is thought to be 1 in 3000–20 000.

Transmission

Almost all cases result from transmission of virus from the genital tract of the mother to her infant. Women with a primary HSV infection occurring late in pregnancy are at greatest risk of transmitting infection. The risk of transmission in the presence of herpetic lesion where there is an expression of reactivation is 3–5%. Virus may be shed from the genital tract in

Table 68.1 The human herpesviruses (HHV)

Virus	Old name	Disease associations
HHV-1	Herpes simplex virus type I	Orolabial herpes*, conjunctivitis, whitlows, meningoencephalitis
HHV-2	Herpes simplex virus type II	Genital herpes*, meningoencephalitis
HHV-3	Varicella-zoster virus	Chickenpox, shingles, encephalitis
HHV-4	Epstein–Barr virus	Glandular fever, Burkitt's lymphoma, Hodgkin's lymphoma, nasopharyngeal carcinoma
HHV-5	Cytomegalovirus	Glandular fever, congenital infection. Retinitis, pneumonitis, enteritis, encephalitis, hepatitis in immunocompromised
HHV-6	–	Exanthem (roseola) subitum
HHV-7	–	Exanthem (roseola) subitum
HHV-8	–	Kaposi's sarcoma

* HHV-1 can also cause genital and HHV-2 orolabial disease.

the absence of any visible lesions. Most genital lesions are type 2, but a small proportion are type 1; very rarely neonatal infection may result from transmission of virus from the cold sore of a mother or medical attendant to the baby.

Incubation period
1–6 days (median 3.5 days).

NATURAL HISTORY AND CLINICAL FEATURES
Illness takes three main forms:

- a generalised systemic infection with respiratory distress from pneumonia and hepatitis
- an encephalitic illness with fits and altered level of consciousness
- localised infection of the skin, eyes and mouth (SEM). The typical skin lesion is the vesicle, which may be seen in the mouth also. Conjunctivitis or keratitis may be seen in the eyes, as well as chorioretinitis. In about one-third of cases, SEM lesions progress to either encephalopathy or systemic infection.

Most cases occur within 1 week of birth but illness may be delayed for up to a month. There is a high mortality from systemic or neurological disease even when antiviral treatment is used. Severe neurological disability occurs in more than half of survivors of the encephalitis. Those infants who developed SEM are likely to have further local recurrences during childhood.

MANAGEMENT

The high mortality and morbidity may be related to the difficulty in diagnosis, particularly when SEM lesions are not present. Most infections in the newborn follow primary genital infection, which may not be apparent. Treatment of established or suspected infection is with aciclovir (20 mg/kg/dose, three times daily, for 21 days in systemic or nervous system disease and 14 days in mild disease).

Appropriate viral studies should be performed; these include cultures of throat and conjunctival swab, blood and cerebrospinal fluid. Vesicle fluid can be cultured or examined under electron microscopy. A number of rapid diagnostic methods are available but none are in general use. When infection is not suspected but an infant is delivered vaginally to a mother with active genital herpetic lesions, aciclovir is recommended when it is thought to be a primary genital infection, after specimens have been taken. Other authorities will treat only if swabs from the baby are positive or the baby is symptomatic. When there are reactivated lesions then it is appropriate to take specimens at 48 hours and observe the infant in hospital for a week, by which time the risk of infection is very low. Infants with active infection should be isolated.

PREVENTION OF INFECTION

When it is known that a mother has active infection, the infant should be delivered by caesarean section once she goes into labour; this should be performed as soon as possible, preferably within 4 hours. It is not considered worthwhile screening mothers for infection in the UK.

Attendants and mothers with facial sores should be very careful to avoid close contact between the affected area and the infant and to wear masks.

CHILDHOOD INFECTION

EPIDEMIOLOGY

HSV-1 infections are common and about 50% of adults are seropositive to this virus. Children may develop gingivostomatitis – labial herpes – from reactivation, ophthalmic infection and herpetic whitlows on fingers. HSV may produce a severe, widespread vesicular rash in children with eczema (eczema herpeticum). Very rarely, herpes encephalitis may occur either as a primary or reactivation of infection. In a child with genital herpes sexual abuse must be considered a probable mode of transmission.

Transmission

Most oral and skin infections result from person-to-person spread from secretions, either from a lesion or, more often, from the oral secretions of an asymptomatic carrier. Virus is present in particularly high concentrations in vesicles during the first 24 hours.

Incubation period

2–14 days.

NATURAL HISTORY AND CLINICAL FEATURES

In many children, primary infection is asymptomatic but reactivation occurs, resulting in vesicles on the lips, which may be painful or itching. Some children develop a painful gingivostomatitis with lesions on the vermilion borders of the lips, the tongue and mucous membranes in the mouth. They may need hospital admission because it may be difficult to drink. The symptoms are at their worst for about 2 days. Eye infection may involve the conjunctiva, cornea and skin around the eye. Dendritic ulcers may form on the cornea and can leave permanent scarring. Children with eczema may develop multiple vesicles over the affected areas of skin.

Herpes encephalitis should be considered in any child with an acute encephalopathy. The signs include fever, an altered level of consciousness and focal fits. There is sometimes a history of previous herpes infection. Cerebrospinal fluid may be normal, bloodstained or show a lymphocytosis or increased protein levels. A CT scan may show features of temporal lobe ischaemia and inflammation. Although encephalitis does not appear to be any more common in the immunosuppressed, other herpetic infections may be more severe and require urgent treatment.

Diagnosis

As for neonatal infection, electron microscopy of vesicle fluid; culture of blood, respiratory secretions and vesicle fluid. The virus is rarely found in the CSF. The diagnostic method of choice is polymerase chain reaction (PCR) for herpes DNA. It has a high sensitivity and specificity. Brain biopsy is rarely indicated.

MANAGEMENT

This is of particular importance in ophthalmic and encephalitic herpes and in the immunocompromised. The effect of oral aciclovir is only marginal in cases of gingivostomatitis and should be started very early in the course of infection if it is to be effective. Topical aciclovir is of little benefit for recurrent cold sores. Ophthalmological advice should be sought in the treatment of ocular involvement. In children with herpes encephalitis, aciclovir has been shown to be beneficial. This should be given intravenously three times daily and should be continued for at least 14 days, otherwise relapse may occur. Similarly, high doses should be used in the immunocompromised.

PREVENTION OF INFECTION

People with cold sores on their mouths or face should not kiss children. Medical attendants with herpetic whitlows should wear gloves.

OTHER HERPESVIRUSES

HUMAN HERPESVIRUS 6 (HHV-6)

This β-herpesvirus resembles cytomegalovirus (HHV-5) genomically and was first isolated in 1986 from B lymphocytes of patients with lymphoproliferative diseases. Once infection has occurred it sets up a persistent infection in human peripheral blood mononuclear cells, predominantly

CD4+ T lymphocytes. Infection is found worldwide and in most settings virtually all children are seropositive by 12–18 months of age. Virus is detectable in saliva and throat swabs of children and adults alike. It is presumed that spread occurs from parents or siblings by close contact, perhaps via saliva. HHV-6 appear not to be transmitted transplacentally, during delivery or via breast milk.

There are two variants of HHV-6, A and B. HHV-6B is isolated predominantly from infants with exanthem subitum (roseola infantum). Exanthem subitum is a common infectious disease of infants. It presents with a sudden onset of fever, which lasts for 2–3 days. Then an erythematous maculopapular rash appears on the trunk and face that spreads to the lower limbs. This is usually coincident with a sudden defervescence. HHV-6 infection has also been associated with febrile convulsions, and in those rare individuals who do not acquire infection until their teens, has been associated with an infectious-mononucleosis-like illness. However, most infections are asymptomatic. HHV-6A is most often isolated from patients with AIDS or lymphoproliferative disorders. It may contribute to allograft rejection and interstitial pneumonitis or encephalitis in AIDS patients.

Infection can be diagnosed by virus isolation serological response (which cannot differentiate HHV-6A from B) or genome detection. HHV-6 responds in vitro to phosphonoformate, although whether patients need to be treated remains to be clarified.

HUMAN HERPESVIRUS 7 (HHV-7)

This β-herpesvirus was isolated from CD4+ T lymphocytes of a healthy individual in 1990. It is similar to HHV-6 in structure, biology and clinical manifestations. Most infections appear to occur after the second year of life (i.e. later than for HHV-6). It is a cause of exanthem subitum and it is possible for a child to have sequential episodes of exanthem subitum due to HHV-6 and then HHV-7. Laboratory diagnosis is as for HHV-6 and the two viruses can be differentiated serologically (by titre of antiserum).

HUMAN HERPESVIRUS 8

This is a γ-herpesvirus that is associated with Kaposi's sarcoma (both AIDS-associated and endemic), primary effusion lymphoma and multicentric Castleman's disease. It is not clear how the virus is acquired, nor what manifestations there are of primary infection. However, infection is highly prevalent in Mediterranean countries and in low-income countries infection appears to occur in childhood (50% of pre-pubertal Ugandan children are seropositive) with a horizontal transmission pattern similar to other γ-herpesviruses such as Epstein–Barr virus.

INFLUENZA

ORGANISM

An enveloped helical RNA virus, the influenza virus is a member of the orthomyxoviruses with three antigenic types – A, B and C. The A strains show considerable variability. Human influenza A viruses are further sub-classified by the haemagglutinin (H_1, H_2, H_3 and recently H_5 and H_9) and neuraminidase (N_1 and N_2) antigens. Minor changes in antigenic structure are known as antigenic drifts, whereas major changes, e.g. H_2 to H_3, are known as antigenic shifts. H_5N_1 has been known to be highly pathogenic in poultry for some years but it was only in 1997 that, for the first time, it was recognised as causing disease in humans.

EPIDEMIOLOGY

Every winter there is an excess of respiratory deaths due to influenza. At intervals, when a sufficiently different strain arises, there are epidemics. The last epidemic in the UK was in 1989–90. When a major antigenic shift in influenza A occurs a pandemic results. There have been four this century: 1918, 1957, 1968 and 1977. These are thought to originate in the Far East following viral reassortment in animal (pigs and bird) hosts. The disease is highly infectious and outbreaks in schools and other institutions are common. Attack rates are usually 10–20% but may reach 50% in boarding schools.

Transmission is from person to person by droplet or direct contact. The disease is highly infectious for 24 hours before and 48 hours after symptoms appear. In the 1997/98 outbreak in Hong Kong, H_5N_1 was spread from chickens to humans but there was no clear evidence of person-to-person spread. All patients had direct contact with poultry.

Incubation period

1–3 days.

NATURAL HISTORY AND CLINICAL FEATURES

Influenza is predominantly a respiratory illness with a rapid onset of fever, headache, general malaise and generalised aches and pains. Upper respiratory tract symptoms of cough, sore throat and coryza follow soon after but may be absent in young infants, where the clinical picture can be non-specific, resembling sepsis. A secondary bacterial otitis media is not uncommon. Abdominal pain, nausea, vomiting, conjunctival inflammation, croup and pneumonia may also occur. Especially in debilitated patients, the latter may be due to a secondary *Streptococcus pneumoniae*, *Staphylococcus aureus* or *Klebsiella pneumoniae* infection. Primary influenzal pneumonia also occurs. Influenza B, in particular, has been associated with an acute myositis, with calf tenderness and pain on walking. Reye's syndrome may follow influenza, especially influenza B, although this has become less common since many countries have banned the use of aspirin in children. Toxic shock syndrome, myocarditis, encephalitis, Guillain–Barré syndrome and myoglobulinuria have all been reported. There is also some evidence to suggest that meningococcal infection has a higher incidence in the period following influenza.

Except in pandemics, the mortality in children is usually low and particularly involves children with pre-existing chronic disorders, including those with neurodevelopmental problems. Influenza has been noted to alter the metabolism of some drugs, in particular theophylline, producing higher blood levels than would otherwise have been expected.

The H_5N_1 outbreak was atypical. Of the 18 cases, 11 were under 18 years old. Of those over 18 years old, six needed ventilation and five died. Of those under 18 years old, two needed ventilation and one died. The overall mortality was therefore 33%.

Diagnosis

The clinical picture may be similar to that caused by a number of respiratory viruses, including respiratory syncytial virus, parainfluenza viruses types 1, 2 and 3, adenoviruses and Coxsackie virus groups A and B. The white cell count may be normal or show a moderate leukopenia. When it is important to make an accurate diagnosis, culture of the virus from nasopharyngeal secretions (aspirate or swab) can be attempted. It takes 2–6 days to grow in tissue culture. Virus isolation is best done in the first 72 hours as virus shedding decreases markedly after this. Antigen detection by immunofluorescence or enzyme-linked immunosorbent assay (ELISA) is also possible. Complement fixation, haemagglutination inhibition and neutralisation tests to detect rising levels of antibodies only allow the diagnosis to be made in retrospect.

MANAGEMENT

In the majority of cases management is symptomatic, using antipyretics and analgesics. Prophylactic antibiotics are rarely indicated in children but suspected bacterial complications should be appropriately investigated and treated. Until the bacterial pathogen has been identified, antistreptococcal and antistaphylococcal cover should be included in any 'blind' treatment. Amantadine (5 mg/kg as one or two daily doses) may shorten the course of the primary infection if due to influenza A but there is no evidence that it prevents secondary infections, which are the main cause of serious morbidity and mortality in children. It is rarely used in children. Ribavirin has an effect in vitro against influenza A and B and has been used in severe infection in compromised children, i.e. those who are immunocompromised and those with serious cardiac or respiratory problems. However, evidence for its efficacy is not conclusive. A neuraminidase inhibitor, zaminavir, is now licensed in the UK for treatment of influenza but not for use in children under the age of 12.

PREVENTION OF FURTHER CASES

Isolation during the early stages is the only way to prevent the spread of disease. However, even this has only limited effect as the patient is infectious before symptoms appear, as well as after.

Chemoprophylaxis

Amantadine can prevent infection with influenza A; however, it is rarely used in children and immunisation of high-risk individuals is to be preferred.

Immunisation

Immunisation against influenza is recommended for those of all ages with chronic respiratory and cardiac disease; those with chronic renal failure and endocrine disorders; and those who are immunosuppressed. It is recommended for all those over 65 years old. There is also evidence to suggest that it should be given to children with neurodevelopmental disorders, e.g. Down's syndrome and cerebral palsy. It is not usually recommended for healthy individuals. Some would argue that all children in boarding schools should be immunised because influenza spreads rapidly once introduced.

Because of the antigenic drift, each year the WHO makes recommendations as to which virus strains should be covered by the vaccine to be used in the forthcoming year. Vaccination should take place in October or early November. Protective levels of antibody take 1–14 days to develop. There is little difference between the vaccines currently available but not all have a licence for children under 4 years old. Children between 6 months and 12 years old should have two doses of vaccine 4–6 weeks apart if receiving it for the first time. Subsequently, doses should be given at yearly intervals. No vaccine currently has a licence for children under 6 months old. Current vaccines are prepared in hens' eggs and should not be given to individuals with a history of severe hypersensitivity reactions to egg products.

Because the interval between recognition of the threat of a pandemic and its arrival may only be a few months, all countries should have in place a plan to cover such eventualities.

PARAINFLUENZA

ORGANISM

There are four types of human parainfluenza virus within the Paramyxoviridae family. Types 1 and 3 are paramyxoviruses whereas types 2 and 4 are rubulaviruses. All contain RNA. Unlike the influenza viruses, they have a single HN surface spike for both haemagglutinin (HN) and neuraminidase (NA) antigens. It is unclear whether type 4 is pathogenic, but it is probably a cause of mild upper respiratory tract infections.

EPIDEMIOLOGY

Types 1, 2 and 3 are the commonest causes of croup, the latter being the most important. Type 1 and 2 occur in winter and type 3 in summer. They may also be responsible for some cases of bronchitis, bronchiolitis (type 3 is second only to respiratory syncytial virus) and pneumonia. Occasionally, rhinitis and pharyngitis may also be due to parainfluenza virus. Illness with type 3 tends to take place in the first year of life whereas that due to types 1 and 2 occurs in the first 3–5 years. The presence of antibodies does not prevent reinfection but the illness is often mild or even asymptomatic.

Transmission
From person to person by droplet or direct contact.

Incubation period
3–5 days.

NATURAL HISTORY AND CLINICAL FEATURES
See Chapters 15 and 16 for details of the illnesses caused by parainfluenza viruses in the respiratory tract.

Diagnosis
Virus can be isolated from nasopharyngeal swabs and is relatively easily grown in tissue culture. It has also been cultured from peripheral blood mononuclear cells in four of a series of 11 cases.

MANAGEMENT
See Chapters 15 and 16 for details of the management of illnesses caused by parainfluenza viruses in the respiratory tract.

PREVENTION OF FURTHER CASES
Respiratory precautions should be taken for inpatients but are not otherwise necessary.

Chemoprophylaxis
Amantadine is ineffective against parainfluenza viruses.

Immunisation
There is no vaccine against parainfluenza viruses.

70 Kawasaki disease

Named after the paediatrician who first described it in Japan in 1967, this condition is also known as the mucocutaneous lymph node syndrome

ORGANISM
Unknown. Many features of the illness suggest that it has an infectious aetiology but, to date, a causative agent has not been identified.

EPIDEMIOLOGY
The disease is particularly common in Japan, affecting 1 in 1000 children. It is less common in western countries, although probably under-reported.

Young children are predominantly affected, with the peak incidence occurring in the second year of life and most cases before the fifth birthday. Asian children show the highest incidence. Male:female ratio is 1.6:1. Second attacks are occasionally seen. Clusters of cases have been described, often in the winter months. The epidemiological pattern of the disease, as well as the clinical features, are what first led to the suggestion that the disease has as infectious aetiology. Arterial damage in this condition may be a long-term risk factor for atherosclerotic coronary artery disease.

Transmission

Direct case-to-case spread has not been demonstrated. The disease is more common in siblings, but this indicates a probable genetic susceptibility.

Incubation period

Unknown.

NATURAL HISTORY AND CLINICAL FEATURES

The illness begins with an abrupt onset of fever, which can rise to 40°C, generally has an unremitting pattern and can last up to 15 days or occasionally longer. The child is usually miserable and may also be irritable. Empirical antibiotic therapy has no effect on the fever. The disease induces a vasculitic process and most of the clinical features can be explained on this basis. The characteristic features develop at around the third day of the illness. They include:

- Eyes – nonexudative conjunctivitis
- Mouth – mucositis with intense erythema; swollen, fissured lips and strawberry tongue
- Lymph nodes – cervical lymphadenopathy, bilateral or unilateral, with glands > 1.5 cm in diameter and sometimes much larger
- Skin – generalised intensely erythematous rash, which may be maculopapular or produce a blotchy or confluent erythema
- Hands and feet – palmar and plantar erythema often with oedema. As the illness subsides in the second to third week characteristic peeling of fingers and toes occurs (see Plate 5).

While classical disease produces fever associated with at least four of the above features, atypical cases with fewer features can occur. Other features of the disease may include diarrhoea, sterile pyuria, arthritis, uveitis, aseptic meningitis, hepatitis and hydrops of the gallbladder. Cardiac involvement is potentially the most serious. In the acute phase a myocarditis or pericarditis may occur, leading to heart failure or arrhythmias. Damage to the coronary artery walls by the vasculitic process can lead to aneurysm formation and this usually occurs in the convalescent phase of the illness. This complication has been reported as occurring in up to 20% of untreated cases. Coronary thrombosis may complicate aneurysm formation. In most cases, aneurysms resolve over the succeeding 12 months. However, particularly in cases developing very large (so-called giant) aneurysms, there may be no resolution and such patients are at high risk of subsequent myocardial infarction. There is increasing concern that, even with resolution of aneurysms, the arteries may not return entirely to normal, resulting in a greater risk of coronary artery disease later in life. The acute mortality rate (usually from cardiac involvement) is between 0.5% and 2%.

Diagnosis

This is based on the clinical features, which become more characteristic as the illness progresses. During the acute phase there is usually a neutrophil leukocytosis, raised acute phase reactants and increased sedimentation rate. Thrombocytosis occurs in the convalescent phase and may reach alarming levels ($> 1 \times 10^{12}$). Electrocardiography and echocardiography (ECHO) during the acute phase may show cardiac involvement. False reassurance should not be derived from the finding of a negative ECHO at this stage since most coronary aneurysms occur later on.

The differential diagnosis of Kawasaki disease is wide. Staphylococcal/streptococcal toxin-mediated diseases such as scarlet fever or toxic shock syndrome have many similar initial features. Since many children will have received empirical antibiotics, drug hypersensitivity reaction may need to be considered. Other differential diagnoses include measles, other viral exanthems, Stevens–Johnson syndrome and systemic onset juvenile idiopathic arthritis.

Management

Though the disease is self-limiting, early diagnosis is important since treatment with intravenous immunoglobulin (IVIG) within the first 10 days of the illness has been shown to reduce the incidence of coronary artery involvement. High-dose IVIG (2 g/kg) is given usually as a single infusion over 12 hours. At the same time, high-dose aspirin therapy (80–100 mg/kg in four divided doses) is commenced and continued until the acute inflammatory phase has subsided. Salicylate levels should be monitored. In the convalescent phase aspirin is continued in low (antithrombotic) doses (3–5 mg/kg as a single daily dose). This is continued for at least 3 months or, if coronary aneurysms have occurred, until these are shown to have resolved on echocardiogram. In those considered to be at very high risk of thrombosis (platelet count $> 800 \times 10^9$/L and/or presence of persistent large aneurysms), dipyridamole (3–4 mg/kg in three divided doses) is added. An electrocardiogram and an echocardiogram should be performed in the acute phase of the illness and the latter repeated at approximately 3 weeks and again at 8–12 weeks after onset of the illness. In those children shown to have abnormal coronary arteries referral should be made to a paediatric cardiologist for further management and follow-up. It should be borne in mind that high-dose IVIG may interfere with subsequent immunisation with live viral vaccines for several months.

PREVENTION OF FURTHER CASES

Until the identity of the aetiological agent is established this is not feasible. Increasing awareness of the possibility of this disease in young febrile children and early institution of specific therapy should help reduce its morbidity and mortality.

71 Legionnaires' disease

ORGANISM

Legionella spp. are a group of Gram-negative bacilli species, but 90% of infections are caused by Legionella pneumophila. Within L. pneumophila there are multiple serogroups, of which 1, 4 and 6 cause most human infections.

EPIDEMIOLOGY

Legionella spp. disease has two manifestations: Pontiac fever, a self-limiting influenza-like febrile illness, and Legionnaires' disease, a severe pulmonary and multisystem infection. It is suggested, but not proved, that Pontiac fever is the result of inhalation of inactive organisms. Infection with Legionella in normal children is probably uncommon and usually results in a mild and self-limiting illness, which would rarely be noticed. However, disease can be severe in immunocompromised children and has been recorded as being acquired in hospital by teenage children who had received kidney transplants. The effects of Legionella species are considerably commoner in adults, among whom Legionnaires' disease is frequently fatal (around 10% in reported cases in Europe).

Legionella can exist long-term in domestic and industrial water systems. It is considered that domestic water systems cause most cases; however, of more community concern are water systems producing aerosols, such as incorrectly maintained air conditioning and water cooling towers. Outbreaks occur among adults because of exposure of numbers of individuals to common sources of infection, such as water from unmaintained cooling towers, within hotels and from poorly maintained machines producing sprays and mists, e.g. jacuzzis. Legionnaires' disease was first recognised in 1976 when a hotel outbreak affected 221 adults in the USA, causing 34 deaths. Nosocomial infections also occur especially among debilitated patients.

Transmission

Inhalation of organisms. Person-to-person spread has never been demonstrated.

Incubation period

This is unknown in children. In adults it is 1–2 days for Pontiac fever and 2–10 days for Legionnaires' disease.

NATURAL HISTORY AND CLINICAL FEATURES

In the normal child an infection may be asymptomatic. In the immunocompromised child (e.g. a child on chemotherapy), a pneumonia and/or systemic infection can occur. This may include central nervous system, liver, gastrointestinal and renal problems. Pontiac fever is the occurrence of systemic illness without pneumonia and is usually self-limiting.

Diagnosis

Diagnosis of Legionnaires' disease requires a diagnosis of pneumonia and laboratory evidence of infection with *Legionella* sp. The latter is by direct recovery and culture, seroconversion (a fourfold rise or greater in titre of antibody) or antigen tests on urine or respiratory specimens. Care needs to be taken with serology as a single positive specimen may reflect prior infections and the rise in titres can be delayed for weeks after infection. DNA probes and monoclonal antibodies are used for further characterisation of clinical isolates. They need to be carried out at a reference centre in order to determine whether a case is sporadic or can be linked to a common source of infection.

MANAGEMENT

Erythromycin is the drug of choice. In immunocompromised children prompt therapy with high-dose intravenous therapy is required and the addition of another agent such as rifampicin or ciprofloxacin may be beneficial. Treatment should be given for 3 weeks.

PREVENTION OF FURTHER CASES

In all cases of Legionnaires' disease, the Consultant in Communicable Disease Control or Director of Public Health should be informed so that epidemiological and laboratory investigations can be undertaken if appropriate. Cases in England and Wales should be reported to the National Surveillance Scheme for Legionnaires' Disease at the PHLS Communicable Disease Surveillance Centre, which coordinates a multicountry surveillance scheme supported by the European Union. This has proved particularly useful in detecting hotel-associated outbreaks.

Regular maintenance of air conditioning/hot water systems in public buildings, including hospitals, is essential to prevent outbreaks of this infection.

72 Leishmaniasis

Leishmaniasis is a spectrum of disease caused by parasitic protozoan *Leishmania* species, which live between mammalian hosts (including humans) and phlebotomine sandflies. Leishmaniasis results in a spectrum of clinical manifestations in children and adults the nature of which is determined in a complex manner according to the parasite pathogenicity, tropism and host factors. However, clinically it is divided into visceral, cutaneous and mucosal syndromes.

ORGANISM

Visceral leishmaniasis – *Leishmania donovani*. Cutaneous leishmaniasis – *Leishmania major* (Old World), *tropica*, *braziliensis* or *mexicana* (New World).

EPIDEMIOLOGY

Leishmaniasis is a vector-borne zoonosis. The reservoir is a variety of warm-blooded animals, including dogs and rodents, and the vector to humans is sandflies.

Visceral leishmaniasis is commonly found in rural areas of most tropical and many subtropical countries, including parts of Asia, the Middle East, Africa, South and Central America, Russia, the Iberian peninsula and the Mediterranean islands.

Cutaneous leishmaniasis is also found in both the Old and the New World – the Indian subcontinent, all of Africa except southern Africa, the Mediterranean, Central and South America. Mucosal leishmaniasis occurs predominantly in the New World, caused by *L. braziliensis*. Rarely it may follow cutaneous infection with other species all over the world.

Transmission

By the bites of sandflies infected by mammals. Man is considered an end host and no further transmission has been reported.

Incubation period

Visceral – varies from a few weeks to 6 months after a sandfly bite, although longer periods have been reported. Cutaneous – a few weeks after the sandfly bite.

NATURAL HISTORY AND CLINICAL FEATURES

Visceral leishmaniasis

Following penetration of the skin by the sandfly, *L. donovani* move through the reticuloendothelial system but concentrate in the bone marrow, liver and spleen. There is malaise, fever and loss of appetite and weight. Signs include enlargement of lymph nodes, liver and spleen. Reticuloendothelial failure causing anaemia, leukopenia and thrombocytopenia may occur. If untreated, haemorrhage and secondary infections are common and may be fatal.

Cutaneous leishmaniasis

Local proliferation in the skin results in a red nodule where the bite took place. Hence these are usually on exposed areas, especially the face. The nodule usually ulcerates later. There may be satellite lesion and regional lymphadenopathy.

Mucosal leishmaniasis

Following cutaneous infection (often years later in adulthood) there may be spread to the mucosa of the nasal and oropharyngeal cavities. Persistent nasal sniffles often occur. Destruction of the facial bones may occur, leading to severe disfigurement.

Diagnosis

Visceral leishmaniasis Diagnosis is difficult as the clinical picture in a child or adult can be indistinguishable from a number of other infections, including malaria, typhoid, schistosomiasis and miliary tuberculosis. Diagnosis is by taking samples from affected tissues (e.g. liver biopsy, bone marrow or lymph nodes) and looking for typical Leischman–Donovan bodies using Giemsa stain.

Cutaneous and mucosal leishmaniasis By taking samples by scraping or a punch biopsy taken from the edge of the lesion and looking for *Leishmania* spp. using Giemsa stain.

Serology and culture might be of value but are only carried out at special centres in the UK (London School of Hygiene and Tropical Medicine and Liverpool Schools of Tropical Medicine), from whom advice should be sought if a diagnosis is suspected.

MANAGEMENT

Specialist advice should be sought (see Diagnosis, above)

Visceral leishmaniasis

Liposomal amphotericin up to a dose of 30 mg/kg over 10–21 days is the treatment of choice. A potentially more toxic alternative is pentamidine isethionate given as a series of **deep** intramuscular injections; 3–4 mg/kg given on alternate days for up to 10 injections.

Cutaneous and mucosal leishmaniasis

Many skin lesions heal spontaneously and a conservative approach is recommended if the lesion is not severe and follow-up is possible. Topical paromomycin may be used. If systemic treatment is needed it should be with liposomal amphotericin.

PREVENTION OF FURTHER CASES

Prevention of insect bites (see Chapter 26).

73 Leptospirosis

Notifiable disease

ORGANISM

Leptospira interrogans is a tightly coiled spirochaete with pointed ends usually bent into the shape of a hook. There are approximately 200 serovars of *L. interrogans* split up into 23 serogroups (including *ictero-haemorrhagiae*, *hebdomidis*, *canicola* and *pomona*).

EPIDEMIOLOGY

Leptospirosis is a zoonosis with a worldwide distribution. It has a higher incidence in warmer climates and in summer in temperate climates. This is because leptospires survive for longer in damp soil with high humidity and ambient temperatures between 25°C and 30°C. Infection is more common in adults but paediatric and congenital infections are described. There are three epidemiological patterns of infection: a) associated with farming of cattle and pigs in temperate climates; b) in tropical climates where disease is not occupational; and c) related to rodents in urban environments.

Transmission

A variety of animals excrete leptospires asymptomatically in their urine. Thus dairy cattle harbour serovars *hardjo* or *pomona*, pigs *pomona*, *tarrasovi* or *bratislava*, dogs *canicola* and rats *copenhagen* or *ballum*. The normal portal of entry is through sodden or abraded skin and mucous membranes (especially conjunctivae). Point contamination of water supplies has resulted in outbreaks of leptospirosis. Person-to-person spread does not occur except for rare cases of transplacental or perinatal spread.

Incubation period

This varies from 2 to 21 days (usually 3–10 days), depending on the infective dose and the virulence of the leptospire.

NATURAL HISTORY AND CLINICAL FEATURES

Leptospirosis can vary in severity from asymptomatic infection to severe Weil's disease. The disease is biphasic with an initial septicaemic phase lasting for about a week, followed by a second phase when leptospires localise to organs. The first phase begins suddenly with fever, chills, headache, myalgia, conjunctival injection and occasionally a rash. Aseptic meningitis may occur in this phase. The second or immune phase is related to the production of antibodies and during this leptospires are excreted in urine. Liver involvement produces icteric leptospirosis, which can be life-threatening (5–15% mortality). It does not produce liver cell necrosis so liver function is not permanently damaged.

Diagnosis

Leptospires can be detected in blood or cerebrospinal fluid by dark ground microscopy (low sensitivity), culture (in serum free liquid media) or genome detection during the first phase, although it is unlikely to be high in the list of differential diagnoses of 'flu-like' illness.

Serology is the way in which most infections are diagnosed, although the bacteria can be cultured from urine in the second phase. The gold standard for serology is the microscopic agglutination test.

MANAGEMENT

In the early stage penicillin (or erythromycin) is the treatment of choice. Antibiotics given late do not effect the duration or severity of the icteric disease but do decrease the period of leptospiruria.

PREVENTION OF FURTHER CASES

Prevention is by decreasing the risk of transfer from animals to humans by education on sources and modes of spread, by control of cattle and porcine infection (immunisation, chemotherapy and culling), environmental control (improving soil drainage) and rodent control.

74 Listeriosis

See also Chapter 4

ORGANISM

Listeria monocytogenes is a Gram-positive rod with the ability to grow at low temperatures. There are 13 serotypes. Early infection is normally associated with 1/2a and 1/2b, with late disease caused by 4b.

EPIDEMIOLOGY

L. monocytogenes is found in cattle, other animals and silage. On occasions it enters the food chain and food-borne transmission is a frequent source of infection, with sporadic cases and common-source outbreaks occurring. *Listeria* has been isolated from unpasteurised soft cheeses, pate, salads and microwave-ready meals. Outbreaks of infection have been traced to pasteurised soft cheese contaminated during processing and to silage through occupational exposure. Groups of patients at risk of severe consequences from infection are pregnant women and neonates, immunocompromised patients and the elderly. Mothers can exhibit vaginal, faecal and urine carriage, which can be asymptomatic, and as a consequence neonatal infections occur. There was an increase in neonatal infection during 1988 as a result of contamination of pate manufactured in Belgium and a major outbreak associated with soft cheese in France in 1993.

Transmission

Transplacental transmission to the fetus can occur during acute bacteraemia in the mother. *L. monocytogenes* may colonise the genital tract so that the neonate may acquire the organism during delivery and ascending infection can also occur. Transvaginal spread is thought to be unusual. Most late-onset neonatal cases result from hospital cross-infection, although they may be acquired from the mother during birth. Nosocomial transmission has been described in day-care centres.

Incubation period

For both neonatal and adult food-borne transmission the incubation period is variable from a few days to 10 weeks. Shorter periods, with development of symptoms in the few days after birth, are more characteristic of neonatal infection; however, neonates can also develop illness late after birth and longer incubation periods are more typical in adults.

NATURAL HISTORY AND CLINICAL FEATURES

Congenital infection may result in stillbirth or a septicaemic illness, normally within 48 hours of delivery, with meningitis being the most severe complication. Meconium staining of the liquor is said to be associated with infection even in the preterm infant. Infants may develop respiratory distress as a result of pneumonia, with a similar presentation to group B streptococcal infection. A characteristic feature of the illness is a red papular rash (roseola) seen on the face, trunk and pharynx. Meningitis may occur. The prognosis is better with later-onset infection. In adults (including pregnant mothers) the infection may result in an influenza-like illness with headache, backache, diarrhoea and abdominal pain. Meningitis also occurs in the immunocompromised and elderly patients.

Diagnosis

Early-onset infection may be characterised by leukopenia. In meningitis either neutrophils or mononuclear cells predominate in the cerebrospinal fluid (CSF). The organism can be isolated from blood, CSF, meconium, placenta and gastric washings, although it may take several days for the isolate to be confirmed because of the difficulties in distinguishing *Listeria* from other bacilli found in nonsterile sites.

MANAGEMENT

Ampicillin and gentamicin, when combined, have a synergistic effect and are the recommended antibiotics in children. Cephalosporins are ineffective. The organism is intracellular and therefore long courses of treatment should be used: 14 days for septicaemia and 21 days for meningitis.

PREVENTION OF FURTHER CASES

Pregnant women should avoid foodstuffs carrying a risk of *Listeria* infection. These include pate, pre-washed salads, and unpasteurised cheese and other milk products. They should ensure that microwave-ready meals are adequately cooked. Pregnant women should also not work with silage. When cases occur a careful history should be taken so that common-source outbreaks can be detected and the Consultant in Communicable Disease Control must be informed promptly. Isolates of *Listeria* must be referred centrally* to permit the further characterisation of organisms and the detection of common-source outbreaks occurring through contamination of the food chain.

Domestic refrigerators should be well maintained to ensure correct temperature control.

75 Lyme disease and other borrelioses

ORGANISM

A spirochaete, *Borrelia burgdorferi*, causes Lyme disease, *B. recurrentis* causes louse-borne relapsing fever and *B. turicatae*, *B. hermsii*, *B. parkeri* and *B. duttonii* cause tick-borne relapsing fever.

LYME DISEASE

EPIDEMIOLOGY

This is a rare infection in the UK but it is endemic in parts of the USA, where it is to be found predominantly on the eastern seaboard and in California and Oregon. In the UK, several cases have been reported from the New Forest in Hampshire.

Transmission

From tick vectors (*Ixodes* species). In the UK these are found on deer and then pass to human beings. It is thought that they need to feed on the human for several hours before the spirochaete is transmitted. Person-to-person transmission does not occur, except for rare cases of transplacental infection.

Incubation period

3–20 days (median 12 days).

NATURAL HISTORY AND CLINICAL FEATURES

Infection is usually manifest by a macular or papular skin lesion (erythema migrans or erythema chronicum migrans), red in colour, which expands to

---

* **In England and Wales to the Food Hygiene Laboratory, Central Public Health Laboratory, 61 Colindale Avenue, London NW9 5EQ, tel. 020 8200 4400.**

become a large, irregular circular lesion. It is found at the site of a recent tick bite, although this may be inapparent, especially in children who have no recollection of a bite. Similar skin lesions may also occur away from the site of the bite. In the early phase there may be many other less specific features, including fever, arthralgia, headache and neck stiffness. A second phase occurring weeks to months later may manifest as central nervous system (especially VIIth nerve palsy and aseptic meningitis), cardiac and joint symptoms. Chronic arthritis is a late manifestation.

Diagnosis

A clinical diagnosis may be possible in the presence of the distinctive skin lesion. Occasionally, *B. burgdorferi* can be cultured from a biopsy of the perimeter of the erythema migrans rash or from blood, or from cerebrospinal fluid if there are central nervous system symptoms. Serological tests can be made using an enzyme-linked immunosorbent assay (ELISA), or Western blot analysis. IgM antibodies may not rise until 3–6 weeks after the onset of disease and IgG titres are very slow to rise; hence serology is not always helpful because of the frequency of borderline-positive results.

MANAGEMENT

This is with doxycycline 100 mg twice daily or amoxycillin 500 mg three times daily for the child over 9. For the younger child amoxycillin (25–50 mg/kg/day) is recommended. Erythromycin can be used as an alternative where there is a history of penicillin allergy. A 3-week course is necessary. Some authorities recommend the use of probenecid with the penicillin-containing regimens. Ceftriaxone (100 mg/kg as a single daily dose) should be used for later complications, including meningitis.

PREVENTION OF FURTHER CASES

This is difficult, but people walking in endemic areas should keep their skin well covered by clothing to avoid tick bites and inspect themselves for ticks afterwards. Any found should be removed as soon as possible.

RELAPSING FEVERS

EPIDEMIOLOGY

Epidemic relapsing fever is carried by the human body louse. It is found worldwide but especially when there is poverty, crowding and poor hygienic conditions, e.g. in mass movement of refugees. Ethiopia has a particularly high incidence, with 10 000 cases per year.

Tick-borne relapsing fever is endemic in certain foci and is spread by *Ornithodoros* ticks, the different species of which give the species name to the bacteria. *B. duttonii* is found in Africa, *B. hermsii*, *B. parkeri* and *B. turicatae* in America.

Transmission

Epidemic louse-borne relapsing fever is transmitted when body lice carrying *B. recurrentis* are crushed. The released bacteria then penetrate skin or mucous membrane. Tick-borne relapsing fever is transmitted by the bite of a tick that has previously fed on a reservoir host (e.g. squirrels, chipmunks, rats, mice, rabbits, lizards or birds). However, the bacteria can be maintained in tick populations by transovarial transmission down the generations. Infection is not directly transmissible from person to person.

Incubation period

For each, the incubation period is 4–18 days with a mean of 7–8 days.

NATURAL HISTORY AND CLINICAL FEATURES

Relapsing fever, as its name implies, is characterised by repeated episodes of fever and defervescence. Each begins with an acute onset of fever, which lasts 5.5 days in louse-borne relapsing fever (LBRF) and 7 days in tick-borne relapsing fever (TBRF), with rigors, headache, myalgia, arthralgias and cough.

Diagnosis

This is by demonstration of *Borrelia* in peripheral blood films stained by Giemsa or by wet films examined by dark ground microscopy.

MANAGEMENT AND PREVENTION

Successful treatment has been achieved with tetracycline, chloramphenicol or erythromycin. The mortality of treated relapsing fever is 5% and of untreated LBRF 40%. Antibiotic therapy will usually induce a Jarisch–Herxheimer reaction. Prevention is by avoidance of the vector and use of insecticides.

76 Malaria

Notifiable disease

ORGANISM

Four species of *Plasmodium*: *P. falciparum*, *P. vivax*, *P. ovale* and *P. malariae*. This is a protozoan parasite.

EPIDEMIOLOGY

Malaria is endemic throughout most of the tropics below 1500 m and parts of the subtropics. Occasional outbreaks of *vivax* malaria occur in nonendemic countries adjacent to endemic areas, e.g. in Greece and Singapore. Figures from the PHLS Malaria Reference Laboratory show that malaria cases diagnosed in England and Wales have increased in the 1990s, with over 2000 reported cases per year in the last 3 years, of which over 10% were in children under 15. Nearly 90% of malaria cases in children affect members of ethnic minority groups travelling with their families to sub-Saharan Africa or the Indian subcontinent. The proportion caused by *P. falciparum* has increased, largely because of the increasing numbers of cases originating from India and other Asian countries, where *P. vivax* cases were previously in the majority. Between three and 11 fatalities per year are reported, almost all due to *P. falciparum* infection.

The type of malaria acquired is related to the country visited. *P. falciparum* accounts for 85% of malaria contracted in Africa, but only 40–75% of cases contracted in south Asia (including the Indian subcontinent) are caused by *P. falciparum*, although this proportion continues to increase. *P. ovale* is uncommon, causing only 6% of all infections, almost invariably related to African travel. *P. malariae* is rare (1% of all cases).

Transmission

Transmission is vector-borne, through the intermediary of the female *Anopheles* mosquito when it takes a human blood meal. The main reservoir of infection is the chronically infected human. Rare cases occur following transfusion or needlestick transmission from infected donors. Airport-related cases have occurred when mosquitoes have survived an air journey from an endemic country.

Incubation period

This can be as short as 8 days and as long as 5 years or more. Some 90% of *falciparum* malaria presents in the first month after exposure, with most of the remaining 10% being seen in the following 4 months. A small minority with *falciparum* malaria (< 1%) present more than 6 months after leaving the endemic area. The picture is different for the benign malarias, with 25% seen in the first month, 30% in the next 4 months, 35% between 6 and 12 months after return and 10% presenting more than a year after travel.

NATURAL HISTORY AND CLINICAL FEATURES

Any child with a fever who has visited a malarious area, especially within the past year, should be considered to have malaria until proved otherwise. Malaria can present with any one of a number of symptoms or signs. These include myalgia, rigors, headache, cough, diarrhoea and vomiting, abdominal pain and jaundice. Consequently, common misdiagnoses in the child with malaria include flu, hepatitis or gastroenteritis. Other than fever, there are no consistent clinical signs. Splenomegaly occurs in less than 50% and hepatomegaly is even less common. Periodic (tertian or quartan) fever is also uncommon and is virtually never seen in travellers with *falciparum* malaria. Only 30–50% of patients with a benign malaria have a discernible pattern to their fever.

Ominous signs are loss of consciousness, especially if associated with decerebrate posturing, fits or focal neurological signs (cerebral malaria). Hypoglycaemia is also a common complication and is especially likely in children given intravenous quinine therapy. Other complications include hypotension and diarrhoea with Gram-negative septicaemia (algid malaria), haemolytic anaemia, haemoglobinuria and renal failure (blackwater fever), disseminated intravascular coagulation, pulmonary oedema, acute renal failure and severe anaemia. The mortality from malaria in the UK is approximately 1% and is usually related to delayed diagnosis. Children who are immunocompromised, asplenic or have homozygous sickle-cell disease are especially prone to severe disease when they contract malaria.

Two chronic malaria syndromes are recognised in children who have lived for prolonged periods in an endemic area. Nephrotic syndrome can complicate *P. malariae* infection. Tropical splenomegaly syndrome, a combination of splenomegaly (which can be massive), pancytopenia, hypergammaglobulinaemia (especially IgM) and a strongly positive malaria antibody test, is related to recurrent exposure to *P. falciparum*.

Diagnosis

The diagnosis cannot be ruled out unless at least three sets of thick and thin blood films, each set taken as the fever rises, have been examined by someone experienced in the recognition of parasites. Fluorescence microscopy using an acridine orange stain (QBC system) is sensitive but nonspecific. Dipstick tests for *P. falciparum* parasitaemia are highly sensitive, as they detect the histidine-rich protein (HRP2) or enzyme components of the parasite. In rare cases the blood film can be negative, especially if the patient has taken antimalarial drugs in the recent past. It is also important to consider alternative and additional diagnoses such as typhoid and meningococcaemia. Malaria antibodies can be measured to confirm the diagnosis of a chronic malaria syndrome or may be used retrospectively in the rare instances of 'slide-negative' malaria.

MANAGEMENT

All children with confirmed or suspected *falciparum* malaria should be hospitalised. The treatment used and the route of administration are dictated by the species of malaria, the country where the infection was acquired and, for *falciparum* malaria, the degree of parasitaemia. Glucose-6-phosphate dehydrogenase (G6PD) deficiency should be sought as its presence may contraindicate some medications.

Infection with *P. vivax*, *P. ovale* or *P. malariae*

Oral chloroquine, 10 mg/kg initially, 5 mg/kg after 6–12 hours then 5 mg/kg daily for 2 more days, will eradicate the acute infection. Primaquine 0.25 mg/kg daily for 14–21 days is subsequently given to eradicate the liver forms of *ovale* and *vivax* malaria if the child is not G6PD-deficient. There are rare reported cases of chloroquine-resistant *vivax* malaria from New Guinea, in which case quinine or possibly mefloquine may be used. Halofantrine is used in some African countries but carries a risk of idiosyncratic tachydysrhythmias, particularly in patients receiving drugs that may prolong the QT interval. Primaquine-tolerant *P. vivax* is also described from that region – this responds to 4 weeks primaquine therapy.

Uncomplicated *falciparum* malaria

Providing the parasitaemia is less than 5%, give oral quinine (10 mg/kg 8–12-hourly) for 5 days. This is followed by sulfadoxine plus pyrimethamine (Fansidar) (0–4 years, half a tablet; 5–6 years, 1 tablet; 7–9 years one and a half tablets; 10–14 years, 2 tablets; over 14 years, 3 tablets), which is normally administered as a single dose. If Fansidar is contraindicated (e.g. in G6PD deficiency), the quinine may be given as a single agent for 10–14 days. Otherwise mefloquine (20 mg/kg in two divided doses, 12 hours apart, starting 12 hours after the last quinine dose) or tetracycline (e.g. doxycycline 200 mg day 1, then 100 mg days 2–7 for children over 12 years) may be substituted. Atovaquone plus proguanil (Malarone) can be used to treat uncomplicated malaria in children over 11 kg. The dosages are: 11–20 kg, 1 tablet daily; 21–30 kg, 2 tablets daily as a single dose; 31–40 kg, 3 tablets daily as a single dose. For children over 40 kg the dose is 4 tablets daily as a single dose (as for an adult). All these are given consecutively on 3 days. Intramuscular and rectal artemesin derivatives are used to treat *falciparum* malaria in the Far East, but are not available in the UK.

Severe *falciparum* malaria

Intravenous quinine 10 mg/kg, up to 600 mg, in an infusion of 5% dextrose (50–250 mL) over 4 hours and repeated every 8–12 hours should be given if the parasitaemia is 5% or higher and there are complications such as cerebral malaria, or if the patient cannot tolerate oral quinine. This is ideally undertaken in a paediatric intensive care setting. Some authorities recommend an initial loading dose of quinine (20 mg/kg over 4 hours), especially for *falciparum* malaria acquired in south and east Asia and the Pacific islands. Dose reduction after the first 24 hours may be required if there is hepatic dysfunction, often related to severe malaria, or severe side-effects (tinnitus, deafness, nausea and vomiting – cinchonism). It is normal for most patients to have mild cinchonism at therapeutic blood levels of quinine. Close monitoring is very important, watching for hypoglycaemia, hypoxia or seizures, all of which adversely affect the prognosis.

The quinine can be given orally at the same dose after 1–2 days to complete 5 days' treatment, followed by Fansidar or one of the alternative drug regimens listed above.

Complications such as renal failure, anaemia, Gram-negative septicaemia and disseminated intravascular coagulation are managed conventionally. Some experts recommend exchange transfusion for very high parasitaemias (> 20%), or high parasite counts (> 10%) in the presence of complications, although this practice is not universally accepted. Some also advise fluid restriction to prevent pulmonary oedema.

PREVENTION OF FURTHER CASES

Mosquito bite avoidance. Advice to parents should include: the use of insect repellents such as diethyltoluamide (DEET); long clothing to be worn, especially at dawn and dusk; insecticide-containing mosquito coils or vaporisers; mosquito meshing for non-air-conditioned rooms and the use of bed nets treated with permethrin insecticide.

Table 76.1 Summary of drugs recommended for antimalarial prophylaxis

Geographical location	Preferable regimen	Alternative
East, central and southern sub-Saharan Africa* *except for*	Mefloquine†	Proguanil + chloroquine
Botswana, South Africa, Namibia, Mauritania, Zimbabwe	Proguanil + chloroquine	Mefloquine
North Africa and Middle East*	Proguanil + chloroquine	Proguanil or chloroquine
Indian subcontinent‡ and south Asia *except for*	Proguanil + chloroquine	
Bangladesh	Mefloquine†	Proguanil + chloroquine
SE Asia (mainly nontourist areas)* (including Yunan and Hainan in China)	Mefloquine†	
Papua New Guinea, Solomon Islands* and Vanuatu	Mefloquine†	Maloprim + chloroquine
Latin America‡ and Caribbean*:		
Amazon Basin of Brazil, Bolivia and Venezuela, Guyana, Surinam, French Guiana and Colombia	Mefloquine†	Chloroquine + proguanil
Bolivia, Equador, East Panama, Peru, Venezuela	Chloroquine + proguanil	Mefloquine
Argentina, Belize, Costa Rica, Dominican Republic, El Salvador, Guatemala, Haiti, Honduras, Nicaragua, West Panama, rural Paraguay	Chloroquine	Proguanil

* No chemoprophylaxis is considered necessary, although mosquito bites should be avoided, in Abu Dhabi, Algeria, Bali, Brunei, Brazil outside the Amazon Basin, Cape Verde, China (main tourist areas), Egypt (tourist areas), Hong Kong, Jamaica, Libya, Malaysia (except Sabah), Mauritius, Morocco, Sarawak, Singapore, Thailand (Bangkok and main tourist areas), Trinidad, Tunisia, Turkey (tourist areas).
† Proguanil + chloroquine for children < 2 years old.
‡ Prophylaxis may not be needed above certain altitudes (see Further reading – these guidelines are subject to change and travellers and those advising them are recommended to consult current authorities).

Antimalarial chemoprophylaxis

Recommendations as of the time of going to press are shown in Table 76.1 and doses in Table 76.2. The regimen may change with emerging patterns of resistance and current advice should be sought from an expert source such as the Malaria Reference Laboratory at the London School of Hygiene, tel. 020 7636 8636.

Table 76.2 Summary of drug regimens recommended for antimalarial prophylaxis

Age	Weight (kg)	Dose and frequency				
		Chloroquine base once weekly	Proguanil hydrochloride once daily	Mefloquine once weekly	Doxycycline once daily	Maloprim® once weekly
0–12 weeks	Under 6	37.5 mg	25 mg	–	–	–
12 weeks–11 months	6–9.9	75 mg	50 mg	62.5 mg	–	¼ tablet
1–3 years	10–15.9	112.5 mg	75 mg	62.5 mg	–	¼ tablet
4–7 years	16–24.9	150 mg	100 mg	125 mg	–	½ tablet
8–12 years	25–44.9	225 mg	150 mg	187.5 mg	Over 12 years, 75 mg*	¾ tablet
Over 13 years	Over 45	Adult dose (300 mg)	Adult dose (200 mg)	Adult dose (250 mg)	Adult dose (100 mg)	Adult dose (1 tablet)

* No suitable formulation available.

Note: Weight is a better guide than age. Specialist advice should be obtained for use of Maloprim® in children under 1 year of age. Prophylaxis is required in breast-fed infants; although antimalarials are excreted in milk, the amounts are too variable to give reliable protection.

Source: *British National Formulary*, September 2000.

FURTHER READING

Bradley DJ, Warhurst DC on behalf of an expert group of doctors, nurses and pharmacists (1997) Guidelines for the prevention of malaria in travellers from the United Kingdom. CDR Rev 10: R138–151.

Department of Health (2000) Health information for overseas travel. HMSO, London.
For updated country-by-country guidelines and information on newer drugs.

77 Measles

Notifiable disease

ORGANISM

The measles virus is the only human pathogen of the genus *Morbillivirus* of the Paramyxoviridae family. The single-stranded enveloped RNA virus is sensitive to heat and cold, ultraviolet light, ether and formalin. Only one serotype is known to cause human infection.

EPIDEMIOLOGY

Humans are the only host. Measles is endemic in most large countries and globally it is estimated that 1–2 million children die from measles annually, mostly in low-income countries. To interrupt transmission requires a protection rate from immunisation of 95% or greater for the whole population of susceptibles. In the UK a pattern of epidemics every 2 years was temporarily interrupted following the introduction of measles, mumps and rubella (MMR) vaccine in 1988 (see Appendix I, Fig. I.5). Because of poor immunisation uptake in children born before then, and the incomplete protection afforded by immunisation, the numbers of susceptible individuals increased in the 1990s, especially among older children. The proportion of measles notifications from older children increased and school outbreaks began to occur. This suggested that a major outbreak was increasingly liable to occur and led to the decision to immunise all school-age children with measles and rubella vaccine in the autumn of 1994. Because 5–10% of recipients do not develop protective antibodies after a single dose of MMR, a second dose has become part of the routine immunisation schedule in the UK. It is recommended that this is given with the preschool booster but it may be given earlier as long as at least 3 months has elapsed after the first dose.

Although notifications of measles are still measured in thousands, usually only 1–2% are confirmed when checked ny saliva testing. Since the

MR campaign in 1994 there have been occasional outbreaks. The largest comprised 150 cases in four connected communities in 1997. All but six were between 1 and 15 years old; 146 were known to be unimmunised and two immunised. The immunisation status in two was unknown.

Owing to the presence of maternal antibodies, the disease is unusual in infants and very uncommon in those under 6 months old. This pattern may change in an era when most mothers have been vaccinated. Antibody levels are lower and persist for a shorter time in the babies of vaccinated mothers. Prior to the introduction of immunisation in the UK, over 90% of individuals had the disease by the time they reached their 10th birthday. The disease is more severe in those exposed to large infecting doses, and overcrowded housing is therefore a recognised risk factor. The prognosis is worse in very young children and children at secondary school. Second attacks have been described but are rare.

Immunosuppressed individuals are particularly susceptible to complications (at least five of the 36 people who died from measles in the USA in 1991 were infected with human immunodeficiency virus, HIV).

Subacute sclerosing panencephalitis is one of the most severe sequelae of measles infection. From 1970 to 1989 in England and Wales 290 confirmed cases were reported. The incidence seems to have declined, with only three confirmed cases being reported in 1993.

Transmission

The disease is highly infectious and transmission is primarily by droplet spread. Contact with fresh nasal or oral secretions may also cause infection. Patients are infectious from 3–5 days prior to the appearance of the rash and until 4 days after its appearance.

Incubation period

Family studies have shown that the rash may appear from 6 days to 19 days (median 13 days) after exposure. The rash appears on the fourth day of the illness and the median incubation period to first symptoms is therefore about 9 days.

NATURAL HISTORY AND CLINICAL FEATURES

Fever, cough, conjunctivitis and coryza are the initial symptoms. In some cases the pathognomonic Koplik's spots (white spots like grains of sand on a red background) appear on the buccal mucosa a day or two later and are followed on the third or fourth day by an erythematous maculopapular rash. The rash begins at the hairline and progresses down the body over the next 3 days. The rash on the upper part of the body tends to become confluent. After 3–4 days, the rash may have a brownish appearance and then begins to fade in the order in which it appeared. The fever usually declines before the rash disappears. While it is present the child tends to be miserable ('measles miseries') with anorexia, coryza, coughing and conjunctivitis. There is often a mild generalised lymphadenopathy.

Complications

In low-income countries the case fatality rate is around 5–10%. Though this rate is far lower in the industrialised world, complications still develop in 5–10% of recognised cases in the UK and about 1 in 70 affected children are admitted to hospital. Severe complications are more common in older children and adults. The most important complications are listed in Table 77.1. The rates are derived from reported cases in the USA. The data may be subject to undernotification or overdiagnosis; however, the relative rates of the various complications at different ages provide a useful indication of the different risks at different times in childhood.

- **Otitis media**: 5–7% of children with measles develop acute otitis media.
- **Pneumonia** is due to the primary virus infection or bacterial superinfection (*Streptococcus pneumoniae*, *S. pyogenes*, *Staphylococcus aureus* and *Haemophilus influenzae*). It is about as common as otitis media.
- **Croup**: A mild laryngotracheobronchitis is a normal part of measles. Some children may go on to develop a severe obstruction requiring intubation.
- **Convulsions and encephalitis**: Convulsions occur in 0.5% of cases and an acute encephalitis develops in approximately 0.1% of cases, usually between the second and sixth day after the development of the rash. Some 60% of cases of encephalitis recover completely, 15% die and 25% are left with neurodevelopmental sequelae.
- **Subacute sclerosing panencephalitis** (SSPE) is a rare neurodegenerative condition with an onset many years after measles infection. Occurring in 1 in 250 000 cases, it is invariably fatal. There is a male: female ratio of 2.8:1. The median period between measles and onset is about 8 years, with a wide range of 3 months to 20 years. It seems somewhat more common in cases where the primary infection has occurred at an early age. Initially there is deterioration in intellectual function, followed by incoordination and falling. Myoclonic seizures follow, and death may occur within 6 months of onset or the course can be prolonged.

Table 77.1 Complication rates (%) derived from reported cases of measles in the USA

Complication*	Age group			
	< 5 years	5–19 years	≥ 20 years	Total
Otitis media	23	5	3	14
Diarrhoea	16	7	13	12
Pneumonia	11	3	11	8
Encephalitis	0.1	0.1	0.4	0.1
Hospitalisation	32	11	36	26
Death†	0.37	0.16	0.43	0.32

* Data for 1991. † Data for 1990.

- **Death**: In industrialised countries the case fatality rate is of the order of 1 in 1000 overall and 1 in 2500 in older children. In the immuno-compromised child, such as those with leukaemia or HIV infection, measles can produce an atypical pneumonia characterised by giant cell formation in the alveoli. In such cases the rash does not appear and there is a high mortality.

Diagnosis

This is usually on clinical grounds. However, when incidence is low, the clinical diagnosis is frequently erroneous. Isolation of virus is technically difficult and rarely performed. Serum antibodies appear within 1–3 days of the onset of the rash and peak at 2–4 weeks. Neutralising and haemagglutination inhibition (HI) antibodies may persist for many years. The presence of measles-specific IgM (detectable from 2 days to 5 weeks after the onset of a rash) or a fourfold rise in antibody titres indicates acute infection. Noninvasive salivary tests detecting antimeasles IgM have now become available and are considered the tests of choice.* PCR on saliva, throat swab or urine can be used to characterise the virus. The characteristic electroencephalogram and the detection of oligoclonal measles antibody in the cerebrospinal fluid confirm diagnosis of SSPE.

MANAGEMENT

There is no antiviral therapy suitable for management of uncomplicated cases. Treatment is symptomatic unless complications develop, when these should be managed appropriately. For secondary bacterial infections antibiotics should be given. Intubation may be necessary for the child with severe laryngotracheobronchitis. Steroids have been used with benefit in encephalitis. Ribavirin and interferon-alpha have been used in immunocompromised children with giant cell pneumonia but without great success. In low-income countries lack of vitamin A is associated with severe measles and its administration to infected children has reduced morbidity and mortality from this infection. A case for routine use of vitamin A for children exposed in measles in industrialised countries has yet to be established.

PREVENTION OF FURTHER CASES

Isolation of cases is of little value as the period of infectivity includes a significant period before the diagnosis will have been made, although hospitalised children should be nursed with respiratory precautions until 4 days after the onset of the rash. In the community, children should also be kept away from nursery or school until they are no longer infectious.

Vaccination following exposure

If given within 72 hours of contact, measles vaccination reduces the chances of developing the disease. For those in whom vaccination is con-

---

* **In the UK contact the local Consultant in Communicable Disease Control.**

traindicated (immunocompromised children, see Appendix VI for definition) and in whom the disease is likely to be severe (e.g. children with severe heart or lung disease or who are immunosuppressed), human normal immunoglobulin (HNIG – for dosage see Appendix VI) can be used within 6 days of contact. It may also be of value if given later in severely immunocompromised children.

Routine vaccination

A live attenuated vaccine in the form of MMR vaccine is recommended for all children as soon after their first birthday as possible. Immunisation is highly effective in giving protection to any individual; however, because vaccine failures occur for a variety of reasons (an estimated 5–10% of cases), a single-dose schedule inevitably leads to a slow accumulation of susceptibles. A number of countries have introduced a two-dose schedule to interrupt transmission. The UK introduced a second dose in 1996. This is usually given at the same time as the preschool booster but may be given earlier as long as at least 3 months has elapsed since the time of the first dose. Conventional contraindications for a live vaccine apply, except that MMR should be given to children who are HIV-infected. Following the administration of HNIG for any reason, 3 months should elapse before immunisation.

Side-effects of MMR immunisation occur; typical frequencies are shown in Table 77.2. Fever generally starts 7–10 days following immunisation, is mild and lasts for a day or so. An unusual side-effect is transient thrombocytopenia; reports of encephalitis following immunisation are extremely rare (less than 1 per million doses) and are probably coincidental. Arthralgia occurs in approximately 3% of children and arthritis in 11% of adolescents and adult women. Lasting effects are uncommon. In the UK, a group of researchers has proposed a link between MMR vaccination and the development of autism and inflammatory bowel disease. Independent studies have shown no support for such hypotheses.

In low-income countries much of the morbidity and mortality due to measles takes place in the first year of life, when conventional immunisation is relatively ineffective. High-titre vaccines have been developed to overcome these problems but have been dogged by association with increased late mortality in recipients and are not in regular use.

Table 77.2 Frequency of side-effects of MMR vaccination

	Children aged 1–2 years	Children aged 5 years	Teenagers
Fever	1 in 5	1 in 14	1 in 25
Rash	1 in 5	1 in 17	1 in 14
Febrile convulsions	1 in 1000	Nil	Nil

78 Meningococcal disease

Meningococcal disease (both meningitis and septicaemia) is notifiable

ORGANISM

Caused by *Neisseria meningitidis*, the meningococcus, a Gram-negative diplococcus. Strains are divided into serogroups by the surface capsular polysaccharide. Groups B, C, A, Y and W135 account for most invasive disease; B and C have been most prevalent in the UK in the last decade, with C increasing.

EPIDEMIOLOGY

Across Europe incidence varies from 0.1–6 per 100 000 population per annum, with higher incidences in northern Europe. In the UK overall incidence (all ages) is 5–6/100 000, with 2831 laboratory reports in England and Wales in 1999. There are around 250 deaths per annum. There are geographical variations even inside the UK (incidence is higher in the north and west). Attack rates are highest in the under-5 age-group, peaking in infancy; half of all cases are in children aged less than 2 years, in whom incidence can reach 50–100/100 000. A second peak occurs in teenagers aged 15–19 years. Infections are commoner in winter. Males outnumber females 3:2. Incidence fluctuates over time (see Appendix I, Fig. I.6). There have been recent rises in incidence in the UK and other parts of northern Europe, with an increasing proportion – around 40% – of cases in adolescents attributable to group C. The rise in group C seems to have been confined to the UK, where numbers are now declining following the introduction of a conjugate meningococcal C vaccine in the autumn of 1999. There is an ecological association between influenza and meningococcal infection, with more cases of the latter occurring when influenza is epidemic.

The annual incidence has risen since 1985 and has not yet returned towards pre-outbreak levels. Among notifications of meningococcal disease to the Communicable Disease Surveillance Centre there was a slight preponderance of meningococcal septicaemia (1828 of 3075 notifications of meningococcal disease overall in 1999). These notifications still underestimate the true number but are now far higher than the total isolates of *N. meningitidis* submitted to the Public Health Laboratory Service Meningococcal Reference Unit for England and Wales, which have fallen because of penicillin pretreatment.

At-risk groups include those in poor general health, living in overcrowded conditions and with sickle cell disease. Active and passive smoking increases the risk of disease. Specific immunodeficiencies (terminal components of complement, properdin and IgM deficiency) increase susceptibility to infection with unusual serogroups, e.g. X, Y and W135.

Transmission

Through close contact with nasopharyngeal droplets or respiratory secretions. Persons living in the household or 'kissing contacts' are most at risk.

Nasopharyngeal colonisation is found in 4–25% of the population. Carriage varies with age. It is low in young children, peaks in adolescence (up to 25%) and is about 10% in adults. Carriers spread infection and disease but incidence and outbreaks are not directly related to crude colonisation rate. For example, the highest rates of disease are in young children, in whom colonisation rates are low.

Invasive disease depends on organism and host factors, although the precise mechanism is obscure. Organism factors include capsulation (protective against host defences), piliation (which aids bacterial adhesion to the nasopharynx) and presence of outer membrane proteins (which influence epithelial penetration). Host factors include prior respiratory tract or viral infection (e.g. influenza), smoking (including passive), secretor status and reduced mucosal and systemic immunity. After invasion, the host response to infection may be important. Genetic predisposition may determine crucial aspects of immunity and the resulting inflammatory cascade, e.g. TNF receptor, mannose binding protein and other cytokine receptor polymorphisms.

Incubation period

Usually 2–10 days. Carriers can retain the organism in the nasopharynx for several weeks, making the time of transmission, and hence intervals between cases, difficult to ascertain or predict. The period of communicability is unknown. NB. Not all systemic antibiotics eradicate nasopharyngeal carriage in a child with invasive disease. Ceftriaxone is an exception and is highly effective at eradicating carriage.

NATURAL HISTORY AND CLINICAL FEATURES

The meningococcus is the commonest cause of bacterial meningitis in the UK, but only 15% of those with meningococcal disease present with pure meningitis: 25% have septicaemia with septic shock; the remaining 60% have mixed features of septicaemia and meningitis. Arthritis, pneumonia, occult bacteraemia, conjunctivitis, endocarditis, endophthalmitis and chronic meningococcaemia are rare presentations.

Most children present with features of early septicaemia or mixed septicaemia and meningitis. A nonspecific prodrome with coryzal symptoms and fever may last a few days; children with the most fulminant disease may become severely unwell in only a few hours.

The characteristic rash with petechiae and purpura may evolve extremely rapidly. Clusters of petechiae are often localised: purpuric elements can appear at any stage. Vasculitic spots with central areas of necrosis usually develop later.

A rapidly appearing red, macular rash precedes the typical petechial rash in 38% of cases. An ill child with an erythematous macular rash of large spots should be examined (and reviewed) for evidence of the typical rash elsewhere, although petechiae or purpura will not always coexist.

This maculopapular rash may mislead doctors into a diagnosis of viral infection.

Other features of the septicaemic presentation include (in decreasing order of occurrence) vomiting, drowsiness, diarrhoea, muscular aches, irritability, confusion, headache, poor feeding, high-pitched cry and fits (may be febrile in origin).

Meningococcal meningitis is clinically indistinguishable from other meningitides. Its features usually develop over several days. Symptoms (see Chapter 10) include fever, vomiting, headache, anorexia, drowsiness, lethargy and high-pitched cry. Photophobia and meningism are present. Patients with severe meningitis may present with convulsions, focal neurological signs and deteriorating level of consciousness, progressing to coma. The petechial rash may not be present.

Septic shock

Septic shock (see Chapter 8) occurs in 30% of meningococcal septicaemia. It may be heralded by signs of impaired peripheral perfusion, including tachycardia, cold peripheries, prolonged capillary refill time, a wide skin-core temperature difference (best measured with thermistor probes on a toe and in the rectum), tachypnoea, oliguria and low blood pressure. Hypotension is a late sign of septic shock in young children who maintain blood pressure by intense vasoconstriction despite severe hypovolaemia. A rapidly progressive haemorrhagic rash may occur, followed by rigors and prostration, coma and death.

Diagnosis

A petechial/purpuric rash in a feverish, ill child is virtually pathognomonic of meningococcal disease (see Plate 7). Diagnosis is rarely difficult but may be delayed if a careful search of all skin areas, including palms and soles, is omitted. The petechial nature of a rash may be confirmed by its failure to blanch with local pressure (e.g. beneath a drinking glass – the 'tumbler test' – see Plate 8). Public awareness of the features of meningococcal disease is now high and parental enquiry about the possibility of meningitis or septicaemia should prompt a careful assessment of the child.

Bacteria that occasionally (< 1%) cause a similar clinical picture include *Streptococcus pneumoniae*, Gram-negative organisms and (rarely since the Hib immunisation programme) *Haemophilus influenzae* type b. Other differential diagnoses include: Henoch–Schönlein purpura (rash not on trunk, child afebrile and generally well); idiopathic thrombocytopenic purpura (ecchymoses, purpura and petechiae of different ages in a generally well child); acute leukaemia (child usually afebrile and nontoxic with evidence of lymphadenopathy and hepatosplenomegaly); and nonaccidental injury (child afebrile with suggestive features in history and examination). Petechiae on the face and neck may be caused by vomiting or coughing but caution should be exercised in making this attribution and so overlooking the diagnosis of meningococcal disease. Other causes are rare. Diagnostic confusion with the rashes of varicella or measles has occurred but is rarely justified. If the diagnosis is in doubt, treat as meningococcal disease until disproved.

Investigations

Blood for: full blood count and differential white cell count; clotting studies; blood culture; blood group and save serum (for serodiagnosis); blood for polymerase chain reaction (PCR) detection of meningococcus (EDTA bottle); urea and electrolytes; throat swab. Typical findings include a neutrophil leukocytosis and thrombocytopenia. Neutropenia is a poor prognostic sign.

Meningococcus can be grown from blood in approximately 50% of all meningococcal disease. Isolation rate is higher in septicaemia but only 5% if pretreated with antibiotics. The organism may also be seen in and grown from aspirates of the skin lesions. All isolates should be sent for serogrouping and typing to the PHLS Meningococcal Reference Unit (Manchester PHL, tel. 0161 291 4628 – 0161 445 8111 out of hours) or the Meningococcal Reference (Scottish) Laboratory (0141 211 0080).

Lumbar puncture (LP) should be considered in children with a meningitic presentation. If children have a petechial or purpuric rash LP may not add to the diagnosis and can delay antibiotic treatment. Defer LP if the child is shocked or has predominantly septicaemic features to avoid deterioration during the procedure. If there are signs of raised intracranial pressure (grossly bulging fontanelle or papilloedema, reduced level of consciousness, focal neurological signs) and no rash is present, defer LP at least until computed tomography or magnetic resonance scan has excluded cerebral abscess or space-occupying lesion. Antibiotics should not be delayed while an LP is performed or when it is deferred.

Cerebrospinal fluid (CSF) findings are those of bacterial meningitis (see Chapter 10). Meningococci may be seen within neutrophils and cultured from the CSF in 80–90% of cases. Bacterial antigen detection may confirm diagnosis when prior penicillin treatment renders blood and CSF cultures negative. PCR testing may detect meningococcal DNA in CSF. Group-specific meningococcal antigens may be detected in CSF, blood and urine by latex-particle agglutination and counter-immunoelectrophoresis, although these are less routinely used. Biopsy (or aspiration) of necrotic skin spots may reveal Gram-negative intracellular diplococci on microscopy. Serology may occasionally give a retrospective diagnosis and it is important to take throat swabs in any pretreated case. Culture stays positive in the early stages of antibiotic treatment and is nearly always the same strain as the one causing invasive disease.

MANAGEMENT

Emergency antibiotic treatment

If meningococcal disease is suspected, give antibiotics urgently. Current evidence shows that this reduces mortality. In primary care use penicillin (Table 78.1), and transfer the child rapidly to hospital. Paediatricians accepting an admission of suspected meningococcal disease should check that penicillin has been given.

Table 78.1 Dose of benzylpenicillin for initial treatment of meningococcal disease in primary care

Age	Dose
> 10 years	1200 mg intravenously (or intramuscularly)
1–10 years	600 mg intravenously (or intramuscularly)
< 1 year	300 mg intravenously (or intramuscularly)

Children who are allergic to penicillin may be given cefotaxime 50 mg/kg intravenously or chloramphenicol 20 mg/kg intravenously.

In hospital the first doctor who sees the child should give cefotaxime (or penicillin) urgently, after taking blood tests. Treatment should not await transfer to a ward area: some children deteriorate despite rapid intervention.

Initial treatment

A senior, experienced paediatrician should be called to assess the child as soon as possible. Establish venous access during venepuncture. Give cefotaxime 200 mg/kg/day intravenously 6-hourly to cover meningococcus and other possible pathogens. Ceftriaxone 80 mg/kg intravenously once daily is an alternative. (Some still add penicillin 300 mg/kg/day intravenously, given 4-hourly.)

Fluid and other management

Assessment of fluid balance may be extremely difficult because of the extensive capillary leak that accompanies septicaemia. Severe hypovolaemia may coexist with increasing oedema.

Treat shock vigorously. Commence 4.5% albumin 20–40 mL/kg over 10–30 minutes, followed by 20–40 mL/kg 4.5% albumin over the next hour. Follow guidelines for management of septic shock (see Chapter 8). Commence maintenance intravenous fluids after restoration of the circulating volume.

Give antipyretics, but avoid sedatives. Corticosteroids should not be used in either pharmacological or physiological dosage in meningococcal disease without careful consideration. In septicaemia they may be detrimental. There is no direct evidence of their efficacy in meningitis but, if they are to be given, it is best to administer them before the first dose of antibiotics.

The first hours

Children who are alert and haemodynamically stable should be nursed in a high-dependency area on a paediatric ward and observed carefully. Noninvasive monitoring of blood pressure, respiratory rate and pattern, pulse, percutaneous oxygen saturation, perfusion (by core–peripheral temperature difference), and urine output should be undertaken.

The initial course of meningococcal disease is unpredictable and apparently stable children may deteriorate rapidly. There is now evidence that intensive care improves the prognosis. Approximately 25% of children with meningococcal disease require admission to a Paediatric Intensive Care Unit (PICU). Early selection for transfer is vital. Transfer to PICU is needed for children in shock who fail to respond to initial resuscitation or those who deteriorate despite adequate fluid and antibiotic treatment. Predictors of poor prognosis include: refractory hypotension, deteriorating conscious level and coma. Weaker predictors include: extreme age, variations in breathing pattern, a spreading rash of more than 12 hours duration, necrotic skin lesions, absence of meningism, seizures preadmission, white cell count $< 10\,000 \times 10^9/L$, thrombocytopenia $< 100\,000 \times 10^9/L$, erythrocyte sedimentation rate < 20 mm/h, disseminated intravascular coagulation, metabolic acidosis (pH < 7.3), CSF white blood cells $< 100 \times 10^9/L$ and antigenaemia.

Several scoring systems have been proposed, aimed at early identification of children with a poor prognosis by a combination of factors. None is universally accepted. The Glasgow Meningococcal Septicaemia Prognostic Score (Table 78.2) is a validated, clinically based scoring system that can be repeated at intervals to identify which children with meningococcal disease should be admitted to a PICU. Children scoring 8 or more have a 20% mortality risk with intensive care and should be transferred to a PICU.

While awaiting the arrival of the PICU team, it is important that resuscitative and stabilising measures are continued (see Chapter 8).

Duration of antibiotic treatment

Rationalise antibiotic therapy when culture results are available. Nearly all strains are very sensitive to antibiotics. Short courses of antibiotics are effective: generally continue treatment intravenously for 5 days for uncomplicated septicaemia and 7 days for uncomplicated meningitis. Antibiotic therapy should not be discontinued until the child has been apyrexial for 48 hours. If penicillin was given, reduce to 200 mg/kg/day intravenously given 6-hourly after 48 hours. If intravenous access becomes difficult and the child is well, use intramuscular ceftriaxone.

Novel therapies

Novel anti-endotoxin and anticytokine treatments may ultimately improve prognosis in severe meningococcal disease: no evidence of their efficacy has yet been produced in randomised, double-blind clinical trials. New therapies may have unappreciated side-effects, are expensive and should not be used outside trial conditions.

CNS involvement

Meningococcal disease may cause cerebral oedema and raised intracranial pressure (ICP). Infarction from vasculitis is an unusual later complication. Intensive care should aim to preserve cerebral perfusion pressure (the difference between blood pressure and ICP). Elective ventilation should aim to keep the $P_a\text{CO}_2$ between 4.0 and 5.2 kPa (30–40 mmHg) to reduce intracranial pressure. Maintain cardiac output by early use of volume-expanders and

Table 78.2 Glasgow meningococcal septicaemia prognostic score (differs minimally from the original description by Sinclair et al (1987) Lancet 2:38)

1.* Systolic blood pressure (see note 1)
If < 75 mmHg (age < 4 years) or < 85 mmHg (age > 4 years) — **Score 3 points**

2.* Skin/rectal temperature difference (see note 2)
If > 3°C — **Score 3 points**

3.* Modified coma scale (see note 3)
If initial score < 8, or deterioration of 3 or more points at any time — **Score 3 points**

4.* Deterioration in last hour
Ask parents or nurses; if yes — **Score 2 points**

5. Absence of neck stiffness — **Score 2 points**

6. Extent of purpura
Widespread ecchymoses, or extending lesions on review — **Score 1 point**

7. Base deficit
If > –8 — **Score 1 point**

Total

* Undertake on arrival and an hour after admission and at any time when deterioration occurs.

Notes:
1. Blood pressure: use Doppler or sphygmomanometer; cuff width not less than two-thirds length of upper arm.
2. Apply skin temperature probe to toe; axillar or rectal temperature taken for 2 min.
3. Modified coma scale:

(i) Eyes open	spontaneously	4
	to speech	3
	to pain	2
	none	1
(ii) Best verbal response	orientated	6
	words	4
	vocal sounds	3
	cries	2
	none	1
(iii) Best motor response	obeys commands	6
	localise pain	4
	moves to pain	1
	none	0

Add scores (i) + (ii) + (iii) to give result.
4. Unspecified and subjective rating.

inotropes but then reduce maintenance fluids to 50–70% of age-related usual. Use intravenous mannitol and corticosteroids only when ICP monitoring is available in a PICU, because of risk of rebound ICP rise. Indwelling ICP monitoring carries risks in severe shock or DIC.

Prognosis

Around 10% of children with meningococcal disease die. Most have haemorrhages into internal organs, especially the adrenals (Waterhouse–Friderichsen syndrome). Endotoxic shock with disseminated intravascular coagulation is the usual mode of death. Hence, meningococcal septicaemia has a higher mortality rate (around 30%) than meningitis alone (around 2%). Cases of mixed septicaemia and meningitis have an intermediate mortality.

Early intensive care, especially elective assisted ventilation, aggressive management of shock and anticipation of complications may improve the prognosis for children with septicaemia. Survival rates approach 70% in high-risk patients requiring intensive care.

Fortunately, unlike other bacterial meningitis, survival is usually accompanied by total recovery. Fewer than 10% of all children with meningococcal disease have sequelae. The commonest complication overall is deafness.

Survivors of intensive care may have greater morbidity. Areas of necrotic skin may need grafting. Necrotic digits or limbs usually autoamputate but surgical intervention is occasionally required. Neurological disability is uncommon but subtle developmental and motor problems, learning difficulties and behavioural disorders can occur.

Aftercare

All children with septicaemia or meningitis should be referred for audiology at time of discharge. All survivors should be followed up. Attention should be paid to psychological sequelae, especially in older children and parents. It is worthwhile investigating children with serogroup X, Y, Z and W135 disease for immunodeficiency.

PREVENTION OF FURTHER CASES

Detailed guidance is available and regularly updated (see Further reading). Prevention rests on three principles:

- Parents, carers for children, the general public and doctors in the primary care services being aware of the early signs of meningococcal disease and the action to take if it is suspected
- Eradication of meningococcal carriage in close contacts of cases
- Immunisation (when cases of serogroup A or C occur, or persons are travelling to endemic areas).

The Consultant in Communicable Disease Control (CCDC) (or an equivalent public health specialist) is responsible for ensuring that antibiotic prophylaxis, or immunisation if appropriate, is offered to contacts at risk. Increased risk of meningococcal disease occurs after close, prolonged contact with the index case during the previous week. Following diagnosis of probable meningococcal disease (septicaemia or meningitis), with or without microbiological confirmation, the CCDC or deputy must be informed urgently by telephone. Cases should also be notified officially in writing, by proforma, according to the predominant clinical picture. Approximately 1% of cases are coprimary, occurring in a contact within 1 week of the index case. The risk to household contacts is 500–1200 times higher than that in the general population. However, even then, the risk of a second case in household contacts within 1 month of the first case is still only 1%.

Antibiotic treatment to eradicate carriage

This should be given within 24 hours. Usually, the hospital provides treatment for those living in the index household to eliminate carriage of potentially pathogenic organisms: the paediatrician notifying the CCDC should have information regarding this household to hand. The CCDC is usually responsible for ensuring that treatment is given to any other close contacts at risk. These are few, by current definitions, and no longer automatically include those in day care or in the same class in a nursery school, where attempted prophylaxis may even eradicate carriage of nonpathogenic strains. Hospital staff do not need prophylaxis unless involved in mouth-to-mouth resuscitation. Oral rifampicin is the agent of choice (Table 78.3). Unless treated with ceftriaxone the index case should receive treatment for carriage: give oral rifampicin before discharge. Recipients should be warned about unwanted effects, including possible interference with the efficacy of oral contraceptives and orange staining of soft contact lenses. Ciprofloxacin (500 mg as a single dose) is an unlicensed alternative (although it will shortly be licensed for older children), while ceftriaxone (250 mg as a single dose) should be used for pregnant women. It should be noted that 'one-off' treatment of a group to eliminate carriage frequently produces only a short-term reduction in carriage rate and that such treatment to eliminate carriage is not effective in treatment of incubating disease.

Nasopharyngeal swabs

Swabbing before treatment for carriage is considered unnecessary, unless it is to gather epidemiological information.

Immunisation

If the strain is group C, W135 or Y A, vaccine should be offered to those contacts given antibiotics (over 18 months age if C). In autumn 1999, an effective conjugate vaccine against serogroup C for any age was introduced. A national immunisation programme against serogroup B awaits development of a satisfactory vaccine. If they have not already received it, conjugate meningococcal C vaccine should be offered to all new students in their first year of higher education.

Table 78.3 Dose of rifampicin for treatment of carriage of meningococcal bacteria

Adult	600 mg twice daily for 2 days
Child	10 mg/kg twice daily for 2 days
Neonate	5 mg/kg twice daily for 2 days

Action in specific circumstances

Single cases in children attending preschool groups

Antibiotic treatment for carriage should be offered to all household contacts of the case and vaccination also offered if indicated. There is no indication for prophylaxis for children or adults attached to the group. Information about the case and meningococcal disease should be given to parents, carers and GPs.

Single cases in pupils/students attending primary or secondary schools, colleges or universities

During term-time Antibiotic treatment for carriage or immunisation should not be offered to these contacts unless the exposure has been comparable to that experienced in a household (e.g. 'kissing contacts' or those sharing dormitory accommodation). Information about the case and meningococcal disease should be given to teachers, parents and GPs and, in secondary and higher education, to the pupils/students themselves.

Out of term-time Antibiotic treatment for carriage or immunisation should not be offered to these contacts. Dissemination of information may not be practical but should be considered when a case occurs within 7 days of the end of term, when rumours abound or when there is press publicity.

Alerting primary care

When cases occur and incidence is high, e.g. in the winter months in the UK, consideration should be given to alerting the public (see below), general practitioners and the community child health services. Written information should remind them of the early signs of meningococcal disease and about the recommendation to give parenteral penicillin to those suspected of having the infection while awaiting hospital transfer. This is usually done after close consultation with the CCDC.

Outbreaks (two or more cases closely connected in place and time)

Detailed advice has been published and is regularly reviewed (see Further reading). It is important to consult the microbiologist and ensure that specimens are sent for grouping and typing. Chemoprophylaxis should be offered to target groups of children and staff if two or more probable or confirmed cases occur within 4 weeks in the same play-group, nursery school or primary school. Clusters in secondary schools, universities and higher-learning institutions often create complex decision, organisational and publicity issues. It is recommended that urgent expert advice is sought from the regional epidemiologist, the Communicable Disease Surveillance Centre (CDSC), the Meningococcal Reference Unit or Gloucester Public Health Laboratory.

Patient, family and public information

Printed information about meningococcal disease must be quickly disseminated to be effective. Family and contacts of the index case must be made aware of the warning symptoms of meningococcal disease and what action to take should they appear.*

General publicity

There is often interest from the media. It is best to have a single point of communication between professionals and press. Statements to the media should come from the CCDC or another authoritative source. Meningococcal disease is still synonymous with meningitis for many members of the public and the medical profession: publicity should emphasise the petechial rash as the cardinal presenting sign of septicaemia and summarise features of meningitis separately. GPs should be prewarned of any press notice. The CDSC or Scottish Centre for Infection and Environmental Health can advise from their previous experience.

Travel abroad

Vaccination should be offered to all those travelling to countries where meningococcal infection with serogroups A and C are endemic (see Chapter 26).

Routine vaccination

A conjugate meningococcal C vaccine, using CRM_{197} (a diphtheria mutant toxoid as used in one conjugate Hib vaccine) has become available for general use in the UK. Others may be available by the time of publication. These use either CRM_{197} or tetanus toxoid as the conjugate. Such vaccines have been shown to be safe and effective down to the age of 2 months.

From late 1999, group C meningococcal vaccine has become part of the routine immunisation schedule in the UK. It is given at 2, 3 and 4 months with the other vaccines due at these times. Booster doses after a full course are not thought necessary. There has also been a 'catch-up' programme, with children between 4 and 12 months being given two doses at monthly intervals and children from 13 months to 17 years receiving only one dose. Young people starting further education for the first time will also be offered the plain polysaccharide vaccine.

FURTHER READING

Cartwright K (ed.) (1995) Meningococcal disease, John Wiley, Chichester. *Particularly relevant chapters are those on 'Treatment of meningococcal disease in childhood' (Nadel S, Levin M) and 'Outbreak control'*

PHLS Meningococcal Infections Working Group and Public Health Medicine Environmental Group (1995) Control of meningococcal disease: guidance for consultants in communicable disease control. CDR Rev 5: R189–195.

---

* **Leaflets for public distribution are available from the National Meningitis Trust, Fern House, Bath Road, Stroud, Gloucestershire, GL5 3TJ (tel. 01453 751738); the Meningitis Research Foundation, 13 High Street, Thornbury, Bristol BS35 2AE (tel. 01454 281811, fax 01454 281094); and the Department of Health (tel. 0800 555777).**

Stuart JM, Monk PN, Lewis DA et al on behalf of PHLS Meningococcus Working Group and Public Health Medicine Environmental Group (1997) Management of clusters of meningococcal disease. CDR Rev 7: R3–5.

See also current guidelines on the PHLS website on http://www.phls.co.uk.

79 Mumps

ORGANISM

Mumps is caused by parainfluenza virus of the paramyxovirus group. There is one serotype and there is no animal reservoir.

EPIDEMIOLOGY

Prior to the introduction of a vaccine, mumps was mainly a disease of children and young adults, with the highest incidence between the ages of 5 and 10 years. Epidemics were commonest in late winter and spring. Both sexes were affected equally. Widespread use of mumps vaccine has been followed by a decrease of approximately 90% in reported cases in the USA and the UK. However, like measles and rubella, there has been a shift in the epidemiology of mumps to an older age group with several outbreaks in colleges or in the workplace. These outbreaks appear to be mainly in unvaccinated individuals rather than resulting from poor vaccine efficacy. When mumps has been introduced into a virgin community, serious outbreaks have affected adults as well as children. Mumps is uncommon in the first 9–12 months of life because of protective maternal antibody, less exposure to infection at this age or other unknown factors.

Transmission

By droplet infection or saliva and possibly urine. Mumps virus can be cultured from saliva, throat-washings, blood (in early stages), cerebrospinal fluid, urine and human milk.

Patients are infectious from approximately a few days before salivary gland enlargement for up to 3 days after they subside. Most children can be regarded as uninfectious 1 week after onset of parotitis.

Incubation period

15–24 days (median 19 days).

NATURAL HISTORY AND CLINICAL FEATURES

Mumps is a systemic disease and 30–40% of infections may be subclinical. Parotitis is the most apparent manifestation but involvement of other organs, e.g. central nervous system (CNS), testes or kidney may occur without parotitis and complications may precede parotitis.

Onset of symptoms is usually related to pain and swelling of the parotid gland. Nonspecific symptoms may precede the development of parotitis and include fever, headache, malaise, myalgia, anorexia and abdominal pain. The temperature usually settles within a week and before swelling of salivary glands subsides. Parotitis is commonly bilateral and one gland usually enlarges 2–3 days before the other. Swelling of the parotid gland is more easily seen than felt and particularly important in diagnosis is the swelling between the angle of the mandible and the sternomastoid muscle, extending backwards beneath the auricle. The earlobe is pushed upwards and outwards. The swelling usually subsides within 7–10 days. Involvement of the submaxillary salivary gland is less frequent and can be very difficult to differentiate from cervical lymphadenopathy. Involvement of sublingual glands is uncommon.

Central nervous system

Involvement of the CNS is common and was the most important cause of aseptic meningitis before routine vaccination became available. Many patients may have cerebrospinal fluid (CSF) and electroencephalogram changes compatible with meningoencephalitis without clinical manifestations. Headache, mental confusion and meningism are the usual symptoms and may occur from a week before to 3 weeks following the onset of parotitis. In the CSF there is increased lymphocyte count, normal to slightly raised protein, uncommonly a slightly reduced glucose and the virus can be readily isolated. Prognosis of mumps meningoencephalitis is good; however, in the rare postinfectious type of encephalitis sequelae and even death may occur. Other CNS complications include facial paralysis (in most cases probably due to local pressure on the nerve), deafness, transverse myelitis, cerebellar ataxia, polyneuritis and hydrocephalus due to aqueductal stenosis or obstruction elsewhere in the ventricular system.

Orchitis

About 20% or more of postpubertal males may develop orchitis. It has rarely been described in young children. It usually develops within a week of parotitis but may occur prior to or without parotitis. Severe local pain and tenderness, often accompanied by systemic symptoms of fever, headache and backache, is usual. A degree of atrophy of the testis is common, which is particularly of concern when orchitis is bilateral (20–30%). However, even in bilateral cases sterility is rare and patients should be reassured.

Pancreatitis

Mild involvement of the pancreas, manifest by upper abdominal pain, tenderness and vomiting, is probably common but severe pancreatitis is rare. Serum amylase levels are usually raised in mumps, which may partly originate from the parotid gland and levels bear no relationship to abdominal symptoms.

Other complications

Other complications include oophoritis, mastitis, thyroiditis, nephritis, arthritis, myocarditis and thrombocytopenic purpura, all of which are usually self-limiting.

Mumps during pregnancy may be associated with increased chance of abortion; no definite evidence of embryopathy has been confirmed. Neonatal mumps infection may occur when the mother is infected around the time of delivery.

Diagnosis

Mumps is usually diagnosed clinically. However, suppurative parotitis, calculus, recurrent parotitis and infection of the parotid glands by influenza and other viruses may cause difficulty in diagnosis. Parotid enlargement is a manifestation of HIV infection.

Mumps virus can be isolated from throat swabs, saliva, CSF and urine. Paired sera for mumps IgG antibody or a single specimen for mumps IgM antibody are reliable methods for diagnosis. Antibodies to soluble (S) antigen that disappear within 6–12 months indicate recent infection whereas those against viral (V) antigen persist.

MANAGEMENT

Management of parotitis and meningitis is symptomatic. Orchitis may be very painful, requiring analgesics; gentle support of the scrotum is helpful.

PREVENTION OF FURTHER CASES

Immunisation with measles, mumps and rubella (MMR) vaccine is highly effective in controlling mumps. There has been a marked decrease in mumps notifications since MMR was recommended for routine use in the USA in 1977 and in Britain in 1988. In the UK only about 3% of notified cases of mumps are now being confirmed serologically. Details of the vaccine are given in Appendix VI. Hyperimmune mumps immunoglobulin has not been shown to be efficacious in preventing or reducing complications. Administration of MMR to contacts, e.g. nonimmune fathers of children with mumps, in the hope of reducing the occurrence of orchitis is not effective in preventing infection or reducing complications.

Reactions to the mumps component of MMR are uncommon. Transient parotitis may develop in the third week and meningoencephalitis 2–3 weeks after vaccination, and rarely deafness. Initially, two types of mumps vaccine were available in the UK, containing the Urabe AM9 and Jeryl Lynn strains respectively. No cases of mild or vaccine-associated mumps meningitis has been reported since 1992, when the Jeryl Lynn strain replaced the Urabe strain in MMR.

FURTHER READING

Gay N, Miller E, Hesketh L et al (1997) Mumps surveillance in England and Wales supports introduction of two dose vaccination schedule. Commun Dis Rep 7: R21–26.

80 Nontuberculous (atypical) mycobacterial disease

ORGANISM

Unlike *Mycobacterium tuberculosis* and *M. bovis*, nontuberculous mycobacteria (NTM) are widely distributed in soil, water and cold-blooded animals and are usually of low pathogenicity for warm-blooded animals. They generally prefer warm climates and their geographical distribution is very varied. Runyon's classification system is most commonly used and is based on pigmentation, rate and temperature of growth and colonial morphology. In children, most infections are caused by closely related slow-growing non-pigment-producing organisms – *M. avium*, *M. intracellulare*, *M. marinum* and *M. scrofulaceum*. It is not clear whether these are really distinct species and they are sometimes referred to as the *Mycobacterium avium* complex (MAC) or the MAIS organisms (*M. avium/intracellulare/scrofulaceum*).

EPIDEMIOLOGY

The epidemiology of infection due to nontuberculous mycobacteria differs greatly from that of tuberculosis. Unlike tuberculosis, NTM infection is rarely, if ever, transmitted from person to person and most cases follow acquisition of the bacilli from the environment. Thus contact tracing and other public health measures are unnecessary. NTM lymphadenitis is almost exclusively a disease of preschool children, possibly because of the relatively poor immunity to mycobacteria found in this age group. It is an uncommon condition, although it may be becoming more common in countries where the incidence of tuberculosis is declining.

Transmission

Person-to-person spread does not occur.

Incubation period

Not known, but probably weeks to months.

NATURAL HISTORY AND CLINICAL FEATURES

Cervical lymphadenitis is the commonest site for NTM infection, with the buccal mucosa as the most likely portal of entry. Typically, children present with firm, unilateral lymphadenopathy, usually high in the neck or close to the mandible but pre- and postauricular nodes and occasionally inguinal nodes may be involved. The nodes are usually relatively painless and firm at first. They then gradually soften, rupture and drain for many months. The surrounding skin may become inflamed (see Plate 1). Despite this, the children remain well without systemic upset or evidence of haematogenous spread. The condition is commonly mistaken for a cervical abscess, while tuberculosis, cat-scratch disease, mumps, salivary stone or a malignancy are other differential diagnoses. Very occasionally children present with disseminated atypical mycobacterial infection; such patients almost invariably have an underlying primary or acquired immunodeficiency.

Diagnosis

Commonly, NTM disease is not suspected and a fine-needle aspiration or incision biopsy is performed. While this usually excludes malignancy, incision often results in sinus formation with superficial skin infection, rendering later surgery more difficult. Furthermore, if histology reveals caseating granulomata with acid-fast bacilli, this does not distinguish *M. tuberculosis* from NTM disease and if culture is performed the diagnosis may not become apparent for some weeks. Differential Mantoux testing with a panel of antigens including tuberculin and antigens from *M. avium*, *M. intracellulare* and *M. malmoense* may be helpful, as the response to *M. tuberculosis* will be small or absent while there will be a much larger response to one of the NTM antigens. It should be remembered, however, that the use of these reagents has not been validated and positive responses must be interpreted with caution and always with reference to the clinical context.

MANAGEMENT

Complete surgical excision of the affected lymph node is the most effective treatment and should be performed if possible. This approach requires the diagnosis to be considered on clinical grounds prior to surgery, which unfortunately does not often happen. The simpler procedure of incision and drainage frequently results in a chronic discharging sinus. Although such sinuses eventually heal, it is only after considerable disruption to the child's life and the healed scar is often very unsightly. If the node is too close to a vital structure, such as the facial nerve, or previous surgical intervention has left a sinus and a significant area of infected skin, total excision may be impossible. In this case, antimicrobial therapy can be attempted, although its efficacy is unproven and as localised disease is not life-threatening the potential toxicity of the agents used has to be balanced against the potential clinical benefit. Treatment with rifampicin, isoniazid and pyrazinamide is usually unhelpful even if in-vitro testing suggests that there is sensitivity to these agents. Infection with NTM may respond to aminoglycosides (in particular amikacin), macrolide antibiotics (azithromycin, clarithromycin) and the quinolones (e.g. ciprofloxacin). Rifabutin and clarithromycin have been successfully used to treat NTM infection in HIV-infected patients and so these agents are usually included in the regimens used for NTM lymphadenitis in normal children. Rifabutin carries a small risk of uveitis. The value of such treatment combinations in reducing residual scarring and the need for further extensive surgery requires proper evaluation. Clinicians confronted with a case should seek expert advice before embarking on either lengthy antimicrobial therapy or radical surgery.

Children with disseminated disease should be referred to a specialist centre for investigation for probable underlying immunodeficiency and for further management.

81 *Mycoplasma* infections

MYCOPLASMA PNEUMONIAE

ORGANISM

Mycoplasma pneumoniae. This bacterium lacks a cell wall. Under the electron microscope, the organism is filamentous and has a terminal organelle used for attaching to respiratory epithelial cells.

EPIDEMIOLOGY

Infections occur worldwide; although endemic epidemics occur at 4–7 yearly intervals. Among children, those of school age and adolescents seem to be the most susceptible. The incubation period is usually 3 weeks with a range of 6–23 days. Man is the only host, and the disease is spread by droplets.

NATURAL HISTORY AND CLINICAL FEATURES

This infection is known as 'primary atypical pneumonia'. Onset of illness is gradual with headache, fever and sore throat. The cough tends to be paroxysmal and may be associated with sputum production. Substernal or pleuritic chest pain may occur. Several days after onset of illness chest signs may occur, such as widespread crackles. The chest X-ray may show patchy consolidation throughout the lung; features such as consolidation of single lobes and pleural effusions may be present. Complications of infection sometimes occurring in the absence of chest disease include erythema multiforme, Stevens–Johnson syndrome, encephalitis and transverse myelitis. Illness tends to be particularly severe in children with sickle cell disease.

Diagnosis

Although the organism can be cultured, the procedure is slow and diagnosis can be established more quickly by serology and identification of cold agglutinins seen in up to 50% of cases. A fourfold rise in complement fixing antibodies is considered diagnostic.

MANAGEMENT

The response to antibiotics is much less dramatic than that seen in pneumococcal pneumonia. However, erythromycin has been shown to be effective and is recommended. There do not appear to be any advantages in using the new macrolides clarithromycin and azithromycin. Ciprofloxacin is also active against this agent.

THE GENITAL MYCOPLASMAS

ORGANISM

Ureaplasma urealyticum and *Mycoplasma hominis*, which, like other members of the *Mycoplasma* family, lack a cell wall.

EPIDEMIOLOGY

The genital mycoplasmas are transmitted sexually and are associated with nonspecific urethritis in males and salpingitis in females. Transmitted to the newborn infant at delivery, both organisms may be a cause of infection, particularly in the premature.

NATURAL HISTORY AND CLINICAL FEATURES

M. hominis is a rare cause of meningitis in the newborn. The clinical signs and cerebrospinal fluid findings are little different from those of cases caused by other bacteria. Research performed over the past 15 years has suggested that in certain populations *U. urealyticum* infection of the respiratory tract is associated with chronic lung disease of prematurity and results in an increased mortality in this group of babies. *U. urealyticum* has been isolated from the cerebrospinal fluid of premature infants with a history of intraventricular haemorrhage, but there is no evidence that it is a cause of ventriculitis.

Diagnosis

This is by culture of secretions. This procedure is expensive and available in only few centres. Frustratingly, even when infection is suspected, lack of resources rarely allows adequate investigation.

MANAGEMENT

Erythromycin is the treatment of choice for genital *Mycoplasma* infections. Both organisms may be resistant to this antibiotic, in which case doxycycline is recommended.

82 Head lice (pediculosis) – 'nits'

ORGANISM

Pediculosis humanus capitis is an arthropod. Humans are the only hosts. Head lice require warmth and human blood to survive.

EPIDEMIOLOGY

Children are the most commonly infected (60% of cases) and some estimates suggest that approximately 9% of school children are affected at any one time. Contrary to popular belief, head lice infect clean and dirty hair and have no preference for long hair. Infestations are found in all social groups, although they are less common in black children as the lice find it harder to hold on to the shaft of their hair.

Transmission

Infestation is predominantly spread by head-to-head contact. Head lice cannot jump or fly. The evidence that fomites and sharing of clothing, combs and hats can transmit infection is not strong.

Incubation period

The eggs take 6–10 days to hatch. The egg-to-egg life cycle is about 25–26 days.

NATURAL HISTORY AND CLINICAL FEATURES

The adult female louse attaches her eggs (nits) to the base of scalp hair. After a week the eggs hatch. The adult louse lives about 2–3 months, feeding on scalp blood, and can survive up to 10 days off the head. Nits can survive for up to 3 weeks. Many infestations are asymptomatic. Pruritus, although rare, is the most common symptom. It is frequently accompanied by enlarged cervical lymph nodes. A maculopapular erythematous eruption, and occasionally urticarial lesions, can occur. Repeated infections are common and many family members may be affected at the same time. Head lice do not transmit other infections, although secondary bacterial infections may occur.

Diagnosis

The presence of live lice is diagnostic. It is important to examine near the base of hair shafts. Nits should not be confused with dandruff, which is easily removed with a comb. Nits only indicate that infection has occurred at some point. They may represent nonviable eggs or empty cases. Only the presence of live lice can be taken as evidence of current infection.

MANAGEMENT

Only when live lice have been found should treatment be initiated. The presence of nits is not enough. The only proven effective treatment is the use of a special insecticidal lotion (shampoos are not as effective as lotions), although intensive repeated wet combing with a special fine metal 'nit' comb without an insecticide is almost as effective. Preparations are available containing malathion, pyrethroids and carbaryl. There is little to choose between them, but carbaryl is only available on prescription. There is no evidence of neurotoxicity if the preparations are used properly. It is important that the instructions are strictly adhered to and two applications are necessary to ensure adequate treatment. The shampoo should be applied very carefully to the hair so that all parts are treated. This will take longer than the usual application of shampoo for washing hair. It is not necessary to comb out the hair after treatment, although many parents choose to do so. All family members and those with close contact should be checked for infection and treated if found. When properly investigated, reports of resistance to treatment are not usually substantiated, although there are some confirmed instances. The reason for failure of the treatment to eradicate the lice usually turns out to be incorrect use of the medication or reinfection from an infected contact. Many instances of so-called resistance are simply the continuing presence of nonviable nits or the slow subsidence of symptoms such as itching. It has been suggested that, so as to prevent resistance arising, treatment should be 'cycled', i.e. one treatment used nationally for some time and then another; however, this policy has been shown to be ineffective and has been abandoned in many areas. Clothing and bedding can be readily disinfected by machine washing, as hot cycles (over 50°C) inactivate lice and eggs. Combs and hairbrushes should be soaked in hot water with a pediculicide for 15 minutes.

There is no need for children to be excluded from school once effective treatment has been given as, although dead lice and eggs will persist in the hair, they are dead and there is no infection risk.

PREVENTION OF FURTHER CASES

It has been suggested that a national 'Bug-busting Day' may be the most effective way to control this pest. Families with children are encouraged to check their hair on the same day throughout the country. Treatment should be given when lice or nits are found. There is little evidence to show that this has any lasting effect and more research is needed.

83 Parvovirus infection – fifth disease

Also known as erythema infectiosum or slapped cheek disease

ORGANISM

Parvovirus B19, a small, nonenveloped DNA virus. (The name does not indicate that there are other types that infect humans; it is an accident of history.)

EPIDEMIOLOGY

Humans are the only hosts. Any age may be affected and 50% or more of adults have evidence of past infection, i.e. half the adult population is probably immune. Outbreaks occur in schools and health-care settings with transmission both to and from susceptible staff.

Transmission

In most cases, the virus is found in respiratory secretions in the early part of the illness and this is thought to be the major route of transmission. By the time the rash appears, virus is no longer present in secretions. The exception to this is the patient with an aplastic crisis, in whom viral excretion may continue for a week or more after the onset of symptoms. The main source of infection is contact with school-age children, either at home or at school.

Incubation period

13–18 days.

NATURAL HISTORY AND CLINICAL FEATURES

About 50% of infections are asymptomatic. The most common disease pattern is of mild systemic upset with fever in 15–30% and a characteristic rash. This usually begins as an erythematous appearance to the face, hence the name 'slapped cheek' disease. It is followed by a symmetrical lace rash on the extremities and trunk. For weeks, and sometimes months, the rash may fluctuate with temperature or exposure to sunlight. The changes may be relatively rapid, with the rash fading over a matter of hours and reappearing a few days or even hours later. Arthropathy is unusual in children, but common in adults, especially women. An acute hepatitis has also been reported.

Parvovirus has been proposed as the aetiological agent in some cases of Kawasaki disease. The virus has a predilection for erythroid precursors and switches off erythropoiesis for up to 7 days. This is of considerable consequence in patients with red cell disorders characterised by reduced red cell survival and increased turnover. Patients with disorders such as sickle-cell disease and congenital hereditary spherocytosis may develop an aplastic crisis. This is usually temporary, lasting 5–10 days, but may necessitate blood transfusion. Virus clearance is only slightly delayed. Patients who are immunocompromised, such as those with human immunodeficiency virus infection, may develop a chronic relapsing anaemia due to marrow aplasia.

Infection in pregnancy may occur in up to 50% of fetuses of infected women. There is a significant increase in hydrops fetalis (caused by fetal anaemia and sometimes myocarditis), fetal death and spontaneous abortion in the second and third trimesters. It has been suggested that the excess risk of fetal death following infection in the first 20 weeks of pregnancy is around 9%. However, this risk is difficult to quantify and may vary between subgroups of women; for example. it appears highest when the mother is asymptomatic. Congenital infection has been reported to have caused thrombocytopenia in an infant. Infection during pregnancy is not teratogenic.

Diagnosis is often made clinically. A slight leukopenia and thrombocytopenia may be present. The main differential diagnosis is rubella and in fact more cases that are clinically felt to be rubella are subsequently found to be parvovirus infection than rubella itself. Where it is necessary to be certain, e.g. in pregnancy, specific IgM can be detected at 2 weeks after exposure, but because the exact time of infection is difficult to determine it may be important to repeat the test following an initial IgM-negative result. When the fetus is affected, ultrasonography may detect hydrops fetalis and serum alphafetoprotein levels may be raised. If cordocentesis is undertaken antigen and polymerase chain reaction tests may be applied, and are also sometimes used with post-mortem material. Detection of specific IgG a year after birth can confirm the diagnosis retrospectively.

MANAGEMENT

Management is symptomatic in most cases. Intravenous normal human immunoglobulin may be helpful in immunocompromised patients. When fetal infection is thought to have taken place specialist advice should be sought. Although interventions such as cordocentesis and intrauterine transfusion have been used, these have their own complications. Where

Diagnosis confirmed in health-care worker
Was the HCW in contact with any patient from the following groups – in the same room for a significant period of time (15 minutes or more), or face-to-face contact during the period from 7 days before the appearance of a rash to the date of appearance of the rash, in the absence of respiratory isolation precautions?
• Pregnant women < 21 weeks gestation
• Immunocompromised
• Haemoglobinopathies

Consider need for action in light of risk assessment

| HCW in contact with pregnant women < 21 weeks | HCW in contact with patients with haemoglobinopathies | HCW in contact with immunocompromised patients |

If the decision is made to investigate, check antenatal/booking serum to identify seronegative susceptible women (40%)

Check serology to identify IgG-negative patients at risk and monitor IgG-negative patients for development of aplastic crisis

Contact reference laboratory for DNA testing as antibody testing may be unreliable. If infected, consider human normal intravenous immunoglobulin (400 mg/kg per day for 5–10 days)

Contact exposed susceptible women or those for whom no previous serum available. Inform them of low risk of infection but need to follow up their serology 21 days after exposure or if a rash develops

Take serum if rash appears or at 21 days after contact. Test for IgG and IgM

| IgG-positive IgM-negative REASSURE – NO RISK | IgG-positive IgM-negative SUSCEPTIBLE BUT NOT INFECTED – need to follow up future rash contacts | IgG-positive INFECTED Refer to specialist follow-up by ultrasound to detect fetal hydrops and intrauterine transfusion if necessary |

Fig. 83.1 Recommended response to parvovirus B19 infection in a health-care worker (HCW): protection of those at risk

pregnant women become aware that they may have been exposed the following course of action is appropriate.

- Ideally confirm the diagnosis in the index case.
- Check antenatal booking serum for parvovirus IgG. If positive, reassure that immune and no further action necessary.
- If negative take blood for parvovirus IgG and IgM 21 days after contact or at appearance of rash, whichever is the sooner. Further action depends on the results.
    - IgG-positive and IgM-negative – reassure that no risk.
    - Both IgG- and IgM-negative – susceptible, but not infected. No action needed this time, but will need testing after any subsequent exposures.
    - IgM-positive – infected. Refer immediately to obstetrician.

PREVENTION OF FURTHER CASES

Studies of individual cases and outbreaks frequently reveal that the source of many infections cannot be traced. Because of this and for practical reasons a policy of protecting all pregnant women from exposure to parvovirus B19 is impractical and probably ineffective. However, women particularly at risk, e.g. pregnant health-care staff, should not be exposed to chronically infectious patients such as patients with aplastic crises. There is comprehensive guidance on management of the situation when a health-care worker is confirmed to have parvovirus virus and patients are at risk (pregnant women at less than 21 weeks, immunocompromised patients and patients with haemoglobinopathies – see Fig. 83.1).

FURTHER READING

Crowcroft NS, Roth C, Cohen B, Miller E (1999) Guidance for control of Parvovirus B19 infection in healthcare settings and the community. J Public Health Med 21: 439–446.

84 Pertussis (whooping cough)

Notifiable disease

ORGANISM

Bordetella pertussis and *B. parapertussis* are Gram-negative bacilli.

EPIDEMIOLOGY

Humans are the only hosts. Pertussis is a very important cause of morbidity and early childhood mortality worldwide, although it seems to be more commonly recognised in temperate countries. In the UK there were three major epidemics in the late 1970s and 1980s following a fall in vaccination uptake in the early 1970s, which itself followed concerns over vaccine safety. The concerns were unfounded; however, vaccine uptake and incidence only returned to pre-1977 levels in the 1990s following a determined drive to improve the immunisation coverage (see Appendix I). Immunisation is currently thought to protect against disease rather than infection; however, the role of asymptomatic infection in transmission is unclear. Although maternal antibody passes across the placenta, no maternal immunity is given to the newborn (indicating that antibodies to *B. pertussis* are not protective) and young infants are most susceptible to severe disease. Infection can occur at any age but in young infants, adolescents and adults pertussis may not be recognised because of its atypical presentation.

Between 1994 and 1997, there were 15 deaths where pertussis was proved to be the cause. All were in unimmunised children: 12 were under 6 months old (mostly under 2 months), two were 6 months and one 16 months. Eight were known to have contact with a case in an older child (seven within the family). The immunisation status of five was known – they were all unimmunised. A study of infants admitted to intensive care units indicates that pertussis is underecognised and underdiagnosed in children with severe lung disease.

Transmission

By droplet spread. Pertussis is highly infectious, with most susceptible household contacts and 50% of school contacts developing the illness. Some 60% of cases will shed organisms for over 2 weeks and 20% for over 6 weeks. Treatment with erythromycin usually renders a sufferer noninfectious within 5 days.

Incubation period

5–21 days, although rarely longer than 10 days.

NATURAL HISTORY AND CLINICAL FEATURES

B. pertussis and *B. parapertussis* produce similar illnesses except that disease due to the former is usually more severe, both in terms of the proportion developing symptoms and their duration. The initial symptoms are coryza and a dry cough. The latter worsens over the next 2 weeks until paroxysms start to occur. The severity and frequency of these increase and the characteristic whoop appears at the end of each paroxysm. This may be accompanied by vomiting. In a severe paroxysm, cyanosis may occur and the child may be utterly exhausted. The paroxysms can be precipitated by feeding, crying or even hearing another person cough. In young infants the typical whoop is usually absent but there may be a period of apnoea at the end of bouts of coughing. The paroxysmal stage continues for 2–6 weeks and may only subside gradually, giving an illness that often lasts 3 months or more. The course of disease is generally more severe in infants. Even in relatively mild cases weight loss occurs and the distress caused to both the child and family is considerable. Subconjunctival haemorrhages are relatively common. The force of the coughing may be sufficient to produce air leaks (surgical emphysema, pneumomediastinum and pneumothorax). Atelectasis is relatively common but, unlike the situation in the preantibiotic era, it now rarely leads to bronchiectasis.

Convulsions may accompany severe cases and an encephalopathy occurs in around 1 in 11 000 cases. There is evidence to suggest that when pertussis is prevalent a proportion of cot deaths are due to undiagnosed pertussis. In adolescents and adults the characteristic whoop is often lacking and sufferers may consider that they have a prolonged cold and cough.

Diagnosis

There is usually a lymphocytosis at 2–5 weeks, which may rise to over 40×10^9/L. This does not occur in *B. parapertussis* infections. For the first 5 weeks of the untreated illness, the organism may be cultured from the nasopharynx, using a pernasal swab plated on to cephalexin charcoal agar. Culture takes at least 5 days. However, bacteria can only be recovered in 50–80% of cases, so alternative methods have been employed, including serology and PCR. The most useful is fluorescent antibody staining of swabs from the nasopharynx but this is still prone to false positives and negatives.

MANAGEMENT

Hospitalisation is sometimes unavoidable if the disease is severe especially for young infants who are prone to apnoea. It can also be necessary when the family is reaching exhaustion from nursing a restless coughing infant. Hospitalised cases should be isolated and subject to respiratory precautions (see Chapter 32). Erythromycin should be given on the basis of a presumptive diagnosis to prevent further transmission. Once the paroxysmal stage has been reached the drug is unlikely to change the course of the illness but it will eradicate the organism in 3–5 days, thus preventing further transmission. No medication has been convincingly shown to reduce the frequency or severity of the paroxysms. The child should be disturbed as little as possible. Vomiting may produce significant dehydration if not treated by nasogastric or intravenous therapy. In a sick infant close respiratory monitoring with pulse oximetry is essential as potentially damaging apnoeic episodes may otherwise go unnoticed.

PREVENTION OF FURTHER CASES

Patients can be infectious for the first 4–5 weeks of their illness if no treatment is given. Once a 5-day course of suitable antibiotic has been completed, there is little danger of transmission. While infectious, the person should be isolated from nonimmune individuals, especially young children.

Chemoprophylaxis

It has been suggested that treating contacts in the presymptomatic or early symptomatic stages with erythromycin may prevent the development of the illness. A recent review of the literature revealed little evidence to support this but there have been few trials. On the basis of this review, guidelines have been drawn up for the management of close contacts of patients infected with *B. pertussis*. Chemoprophylaxis (erythromycin for 10 days) should be considered when:

- the infected patient has an onset of symptoms in the previous 21 days **and**
- there is one or more family or household contact who is not fully vaccinated (or is older than 5 years) and is especially vulnerable because they are immunocompromised or have chronic respiratory or cardiac disease.

Under these circumstances erythromycin should be given to:

- all cases with onset in the previous 21 days to reduce transmission
- newborn infants born to mothers with pertussis
- unimmunised or incompletely immunised contacts with chronic cardiac or respiratory problems
- contacts over 5 years old, whether immunised or not, who have chronic cardiac or respiratory problems.

All pregnant women with suspected or confirmed pertussis should be given chemoprophylaxis for at least 3 days prior to delivery for 10 days.

Vaccination

A highly effective 'whole-cell' vaccine against *Bordetella pertussis* has been in use in the UK for over 50 years. It is available in combination with diphtheria and tetanus as the 'triple vaccine'. Recent studies have shown that a course of three doses of the whole-cell vaccines gives about 90% protection. If a fully immunised individual develops the disease, it is much less severe than in the unimmunised individuals. However, when cases occur, vaccination of contacts is of no value in preventing spread of the disease as a number of doses are needed and immunity takes time to develop.

There are very few contraindications to the vaccine and the Department of Health guidelines are now very clear (see Appendix VI). The current vaccine contains at least six active components but frequently causes minor local and systemic reactions in recipients. Reaction rates are age-dependent, increasing with age of immunisation, and typical rates experienced with the whole-cell vaccine are given in Table 84.1. Reactions are more common

Table 84.1 Rates of reaction to whole-cell pertussis vaccine (%)

	First (2 months)	Second (3 months)	Third (4 months)	Combined*
Fever (> 38°C	5	10	20	4–11
Mild malaise	–	–	–	12–18
Local pain, redness or induration	< 2	5	1–5	

* Combining data for immunisations at 2, 3 and 4 months. A range is stated because of variation according to the particular vaccine manufacturer.

with the second and third immunisations. It remains unclear whether permanent harm ever results from the whole-cell vaccines currently in use. If permanent harm ever does take place it is extremely rare.

Until the end of 1999, 'acellular' (component) pertussis vaccines were not licensed for use in the UK. Trial data from the 1990s suggests that, while in older children they produce less of the mild reactions associated with the whole-cell vaccine, when given at 2, 3 and 4 months there is little difference. As a generalisation, the efficacy of the acellular vaccines is directly related to the number of components, with the five-component vaccine being the most effective. These latter have an efficacy approaching that of the whole-cell vaccines in use in the UK but those vaccines with fewer components are not as protective as current UK whole-cell vaccines.

In 1999 problems with the supply of whole-cell vaccine reached such a point that acellular vaccines were licensed for use in the UK as part of the primary course as alternatives to the whole-cell vaccine.

There is evidence from many sources that the protection from all whooping cough vaccines wears off after the primary course in infancy. While infection in adults is rarely serious, it can produce a cough lasting some months and is an important source of infection of infants too young to be immunised. It has been suggested that boosters of pertussis vaccine should be offered to children prior to starting school and again before leaving.

85 Plague

Notifiable disease

ORGANISM

Yersinia pestis – the plague bacillus, a Gram-negative bipolar bacillus.

EPIDEMIOLOGY

Plague is a zoonosis with humans only accidentally infected. Wild rodents are the natural reservoir of plague with different rodents (not only rats) being the reservoir in different locations. *Y. pestis* is endemic in animal populations in a large number of countries including in sub-Saharan Africa, the Indian subcontinent, China, south-east Asia, Brazil, the Andean region of South America and rural regions of the south-western USA (sporadic cases). In all these regions, outbreaks among adults and children have occurred in the past two decades, contributing a global figure of reported cases of 200–2000 cases annually. Many more cases go unrecognised. Outbreaks are thought to be due to natural occurrences disrupting rodent populations or humans coming into contact with previously isolated rodent populations. A high-profile outbreak of plague took place in 1994 in and around Surat city, Maharashtra State, India. There were thousands of reported cases (many of which were not confirmed), local panic and major international concern in countries having trade and travel links with India. No spread took place to other countries.

Transmission

Bubonic plague is transmitted by the bite of a human by an infected flea from an animal. Pneumonic plague is transmissible by coughing and inhalation of aerosols from a person with acute pneumonic plague so that nosocomial infection occasionally occurs. The period of infectivity is unclear. It is thought that fleas may remain infective only for a few days before they themselves die. Pneumonic plague is considered infective through aerosol in the severe phase but is not thought to be infective prior to symptoms.

Incubation period

2–4 days in pneumonic and 2–6 days in bubonic plague.

NATURAL HISTORY AND CLINICAL FEATURES

There are three forms of plague, bubonic, septicaemic and pneumonic, the latter two usually being complications of bubonic plague.

Bubonic plague

Symptoms and signs include a high temperature, enlarged lymph nodes draining the sites of flea bites, which can enlarge to become 'buboes', restlessness, generalised malaise and shock. Extension may occur elsewhere causing meningitis, septicaemia (septicaemic plague) or pneumonia (pneumonic plague), which are frequently fatal if untreated.

Pneumonic plague

This can be overwhelming and result in a severe productive cough and death in a matter of days through respiratory failure.

Diagnosis

Plague should be considered in febrile children who have been exposed to wild rodents in endemic areas. Definitive diagnosis is by isolation and identification of *Y. pestis* by an experienced reference laboratory. In endemic areas it will be necessary to treat possible cases on the basis of a presumptive diagnosis made on clinical grounds and/or microbiological examination of sputum or bubo material. However, before an outbreak is declared it is important to make the definitive diagnosis. During a confirmed outbreak a presumptive diagnosis can be made by microbiological examination of sputum or bubo material. Care must be taken as this is a highly hazardous organism. It should be cultured and some specimen fixed in alcohol and stained for examination for *Y. pestis* bacilli by an experienced microbiologist. Serology may be of benefit in demonstrating rising titres but is not as useful as isolation of the organism.

MANAGEMENT

Suspected cases should be isolated and admitted to hospital, preferably to a specialist centre. If used early in the infection the drugs of choice are usually effective: streptomycin, gentamicin, chloramphenicol (especially recommended when meningitis is suspected) and tetracycline (not for children under age 7) and streptomycin. Plasmid-encoded multidrug resistance has been described in Madagascar.

PREVENTION OF FURTHER CASES

Travellers should be advised against visiting areas where new infections and human-to-human spread is occurring. Those who have to travel should wear insect repellent. If exposure is suspected those infected should take a course of tetracycline (250 mg four times daily for 7 days). Children between 6 weeks and 12 years may take a week's course of co-trimoxazole and younger babies can have ampicillin (although protection is probably less). In endemic areas control of fleas and rodent populations is important. Currently, no effective vaccine is available in the UK.

86 Pneumocystis carinii

ORGANISM

Formerly thought to be a protozoon, *P. carinii* is now known to be a fungal species.

EPIDEMIOLOGY

This is a ubiquitous organism, which can affect many different animals, including man. Serological studies suggest that most children become subclinically infected within the first few years of life. Clinically significant disease only occurs in those who have immunocompromising conditions affecting cell-mediated immunity. This includes children with congenital immune deficiencies, HIV infection and secondary immune deficiency such as that induced by chemotherapy. It is probable that clinical disease in the first 2 years of life represents primary infection while disease in older individuals is due to reactivation.

The disease has been seen in outbreaks occurring in populations suffering severe malnutrition and occasionally as an opportunist pathogen in severely compromised premature infants.

Transmission

The mode of acquisition of this organism is not clear. It is probable that person-to-person transmission does occur by the airborne route.

Incubation period

Unknown.

NATURAL HISTORY AND CLINICAL FEATURES

P. carinii produces a diffuse pneumonitis (*P. carinii* pneumonia, PCP), usually with an insidious onset. Typically, symptoms build up over a period of
a few weeks, although more acute forms can occur in patients with AIDS.
The symptoms include tachypnoea, fever and dry cough, sometimes
associated with hoarseness. As the disease progresses there are
increasing signs of respiratory distress and of desaturation. There are
usually no abnormal auscultatory findings. Chest radiograph may be relatively normal at the onset of symptoms but diffuse pulmonary infiltrates
soon appear, most marked in the perihilar regions but later spreading to
extensively involve both lung fields.

As the child progresses into respiratory failure the typical arterial blood
gas findings show a reduced oxygen tension with hypocapnia.

Diagnosis

The differential diagnosis is wide and includes viral pneumonitis, atypical
bacterial pneumonia and other fungal pneumonias. Confirmation of the
diagnosis requires demonstration of the organism in pulmonary secretions
or lung tissue. The classical way of confirming the diagnosis is by lung
biopsy, either obtained by thoracotomy or at bronchoscopy (trans-
bronchial biopsy). The organisms can be demonstrated on methenamine
silver stains. Less invasive (although probably less sensitive) techniques
are increasingly used, at least in the first instance. These include examination of bronchial secretions obtained by bronchoalveolar lavage or, in
older children, examination of induced sputum produced following inhalation of hypertonic saline. Newer methods have also been developed for
demonstrating the organism in respiratory secretions using an immunofluorescent technique. Polymerase-chain-reaction-based techniques are
also available but not yet fully evaluated.

MANAGEMENT

Patients will usually require oxygen therapy and in more severe cases ventilatory assistance. High-dose co-trimoxazole (30 mg/kg given four times a
day) should be started as early as possible. It is normal to start this intravenously but provided the patient does not have significant gastrointestinal
disease therapy can be continued by the oral route. For critically ill patients
where it is felt that invasive procedures will not be tolerated this treatment
can be commenced empirically – improvement occurring over the first 36–48
hours being fairly strong confirmatory evidence of PCP. In severe pneumonitis it has been shown, in adults, that adjuvant therapy with corticosteroids is
beneficial. Although there are no studies in children it is recommended that,
in severe disease, treatment with prednisolone is given. A suitable dosage is
2 mg/kg/day for 10 days then tailing off over a further 10 days.

In those who show intolerance of high-dose co-trimoxazole treatment
or fail to show any improvement after 5 days, pentamidine (4 mg/kg/day)

given intravenously or intramuscularly should be used. Immediate side-effects of this treatment include hypotension, hypoglycaemia and arrhythmias. Further problems can include pancreatitis, renal impairment, neutropenia and fevers. Other possible treatment options include atovaquone (40 mg/kg/day in divided doses) or trimetrexate (45 mg/m² daily) with folinic acid (20 mg/m² every 6 hours). Treatment should be continued for a minimum of 2 weeks (3 weeks is becoming standard practice). Thereafter, prophylaxis (see below) should be given indefinitely because of the risk of recurrent disease.

PREVENTION OF FURTHER CASES

Prophylactic treatment has been shown to be effective in preventing PCP in high-risk individuals. The treatment of choice is co-trimoxazole given on three days a week (see Appendix III, p. 470). This treatment should be given to HIV-positive and HIV-indeterminate children (see Chapter 23), children with congenital cell-mediated immune deficiencies and children undergoing chemotherapy, particularly continuous prolonged chemotherapy as in the protocols for acute lymphoblastic leukaemia. Alternative treatments in those intolerant of co-trimoxazole include dapsone (2 mg/kg/day; maximum 100 mg) or inhaled pentamidine (300 mg given monthly). The latter is unsuitable for children under 5 years of age because of the difficulties in administration. In older children, particularly those with an asthmatic tendency, it may induce bronchospasm and pretreatment with nebulised salbutamol is advisable. The potential side-effects and the lack of efficacy data make the use of intravenous pentamidine inadvisable for prophylaxis.

Patients with PCP should not be allowed to come into contact with severely immunocompromised children because of the potential risk of person-to-person spread.

87 Poliomyelitis

Notifiable disease

ORGANISM

Poliovirus, an enterovirus of three antigenic types: 1, 2 and 3.

EPIDEMIOLOGY

Occurs only in humans but can survive in water in favourable conditions for up to 3 months. Because of the success of routine immunisation, transmission of wild virus is not occurring in the UK or elsewhere in western Europe. However, imported infections and vaccine-associated cases (through rare reversion of attenuated forms of the live oral polio vaccine –

OPV) still occur in unimmunised or incompletely immunised persons. From 1985–99, 97 confirmed cases were reported in England and Wales – 27 vaccine-associated (19 recipient, 8 contact), 6 imported – while for 5 the source was unknown.

The WHO committed itself to a goal of global eradication of polio worldwide by the year 2005. That has not been achieved but huge progress has been made. The Americas have been polio-free since 1991 and incidence rates have fallen dramatically in much of Asia, where mass immunisation campaigns have sometime immunised millions of children in a single day. However, polio remains endemic in a few parts of the developing world, notably sub-Saharan Africa and some parts of Asia, especially where there are wars or ongoing civil conflict. Hence there remains a potential hazard to travellers to low-income countries. Outbreaks also have continued to occur in groups avoiding immunisation in industrialised countries, the last being in a religious group in the Netherlands in 1992/3.

Transmission

By the faecal–oral route; transmission by food or water contamination is rare.

Infectivity of wild virus via faeces may be prolonged for several weeks or longer but is highest in the few days around the onset of symptoms. Infectivity of OPV is shorter (rarely more than 2 months). Virus transmission may also be prolonged in the immunosuppressed.

Incubation period

7–21 days for paralytic wild cases. In vaccine-associated cases the period is 7–28 days in recipients and 7–60 days in contacts.

NATURAL HISTORY AND CLINICAL FEATURES

In children most cases are subclinical or simply show as a mild febrile illness. However a minority of infections with wild or reverted OPV proceed to invade the nervous system, causing either an aseptic meningitis (nonparalytic polio) or, more rarely, paralytic polio caused by the virus attacking the motor cells in the spinal cord. Paralysis is of a lower motor neurone type, usually asymmetrical, and may affect only a single muscle group (usually in the limbs) or more extensive groups. If this includes the muscles of respiration and swallowing it can be fatal. Paralysis frequently improves but residual effects are usually permanent. Older children and adults are more at risk of paralytic disease.

Diagnosis

Poliovirus can be recovered from the faeces, throat and, rarely, cerebrospinal fluid by isolation in tissue culture. Two specimens of faeces, separated by 7 days, should be obtained from all patients with acute flaccid paralytic disease (including those in whom Guillain–Barré syndrome is the considered diagnosis) for isolation of the virus, because rectal swabs are insensitive. Culture from two specimens collected within the first 15 days of illness is the diagnostic test of choice. Serological testing of acute and convalescent sera can be performed in patients suspected of having paralytic poliomyelitis. However, interpretation of serological tests can be difficult.

Diagnosis by clinical signs alone is often difficult and indicates the importance of the collection of virological specimens from all children with an unexplained viral meningitis or rapid-onset paralysis. Important differential diagnoses include the other causes of aseptic meningitis and acute flaccid paralytic disease: Guillain–Barré syndrome, acute polyneuritis (other including viruses and toxins), localised paralysis following specific infections (Epstein–Barr virus and infective mononucleosis) and other enteroviruses (Coxsackie A7, echo 3) causing a poliomyelitis-like illness.

MANAGEMENT

There is no specific treatment for the paralytic form apart from bed rest in the acute phase.

PREVENTION OF FURTHER CASES

Informing

When a case of polio is suspected the Consultant in Communicable Disease Control (or the Director of Public Health) must be informed immediately along with the Communicable Disease Surveillance Centre or the Scottish Centre for Infection and Environmental Health so they can institute public health measures. The case should also be notified.

Isolation

For patients suspected of excreting wild poliovirus, enteric precautions are indicated for the duration of hospitalisation or until virus can no longer be recovered from the faeces.

Urgent immunisation

After a single case of confirmed polio due to wild indigenous virus a dose of OPV should be given to all people in the immediate neighbourhood regardless of immunisation history. In previously unimmunised persons the course must be completed.

If it is unclear whether this is a wild or vaccine-associated case it should be assumed that it is wild and control measures should be instituted.

Routine immunisation of infants and children

Two types of trivalent vaccine are available: live oral poliovirus vaccine (Sabin) – OPV – and inactivated poliovirus vaccine (Salk) – IPV – given parenterally. Both are effective in preventing poliomyelitis in individuals. OPV has the additional benefit of often boosting immunisation in other family members through ongoing transmission. There is no evidence of OPV being associated with increased risk of intussusception.

On the basis of consideration of the risks and benefits in the UK OPV is currently the vaccine of choice because it induces intestinal immunity, is simple to administer, results in immunisation of some contacts of vaccinated persons and has eliminated disease caused by wild polioviruses in the UK. Multiple doses of OPV are given to ensure that infection occurs with all three types of poliovirus and induces complete immunity. In the UK, OPV is given at 2, 3 and 4 months with DTP, Hib and meningococcal vaccines, at school entry and school leaving. Some other countries in Europe have chosen to switch to IPV, which is the general policy in North America. In low-income countries it seems to be the case that more doses of vaccine are needed to achieve adequate immunity, perhaps because of the interference in the acquisition of immunity from other enteroviruses. A very powerful contribution to control in low-income countries has come from National Immunisation Days when whole populations of children are immunised. Recommendations on polio vaccination for people travelling abroad should appreciate that polio has been eliminated in the Americas so that vaccination with polio is no longer necessary for tourists to South, Central or North America.

OPV should not be used in households with an immunodeficient person, including those known to be HIV-infected, because OPV is excreted in the stool by healthy vaccinees and can infect an immunocompromised household member, which may result in paralytic disease. Only IPV should be used in such households; this includes those containing HIV-infected mothers. Should a genuinely immunocompromised person or his/her household contact be given OPV they should be given normal immunoglobulin (under 1 year 250 mg, 1–2 years 500 mg, 3 years and over 750 mg). This will not prevent infection but it may prevent or modify any viraemia and reduce the change of reaction or paralysis. Further advice on management is available from the Immunisation Division at CDSC (020 8200 6868).

88 Molluscum contagiosum (MCV)

ORGANISM

Large double-stranded DNA poxvirus. There are 3 subtypes, MCV I, II and III. MCV I accounts for the majority of infections (c. 85%) and MCV III the least number (c. 1%). There is no difference between the presentations of infection due to the three subtypes.

EPIDEMIOLOGY

Humans are the only host. The infection occurs worldwide and is not related to personal hygiene. It is rare under 1 year old, possibly because of the presence of maternal antibody. Data from general practice in Holland showed the condition to be commonest in childhood, peaking between 5 and 10 years old. Some 17% of children had consulted their GP with the infection by 15 years old. There were a number of consultations in older people but these were often in relation to sexual transmission. The incidence is higher in tropical countries, where the peak incidence is at a younger age (1–4 years old).

Transmission

This requires close contact and can also occur by autoinoculation. Spread via shared clothing, towels and gymnastic equipment has also been suggested. In older patients it may be sexually transmitted.

Incubation period

Between 2 and 7 weeks, but may be as long as 6 months. Lesions have appeared in neonates as early as 7 days after delivery.

NATURAL HISTORY AND CLINICAL FEATURES

The typical lesion is a pearly, dome-shaped, smooth papule with a central punctum. It may be flesh-coloured, white, translucent or pale yellow and contains a cheesy material. The papules are usually 1–5 mm across but can be as big as 1–2 cm. Most patients have 20–30 lesions, but there may be over 100. Usually the lesions are asymptomatic, although there may occasionally be some pruritus or tenderness. In as many as 10% of patients, the lesions are surrounded by an eczematous reaction ('molluscum dermatitis' or 'molluscum eczema') and in up to 17% there may be an inflammatory reaction. The lesions usually resolve within 6 months to 2 years and leave no scarring.

Lesions most commonly occur on the face, trunk and extremities. They are also found in the perineal, scrotal, perianal and groin areas, especially when the condition is sexually transmitted, as is often the case in adults. This is less common in children, but when lesions are present in these areas the possibility of sexual abuse should be considered.

Patients with HIV infection, especially those with low CD4+ counts, are not only more susceptible to infection but the lesions are often more extensive and resistant to treatment and have a more prolonged course.

Diagnosis

This is usually clinical as, especially in children, the appearance is characteristic. When there is doubt, the virus can be visualised by electron microscopy of the crushed molluscum body.

MANAGEMENT

As the condition is self-limiting and leaves no scars, it is usually appropriate to let nature take its course. Treatment is usually only necessary in immunocompromised children with extensive disease (often prone to secondary bacterial infection). A number of alternatives are available but rigorous trials of their efficacy are lacking. Curettage, preceded by the application of EMLA cream, is effective, as is cryotherapy. Topical use of the broad-spectrum antiviral agent cidofovir may be useful.

PREVENTION OF FURTHER CASES

Isolation and exclusion from school are not justified as the condition is not very contagious.

89 Prion disease (transmissible spongiform encephalopathy – TSE)

ORGANISM

This is a group of syndromes (Creutzfeldt–Jakob disease, CJD; fatal familial insomnia; Gerstmann–Sträussler syndrome, GSS; and kuru), all of which are characterised by vacuolation of neurones and neuropil in the grey matter of the cerebrum and cerebellum. This leads to the appearance of numerous small holes (spongiform) in the brain on histological examination. There is no evidence of inflammatory changes, hence 'encephalopathy'. The disease is transmissible and several hypotheses of the nature of the infective agent(s) have been propounded. The prion (proteinaceous infectious agent) hypothesis has gained widest acceptance. It proposes that the infectious agent is an indigestible self-replicating form of a normal brain protein. The agent copurifies with a modified host protein (PrP_{sc} in scrapie) and is resistant to conditions that would inactivate conventional viruses (nuclease, 90°C for 30 min, ultraviolet light, disinfectants). There are TSEs described in many other animal species including sheep (scrapie) and cattle (bovine spongiform encephalopathy, BSE). Recently (1996), a new form of CJD termed variant CJD (vCJD) was described (initially this was called new variant CJD, nvCJD). The vCJD prion protein has characteristics distinct from other CJD prions but similar to those in bovine spongiform encephalopathy.

EPIDEMIOLOGY

CJD is the most common of the syndromes (0.5–$1/10^6$ population). Kuru, which was endemic in the Fore language group in Papua New Guinea, has been eradicated. In addition to an infective agent there is a genetic predisposition; for example, 10% of cases of CJD and up to 80% of cases of fatal familial insomnia occur in close relatives. Most cases of CJD occur in adults but some recent cases, usually associated with human growth hormone administration, have occurred in teenagers. Variant CJD has been reported in adolescents. As of October 2000, 85 cases of vCJD have been identified in the UK, 3 in children.

Transmission

The mode of transmission of sporadic CJD is unknown. For iatrogenic CJD modes of transmission are by direct intracerebral inoculation and include neurosurgery, tissue transplantation (cornea, dura mater) and injection of tissue extracts (growth hormone and gonadotrophins). Kuru was transmitted by ritual cannibalism. The possibility of transplacental transmission of CJD has recently been raised. It is thought that vCJD has been transmitted by ingestion of BSE-infected tissue. It is thought that the agent is carried in the blood stream attached to B lymphocytes, whence it may travel to brain and lymphoid organs. Because of this possibility British plasma is no longer used to produce pooled albumin or immunoglobulin products and a variety of measures have been undertaken to prevent transmission from bovine products. All bovine material used in medications and vaccines is sourced from herds in countries where BSE does not occur.

Incubation period

For direct inoculation into brain (neurosurgery or transplantation) the incubation period is 18–54 months and for injection into muscle (growth hormone, gonadotrophins) it is 5–20 years. For kuru the youngest patient was aged 4 years, which sets a minimum known incubation period by ingestion.

NATURAL HISTORY AND CLiNICAL FEATURES

The presentation of iatrogenic CJD differs according to the mode of inoculation. In those infected through neurosurgery or tissue transplantation, mental deterioration is the major presenting feature (70% of cases) with 33% showing cerebellar signs and 20% visual and oculomotor signs. In those infected through tissue extracts (growth hormone gonadotrophin) all presented with cerebellar signs and 15% with visual and oculomotor signs but none with mental deterioration. During the course of disease, which usually lasts 6–18 months, the disease patterns merge with the above features, myoclonus and pyramidal and extrapyramidal signs.

vCJD differs from CJD in presenting at a younger age (range 16–39 years) and having a longer duration of illness. The onset is characterised by personality and behavioural changes and dysaesthesia. Cerebellar ataxia occurs early, with chorea and myoclonus in later stages. On brain histology the prion protein plaques in vCJD are larger and in a pattern more reminiscent of that seen in kuru.

There are none of the usual signs associated with infection and disease progresses inexorably to death.

Diagnosis

The definitive diagnosis is by histological and electron microscopic examination of brain biopsy. Prion protein has also been detected in lymphoid tissue, including tonsils and appendix, and these may be more easily available tissue for biopsy. Immunoassays for detection of prion proteins or proteins expressed during TSE are under evaluation. Characteristic electroencephalographic changes (periodicity) are present in a minority of those with iatrogenic CJD but not in vCJD.

MANAGEMENT

There is no specific therapy and supportive treatment does little to alter the course of the disease. Care must be taken to prevent transmission of disease to others (at post mortem, etc.).

Notifiable disease

ORGANISM

Rabies virus, a virus of the family Rhabdoviridae: genus *Lyssavirus*. Different types of rabies virus occur in some species; for example, the virus responsible in bats is distinct from that in dogs.

EPIDEMIOLOGY

Rabies is a zoonosis with reservoirs of infection in a variety of warm-blooded, usually wild, animals. Important species include foxes in Europe, racoons and bats in the USA and Australia and dogs and foxes in south Asia. A limited number of industrialised countries are rabies-free, including those of Australasia (although recently there have been two deaths from a bat rabies virus in Australia), parts of Europe (the UK, Eire, Albania, Greece, Iceland, Macedonia, Norway, Portugal, Sweden and most of Spain) and a number of islands (including much, but not all, of the West Indies). In Europe no animal cases have been reported in the last 2 years in Austria, Belgium, Denmark, France, the Netherlands and Slovenia but the last reported animal cases were less than 2 years previously. Other European countries either have had animal cases in that period or have not supplied sufficient data. Worldwide by far the most important mode of infection is by bites from domestic dogs that themselves have been infected by wild animals or by other dogs. Human infections from cats, bats and other animals are unusual. UK residents are only at risk when in countries where rabies are endemic, usually from domestic animals. Of the extremely few UK cases recently reported most have been due to dog bites taking place in south Asia and Africa.

Transmission

Transmission is most commonly from a bite. As the virus is present in saliva, licking of injured skin or open mucous membrane also poses a small risk. Person-to-person spread is not recorded except in a very unusual example when rabies infection has taken place through transplantation of corneas following an undiagnosed rabies death. Once a dog or cat is infectious it almost always develops symptoms within 14 days.

Incubation period

Highly variable in humans, from a few days to over a year in children following exposure. The virus is neurotrophic and travels up nerves to affect the brain. Consequently, the closer the site of infection to the brain the more rapid the appearance of symptoms, with bites on the face resulting in the quickest appearance.

NATURAL HISTORY AND CLINICAL FEATURES

An affected patient presents with a fever and a deteriorating neurological condition including confusion and convulsions. There will usually be a history of exposure to a rabid animal. Hydrophobia is a feature.

Diagnosis

Preliminary diagnosis in humans is by history of exposure and then appearance of symptoms. Premortem diagnosis is very difficult but may be possible by specialist laboratories through detection of virus in saliva or cerebrospinal fluid. Definitive diagnosis in an animal is by demonstration of the virus in brain tissue. The PHLS laboratory with special expertise in diagnosis of rabies in humans is the Virus Reference Division, Central Public Health Laboratory, Colindale, tel. 020 8200 4400. It also issues prophylactic treatment, both rabies vaccine and specific immunoglobulin.

MANAGEMENT

Treatment, once symptoms have developed, is supportive, but it is very unusual for the patient to survive (the best treatment is prevention!). Isolation is recommended.

PREVENTION

Pre-exposure immunisation

Some persons require pre-exposure immunisation because of the risk of exposure through their work. These include the following:

- Laboratory workers handling the virus
- Persons whose work is expected to bring them into contact with imported animals, e.g. zoo workers and quarantine kennel workers
- Persons going to work in endemic countries who may be in contact with animals (e.g. veterinary officers).

In addition, some persons travelling to endemic areas where risk is high and postexposure immunisation unavailable choose to have pre-exposure vaccination.

Pre-exposure immunisation consists of three immunisations with the inactivated vaccine at 7- and 21-day intervals. Immunisation is by the deep intramuscular or subcutaneous route (intradermal immunisation is not recommended).

Postexposure prophylaxis

Because of the relatively slow time-course of rabies, involving the organism slowly tracking up nerves to affect the central nervous system, there is usually time to successfully apply postexposure prophylaxis (immunisation and sometimes also rabies-specific immunoglobulin).

Hospital exposure

Following a case of proven exposure, hospital and laboratory staff need immunisation, and also immunoglobulin if their mucous membranes or an open wound have been exposed to saliva, cerebrospinal fluid or brain tissue from a rabid animal.

Community exposure – animal bite

Any animal bite in any country should be flushed immediately with water or the most available clean fluid (any bottled drink will do in the first instance); then the wound should be cleaned with soapy water.* Good drainage is important and stitching should be avoided or delayed unless there are good cosmetic reasons.

Exposures are classified according to the level of risk of the area where it took place.

- No-risk areas: UK, Ireland, Denmark, Norway, Greece, Portugal, Spain (except central areas), Australasia, Malta, Cyprus, Jamaica and Bermuda.
- Low-risk areas: Countries where rabies is present in the wildlife but very rarely in domestic animals and where dogs are routinely immunised. These are the USA, Canada and Europe (except those countries in the 'no-risk' category).
- High-risk areas: Countries where rabies is widespread in both wild and domestic animals. These are most countries in Africa, South and Central America, most of the Middle East (including Turkey), south and south-east Asia and mainland China. Even though the absolute risk from a single dog bite in these areas is probably very low, rabies immunisation is usually given (unless the possibility of rabies can be ruled out, e.g. if the dog is well 10 days after the bite), because of the severity of this illness and its untreatability once established.

It is difficult to make completely firm rules as to who should receive postexposure immunisation or immunoglobulin. A good history will always help in making a rational decision covering the following points:

- **The exposure**: Which country (level of risk as above) and when, where on the body, was the skin broken, was there a pre-existing wound, were the mucous membranes exposed and was local management applied (i.e. was washing undertaken), had pre-exposure immunisation been received (when and was it a complete course)?
- **The animal**: What species (the risk is predominately from dogs), name and contact details of the owner, was the animal provoked or was it behaving oddly? What happened to the animal subsequently? If a dog is known to be alive and well 14 days after the exposure rabies exposure can be ruled out and a phone or fax to a reliable owner can often obviate the need for postexposure prophylaxis.

---

* **Infections from animal bites are unusual. In addition to rabies they include cat-scratch disease and *Pasteurella* from cats, staphylococcal infection from almost any bite and infection with Gram-negative organisms. In general, prophylactic antibiotics are not recommended and it is more important to clean and wash the wound and observe progress of healing. It should be ensured that tetanus immunisation is up to date – see also Animal bites in Chapter 33, pages 220–221.**

Following ascertaining a history, and if there has been any significant exposure, specialist advice must be taken.

Post-exposure prophylaxis consists of the following.

Previously unimmunised individuals

Six doses of vaccine repeated on days 3, 7, 14, 30 and 90, counting the day of the first vaccine as day 0. It may also be considered necessary to give specific immunoglobulin (20 IU/kg; half infiltrated into the wound/exposure site and half given elsewhere by parenteral injection).

Previously immunised individual

Two doses of vaccine at an interval of 3–7 days without immunoglobulin.

Quarantine restrictions

A controversial topic is whether island communities such as the UK should have a strict policy of quarantine for imported animals and, in particular, domestic pet dogs. The UK has dropped its quarantine strategy and is now trying to ensure that all dogs and cats have rabies immunisation prior to entering the country.

91 Respiratory syncytial virus (RSV)

ORGANISM

An RNA paramyxovirus of the genus *Pneumovirus*.

EPIDEMIOLOGY

This has a worldwide distribution with annual epidemics during the autumn, winter and early spring. Infections occur predominantly in infants and young children and the majority of people are infected by their second birthday, although reinfections continue throughout life. The major cause of bronchiolitis, the epidemiology of RSV in older persons is poorly described, but it is probably under-recognised as a cause of adult respiratory disease. The infection is particularly severe in infants with congenital heart disease and those with a history of chronic lung disease following respiratory distress syndrome of prematurity. Passive smoking is a risk factor for infection.

Transmission

Humans are the only source of infection and transmission is mainly person-to-person by droplets from the respiratory tract. The virus is known to be viable for up to 6 hours in secretions outside the body. Infection is communicable for up to 1 week after the onset of symptoms. More prolonged shedding of virus may occur in young infants.

2–8 days.

NATURAL HISTORY AND CLINICAL FEATURES

RSV is the usual cause of bronchiolitis in infancy. In the preterm infant infection may result in apnoea, lethargy or nonspecific signs of sepsis. In term infants signs are more localised to the chest, with tachypnoea and subcostal recession. Auscultation may reveal crackles and wheezes. In the majority of children recovery occurs within 5–7 days, but in the high-risk groups described above respiratory failure ensues, which, if not recognised quickly, may lead to respiratory arrest.

Diagnosis

By immunofluorescence on secretions from the nasopharynx. Such tests have 60–90% sensitivity during the first few days of the illness. This investigation should be available in all paediatric units treating high-risk infants eligible for ribavirin.

MANAGEMENT

Treatment is generally supportive; fluids are given by nasogastric tube or intravenously in sick hospitalised babies. In more severe cases oxygen should be given by headbox or nasal cannula. Where oxygen saturation is measured this should be kept above 90%. Neither inhaled bronchodilators nor oral steroids have been found to be effective. Although recent publications suggest that the antiviral agent ribavirin is not effective, it is still used in some units for severely affected infants. It is administered by a small-particle aerosol generator over 12 hours for 2–4 days, either into a headbox or ventilator tubing. It has been recommended for infants with congenital heart disease, bronchopulmonary dysplasia and cystic fibrosis; those with deteriorating respiratory function – an oxygen saturation of less than 90% – and rising CO_2 and infants requiring mechanical ventilation for RSV infection. Ribavirin has been found to be teratogenic in rodents. There is no evidence of teratogenicity in human beings but it should not be administered by pregnant attendants.

PREVENTION OF FURTHER CASES

Infants with RSV infection should be isolated. Attendants should pay particular attention to hand-washing. There is some evidence that cohort nursing reduces the risk of cross-infection but this is usually difficult to organise. There is a lot of interest in developing an RSV preventive vaccine although much basic works remains to be done before this will be produced.

Recently, passive protection in the form of intravenous RSV immunoglobulin and an intramuscular monoclonal antibody (palivizumab) has become available for groups at higher risk (premature babies, children with chronic lung disease). Both treatments have to be given monthly during the RSV season. There is some evidence of the effectiveness of this approach but it is expensive and the cost-effectiveness as a treatment has yet to be demonstrated. It has been shown to reduce hospital admissions and oxygen requirements in high-risk infants, but there was no reduction in days of ventilation. There has been a trial of treatment in children under 2 years with bronchopulmonary dysplasia requiring medical therapy (oxygen, steroids, bronchodilators or diuretics) and premature infants – under 35 weeks – who were under 6 months at the onset of the RSV season. The dosage of palivizumab is 15 mg/kg intramuscularly monthly, given during the RSV season. Its licence does not extend to infants with congenital heart disease because studies have not been performed with this group. The intravenous immunoglobulin product can interfere with immunisation, e.g. MMR, which may need to be delayed for several months.

FURTHER READING

Simoes EAF (1999) Respiratory syncytial virus infection. Lancet 354: 847–852.

The Impact–RSV Study Group Palivizumab (1998) A humanized respiratory syncytial virus monoclonal antibody reduces hospitalization from respiratory syncytial virus in high-risk infants. Pediatrics 102: 531–537.

92 Rickettsioses

ORGANISM

All are Gram-negative bacteria that are obligate intracellular pathogens. There are at least nine species causing different disease manifestations throughout the world (Table 92.1).

EPIDEMIOLOGY

Spotted fever

Rocky Mountain spotted fever (RMSF – *Rickettsia rickettsii*) is not limited to the Rocky Mountains area but is also present in eastern USA, Canada, Mexico, Colombia and Brazil. In eastern USA it is more common in women and children, whereas in the Rockies it is commoner in male adults. It is transmitted by ticks (four different species), either by bites or if a tick is crushed over abraded skin. Many small animals, including rabbits, rats and dogs, are reservoirs. Most cases occur in late spring and summer when ticks are most active. The infective dose is very low (c. 1 organism) and the incubation period is 3–12 days (mean 7 days), but person-to-person spread does not occur. *Fièvre boutonneuse* (*R. conorii*) is found in coastal Mediterranean countries and increasingly in France and Spain. It is transmitted by the dog tick (*Rhipicephalus sanguineus*) from dogs, rabbits and rodents.

Table 92.1 The rickettsioses

Disease	Species	Syndrome	Reservoir	Vector	Geographical distribution
Spotted fevers	R. rickettsii	Rocky Mountain spotted fever	Various rodents and small animals	Tick	The Americas
	R. conorii	Fièvre boutonneuse	Small animals, dogs	Tick	Mediterranean Europe
	R. conorii	South Africa tick typhus	Cattle	Tick	South Africa, Zimbabwe
	R. australis	Australian tick typhus	Rodents	Tick	Australia
	R. akari	Rickettsial pox	Mice	Mite	USA, former USSR
	R. japonica	Oriental spotted fever	Rodent, dogs	Tick	Japan
	R. sibirica	Siberian tick typhus	Birds, domestic animals	Tick	Siberia, Mongolia, north China
Typhus	R. prowazekii	Louse-borne typhus	Man	Louse	South America, Africa
		Brill–Zinsser disease	–	–	Reactivation of primary infection, thus worldwide as people migrate
		Sporadic typhus	Flying squirrel	Flea (faeces)	USA
	R. typhi	Flea-borne typhus	Rat, cat, possum	Flea (faeces)	Worldwide
Scrub typhus	Orientia tsutsugamushi	Scrub typhus	Rats	Chigger (mite) bite	Asia, North Australia, Pacific islands

Rickettsialpox (*R. akari*) is transmitted by a mite that lives on house and field mice. It is found in eastern USA, Central America, central and southern Africa, the Crimea and Korea. The incubation period is 7–10 days.

Epidemic typhus

Infection is due to *R. prowazekii* and occurs at all ages, although infection in children is less severe. It occurs worldwide and is epidemic when there is overcrowding, poverty and poor sanitary conditions. It is particularly associated with refugees and in war zones. It is transmitted by the human body louse (*Pediculus humanus corporis*), which becomes infected when it takes a blood meal from an infected patient. The bacterium replicates in the louse's intestine and is excreted in its faeces. Patients become infected when they scratch the faeces into their skin. In endemic regions (cooler mountainous regions of the tropics, Serbia and Greece), infections occur most often in winter, when people crowd together for warmth. The incubation period is, on average, 12 days (range 1–2 weeks). Infection does not always result in complete immunity and persistent asymptomatic infection can occur. This can recrudesce (or relapse) years later (Brill–Zinsser disease) to provide unexpected foci of infection in other parts of the world (the original description was in Jewish immigrants to New York from the Balkans).

Endemic typhus

Infection is due to *R. typhi* (previously known as *R. mooseri*), and is found worldwide. It is particularly prevalent in south-eastern USA, Central America, the Balkans, Israel, west Africa, India, Pakistan, south-east Asia, China and Australia. The natural hosts are rats (brown and black) and mice, which are unaffected by the bacterium. Infection is transmitted between rats and mice by lice and mites, but to man by fleas (*Xenopsylla cheopis*), which is a biological vector. The bacteria are excreted in the fleas' faeces and inoculated when the flea bites are scratched. The incubation period is 12 days (range 1–2 weeks).

Scrub typhus

Infection is due to *Orientia tsutsugamushi* and is highly prevalent throughout south-east Asia, including India, Myanmar, Indonesia, Malaysia, Thailand, Indo-China, China, Papua New Guinea and northern Australia. Its reservoir is wild rodents and infection is transmitted by trombiculid mites that feed on them. The mites live on scrub grasses that have grown when primary jungle has been cleared for cultivation. The sharp scrub grasses abrade the skin and inoculate the mites and bacteria. The incubation period is 5–10 days.

NATURAL HISTORY AND CLINICAL FEATURES

Spotted fevers

In RMSF *R. rickettsii* primarily infects endothelial cells, and macrophages occasionally, and the rash is a result of vasculitis. There is rarely an eschar at the site of the tick bite. There is an abrupt onset of fever, severe headache, myalgia and dry cough. After 2–3 days a fine pink macular rash appears, which is most marked on the soles, wrists and forearms. In severe disease it becomes petechial, with large ecchymoses and even gangrene of fingers or toes. Meningoencephalitis is common in severe cases as is disseminated intravascular coagulation. The overall mortality is 7–10% but in young children and the elderly is up to 25%. In the preantibiotic era mortality rates were 23–70%. The differential diagnosis includes meningococcal septicaemia, tick-borne relapsing fever, haemorrhagic measles, tularaemia and Lyme borreliosis. Specific diagnosis is aided by detection of heterophile antibodies to *Proteus mirabilis* strain OX-19 but not OX-2 in the Weil–Felix reaction. Detection of specific IgM or IgG by immunofluorescence, immunohaemagglutination or antibody-capture enzyme-linked immunosorbent assay (ELISA) is more rapidly positive and sensitive.

Fièvre boutonneuse is similar to RMSF but usually far less severe. It is characterised by a primary necrotic lesion at the site of the tick bite (eschar or *tache noire*). Diagnosis is serological. The onset of rickettsialpox is marked by the development of an eschar at the inoculation site. This is followed by fever and 'flu-like' symptoms and a sparse maculopapular rash. These become vesicular (hence pox), then crust and fade. For serological diagnosis the Weil–Felix reaction is negative but other tests such as agglutination are positive in rickettsialpox.

Epidemic typhus

There is an abrupt onset of fever with prostration, severe headaches, limb pain (especially the shins), nausea and vomiting. The fever rapidly rises to 40°C until the patient dies or it resolves by crisis towards the end of the second week of illness. The typhus rash, which consists of small irregular pink macules turning purple, appears on the second to fourth days and is largely confined to the trunk and limbs. There is no eschar but the rash may become petechial and eventually turns brown. Approximately half the patients develop meningoencephalitis. Other complications include myocarditis and acute renal failure. In epidemics the mortality rates are high (10–66%), depending on the health and nutrition of the affected population. The differential diagnosis includes typhoid, viral haemorrhagic fever, meningococcal septicaemia, louse-borne relapsing fever and leptospirosis. Specific diagnosis is aided by a positive Weil–Felix reaction to both OX-19 and OX-2 and detection of specific antibody by immunofluorescence antigen detection (IFA) or ELISA. *R. prowazekii* can be cultured in embryonated duck eggs or guinea-pigs but this is not rapid and the bacterium is a category 3 pathogen, requiring special containment facilities. A polymerase chain reaction (PCR) method has been developed. The recrudescent Brill–Zinsser disease is milder than the initial attack of epidemic typhus. However if the patient is infested with lice this may serve to initiate an epidemic.

Endemic typhus

The illness has a similar pattern to epidemic typhus but is much less severe. Headache and myalgia are the predominant features. There is no eschar and the rash of fine red macules is far less extensive. Neurological and renal complications are rare and the mortality rate is 1–2%. The differential and specific diagnosis is as for epidemic typhus.

Scrub typhus

This begins as an abrupt febrile illness and single or multiple eschars with swelling of draining lymph nodes. This will progress, with headache, conjunctival injection, myalgia and drowsiness, to generalised lymphadenopathy and hepatosplenomegaly. The rash is similar to that of epidemic typhus, occurring mainly on the trunk, arms and thighs. In severe cases there is meningoencephalitis and acute renal failure. Untreated the mortality is 10% but with treatment death is rare. Repeat attacks are common. Specific diagnosis is based on specific serology and PCR.

MANAGEMENT

Specific treatment is with oral or intravenous chloramphenicol or tetracycline for 7–10 days, or a single oral dose of doxycycline (200 mg for adults, 100 mg for children).

PREVENTION OF FURTHER CASES

Prevention is by stopping transmission from reservoir to patient, which involves preventing access of rats, mice and other small rodents, use of insecticides to kill fleas and mites and, in the case of epidemic typhus, delousing patients, close contacts (with lindane or permethrin) and bedding and clothes. There are as yet no safe and effective vaccines.

93 Rotavirus and other viral enteropathogens

ROTAVIRUS

ORGANISM

Rotavirus is a medium-sized nonenveloped RNA virus with a characteristic double-shelled capsid which gives the characteristic wheel shape (rota = wheel). It is a genus within the family Reoviridae and its genome consists of 11 segments of double-stranded RNA. Rotavirus is divided into seven serogroups (A–G). Most infections in children are due to serogroup A although serogroups B and C have been responsible for major epidemics. For epidemiological purposes rotaviruses are further subdivided into G (for glycoprotein) serotypes (1–14), P (this viral protein is activated by proteolysis) serotypes (1–20) and on the migration pattern of the 11 ds RNA segment on polyacrylamide gel electrophoresis (electropherotypes). Most human infections are due to G-serotypes 1–4 and antibodies to these epitopes neutralise infectivity. Recently G8 and G9 have emerged as globally important stereotypes.

EPIDEMIOLOGY

Rotavirus is the most important cause of gastroenteritis and dehydration in children throughout the world. In hospital-based surveys rotavirus is responsible for 20–60% of cases of gastroenteritis in infants and children. In community-based surveys the proportion of cases due to rotavirus is lower, ranging from 6–35%. Estimated hospitalisation rates for rotavirus gastroenteritis in developed countries range from 2.2–8.5/1000 children. In low-income countries rotavirus is responsible for 125 million cases of gastroenteritis per year, 18 million of which are severe, leading to over 800 000 deaths each year. The peak incidence of rotavirus infection is in children aged 3–15 months. Repeated rotavirus infections are frequent but are usually mild or asymptomatic unless due to serogroup B or C virus.

In temperate countries such as the UK rotavirus infection occurs predominantly in the cooler winter months although infections do occur throughout the year. Most mammalian species are infected by rotavirus, and human–animal reassortant rotaviruses have been detected in humans. Most rotavirus infections are community-acquired but sporadic and epidemic nosocomial spread has been described.

Transmission

Person-to-person spread occurs predominantly by the faecal–oral route. However, because the spread is so efficient in both developed and developing countries it has been suggested that transmission might also occur by the respiratory route. During acute infection a child can excrete up to 10^{11} rotavirus particles per gram of faeces. The infective dose is estimated to be as low as 10^2 particles. Infection can be transmitted from symptomatic or asymptomatically infected children and all four major G serotypes (1–4) circulate at a given time, although one serotype tends to predominate.

Incubation period

2–4 days.

NATURAL HISTORY AND CLINICAL FEATURES

Ingested virus first replicates in the proximal small intestine and spreads distally to the terminal ileum. Rotavirus does not infect the stomach or colon. Virus infects mature villous enterocytes but not the crypt enterocytes. The villous enterocytes are killed, leading to blunted villi. This results in loss of absorption and decreased disaccharidase activity and thus to an osmotic diarrhoea. In addition viral NSP-4 (nonstructural protein-4), which is involved in viral assembly, has recently been shown to be an enterotoxin causing watery diarrhoea in infant mice.

Rotavirus gastroenteritis can vary in severity from mild watery diarrhoea lasting 24 hours to overwhelming dehydrating and occasionally fatal gastroenteritis. It is not possible to distinguish rotavirus gastroenteritis clinically from other causes of small intestinal diarrhoea. Vomiting is a frequent occurrence, often preceding diarrhoea. The illness lasts on average 5–7 days in hospitalised children. Virtually all children are febrile and a large proportion have upper respiratory tract symptoms, although the latter association may be coincidental. Infection in neonates is frequently asymptomatic and in outbreaks in neonatal intensive care units only 10–20% of those infected are symptomatic.

Extraintestinal infections with rotavirus have been rarely described and include hepatic abscess, myositis, meningitis and encephalitis.

Immunocompetent children continue to excrete rotavirus for 5–8 days following cessation of diarrhoea. Immunoincompetent children may excrete virus for much longer.

Infection with rotavirus provides some protection from subsequent symptomatic infection. Thus, children who have experienced one, two or three episodes of rotavirus infection have relative risks of experiencing rotavirus diarrhoea of 0.23, 0.17 and 0.08 respectively and of asymptomatic rotavirus infection of 0.62, 0.40 and 0.34 respectively.

Diagnosis

It is not possible to diagnose rotavirus gastroenteritis on clinical features. Although it is possible to grow rotavirus in tissue culture this is not a useful diagnostic procedure.

Electron microscopy

During acute infection sufficient virus is excreted for it to be detected by negative-stain electron microscopy (a minimum of 10^6 particles/mL faeces is needed). This has good sensitivity and high specificity, which can be enhanced by addition of specific antisera to clump virus particles (immunoelectronmicroscopy). Electron microscopy will detect most other viral enteropathogens and is thus a 'catch-all' technique. The remaining techniques are all pathogen-specific.

Antigen detection

There is a variety of commercially available methods for detection of rotavirus antigen in faeces, including enzyme-linked immunosorbent assay (ELISA), radioimmunoassay and latex particle agglutination. The sensitivity and specificity of such tests are high but in general ELISA tests perform best, although all may not detect group B or C rotaviruses.

Genome detection

So much virus is excreted during acute infection that it is possible to extract rotavirus RNA directly from faeces, separate its 11 ds RNA segments by polyacrylamide gel electrophoresis and visualise them by silver staining (RNA-PAGE). This is a sensitive, specific and inexpensive diagnostic test that also provides epidemiological information.

Recently, reverse transcription polymerase chain amplification has been used for diagnosis and to provide information of rotavirus serotypes.

Antibody detection

This is of little value for diagnosis of infection.

MANAGEMENT AND PREVENTION

There is no specific therapy available. Management principally involves assessment of dehydration and replacement of fluid and electrolytes orally or intravenously. Therapy with immune colostrum or gamma globulin has been tried with mixed results and such therapies remain experimental. Breastfeeding may provide protection by providing both specific IgA antirotavirus and trypsin inhibitor. Recently a live tetravalent human–Rhesus rotavirus vaccine has been licensed for routine infant immunisation in the USA. This contains 10 Rhesus rotavirus gene segments and one (encoding G-serotypes) human rotavirus segment. Tetravalent means that it includes the four most important G-serotypes (1–4). In trials this produced 50% protection against rotavirus diarrhoea and 80% protection against severe diarrhoea. In 1999 an association between use of the vaccine and infants developing intussusception was reported in the USA and led to the suspension of the vaccine programme.

ADENOVIRUS

ORGANISM

Adenovirus is a medium-sized nonenveloped DNA virus with eicosahedral symmetry. It has a double-stranded linear DNA genome. Of the 46 serotypes only adenovirus 40 and 41 are associated with diarrhoeal disease. In comparison to other serotypes they do not grow easily in tissue culture ('fastidious adenoviruses').

EPIDEMIOLOGY

Adenovirus 40/41 is the second or third commonest cause of diarrhoeal disease in children under 5 years. It has been found to be responsible for 4–10% of cases of diarrhoea in children in community- and hospital-based surveys. Unlike rotavirus there is no seasonality of endemic infection. Most infections occur in those under 2 years.

Transmission

Infection is transmitted from person to person by the faecal–oral route. Most infection is community-acquired but nosocomial outbreaks occur.

Incubation period

8–10 days.

NATURAL HISTORY AND CLINICAL FEATURES

Little is known of the pathogenesis of adenovirus gastroenteritis but it is presumed to be similar to that of rotavirus. The clinical features are similar to those of rotavirus. The most prominent feature is a watery diarrhoea, which lasts 5–12 days. Vomiting usually occurs after the onset of diarrhoea. The severity is usually less than rotavirus diarrhoea. Virus tends to be excreted in stool for some time (up to 14 days) after cessation of diarrhoea.

Diagnosis

Diagnosis is by detection of virus, its antigens or genome using immuno-electronmicroscopy, ELISA or DNA hybridisation.

MANAGEMENT

This is symptomatic. There is no vaccine available for prevention nor is there information available on determinants of immunity.

ASTROVIRUS

ORGANISM

Astrovirus is a small, round, nonenveloped RNA virus with a characteristic six-pointed star on its surface. Astrovirus is difficult to grow in tissue culture.

EPIDEMIOLOGY

There are eight serotypes but serotype 1 accounts for 80% of cases in Europe and the USA. Astrovirus is responsible for 5–12% of cases of diarrhoeal disease in children under 5 years. The majority of infections occur in children under 2, and antiastrovirus antibodies are detectable in 70% of UK children by the age of 4. Astrovirus has a similar seasonal distribution to rotavirus, with peaks of infection occurring in winter 2–4 weeks prior to the rotavirus peak.

Transmission

Spread from person to person is by the faecal–oral route.

Incubation period

3 days.

NATURAL HISTORY AND CLINICAL FEATURES

Illness commences with 5–7 days watery diarrhoea. Vomiting is also a prominent feature. Astrovirus diarrhoea tends to be less severe than that due to rotavirus.

MANAGEMENT

Specific diagnosis is by negative-stain electron microscopy, ELISA or polymerase chain reaction (PCR) amplification of viral RNA. The latter will also provide information on the serotype.

The management is as for rotavirus diarrhoea. There is no vaccine available for prevention of infection.

CALICIVIRUS

ORGANISM

Calicivirus is a small, round, nonenveloped RNA virus with cup-shaped indentations (calyx = cup) that may lead to the appearance of a 'star of David' on electron microscopy.

EPIDEMIOLOGY

It is responsible for 2–4% of cases of gastroenteritis in children but may affect older children and adults. There is no apparent seasonality of infection. Outbreaks of infection occur in schools, orphanages and hospitals.

Transmission

Infection is spread by the faecal–oral route either directly or indirectly (large water-borne and shellfish-associated outbreaks have been described).

Incubation period

1–3 days.

NATURAL HISTORY AND CLINICAL FEATURES

The illness is clinically indistinguishable from mild rotavirus gastroenteritis. Diarrhoea persists for 4–6 days on average.

Diagnosis

Specific diagnosis is by negative-stain electron microscopy, ELISA or PCR amplification of viral genome.

NORWALK VIRUS

ORGANISM

Norwalk, Southampton and Lonsdale viruses are small, round, structural nonenveloped RNA viruses within the Caliciviridae but without the characteristic cup-shaped depressions in their surface.

EPIDEMIOLOGY

Norwalk virus is responsible for up to 40% of outbreaks of gastroenteritis in recreational camps, cruise ships, communities, schools, nursing homes or hospitals. Infections tend to be more common in older children and adults. The seroprevalence to anti-Norwalk-virus is low in childhood and rises through adolescence to adulthood where 60% are seropositive. In low-income countries infection occurs earlier. There is no seasonality of infection.

Transmission

Person-to-person spread occurs via the faecal–oral route although airborne transmission has been suggested since this is consistent with the explosive secondary transmission seen in outbreaks. Indirect spread via drinking or recreational water and food (poorly cooked shellfish, salads and cake icing) is a common occurrence in outbreaks.

Incubation period

4–77 hours (median 36 hours).

NATURAL HISTORY AND CLINICAL FEATURES

The virus replicates in the mucosa of the proximal small intestine. Gastric emptying is delayed, which probably accounts for the frequent occurrence of nausea and vomiting. Diarrhoea lasts from 3–6 days.

MANAGEMENT

Virus is excreted in vomitus and faeces in large numbers only in the first few days of illness and negative-stain electron microscopy is useful only during that period. Antigen detection by ELISA provides the most useful diagnostic test. There is no vaccine available.

OTHER VIRAL ENTEROPATHOGENS

A variety of other viruses have been associated with gastroenteritis, including small, round, structureless viruses (possibly parvovirus), coronavirus, torovirus (e.g. Breda), pestiviruses and picobirnaviruses. However, the evidence linking them to diarrhoeal disease is not strong and they represent a minority of cases if any.

PREVENTION OF FURTHER CASES

Routine enteric precautions should apply (see Chapter 23). Children with presumed or confirmed viral infection may return to school or day care once symptoms have terminated.

94 Rubella

> Notifiable disease. All children in the UK and Ireland with congenital rubella should be reported to the British Paediatric Surveillance Unit (BPSU).

ORGANISM

Rubivirus is an RNA enveloped togavirus in the Togaviridae family.

EPIDEMIOLOGY

Humans are the only host and the disease is endemic worldwide. It occurs in epidemics about every 6–9 years where rubella vaccine is not in use. In the UK and western Europe, infection is more common in late winter and early spring. A downward trend in the incidence of rubella in England and Wales was reversed in 1993 when there were local outbreaks particularly affecting young adult males.

Transmission

Transmission is by direct contact or droplet spread. The period of infectivity is not known but virus is shed from 7 days before to 6 days (rarely 21 days) after the appearance of the rash. The most infectious period is prior to onset of the rash. Congenital rubella (see below) is contracted by the fetus when the mother is infected at or after the time of conception or in early pregnancy. Infants with congenital rubella may continue to excrete virus for 6 months or longer after birth.

Incubation period
15–20 days (median 17 days).

NATURAL HISTORY AND CLINICAL FEATURES

Between 25% and 50% of cases are totally asymptomatic and in the remainder the disease is rarely serious. In children there is usually little if any prodrome. In adolescents and adults a prodrome of low-grade fever, malaise, headache, conjunctivitis, coryza, sore throat and cough may precede the rash by 1–5 days. At all ages there is a generalised lymphadenopathy, the suboccipital, postauricular and cervical nodes being most affected. This may precede the rash by up to 7 days. An enanthem consisting of small red spots may be present during the prodrome or on the first day of the exanthem. The exanthem itself consists of discrete puckered maculopapules, appearing first on the face. These spread rapidly so that after 24 hours the entire body may be covered. On the second day the rash disappears from the face and may coalesce on the trunk. By the end of the third day the rash has usually gone entirely. The lymphadenopathy may take longer to resolve. The rash may appear similar to that caused by measles, scarlet fever or parvovirus B19. Rubella can be distinguished from measles where the general upset is greater and the evolution of the rash slower than in rubella, while in scarlet fever the rash spares the area around the mouth (circumoral pallor).

Complications are unusual. Adults and adolescents are more likely to develop an arthritis than are children and women are more commonly affected than men. This is often a polyarthritis with a predilection for the small joints of the hands. There is rarely any residuum. In approximately 1 in 6000 cases an encephalitis may occur. Fatalities are rare and the survivors are usually undamaged. Purpura (with normal or low platelet counts) rarely occurs and may be accompanied by serious bleeding, e.g. into the intestinal tract or cerebral substance. It is usually self-limiting and resolves within 2 weeks. Idiopathic thrombocytopenic purpura may follow an attack of rubella.

Diagnosis

Diagnosis is usually made clinically in children. In children under 5 years old, less than 5% of clinically diagnosed cases are confirmed serologically. The corresponding figure in older children and adults is about 50%. In acute infection either a single test for rubella IgM or paired tests with a 10-day interval for rising rubella IgG levels is diagnostic. The virus can also be recovered from the nasopharynx and the urine in the acute phase. Because of the uncertainties in clinical diagnosis a history of rubella should never be accepted without serological confirmation where it is important to be certain, i.e. when a pregnant woman is involved. The presence of IgG specific for rubella indicates immunity due to prior infection or immunisation. Testing for rubella-specific IgM on a single saliva sample is about 80% sensitive and almost 100% specific. Salivary IgG testing is 98% sensitive and 100% specific. All notified cases in England and Wales should be followed up with salivary testing.

MANAGEMENT

Management is symptomatic.

PREVENTION OF FURTHER CASES

Unless a child is likely to come into contact with a pregnant woman, isolation is not appropriate. The main strategy to prevent further cases, especially of congenital rubella, is twofold:

* Ensuring high herd immunity in children of both sexes through rubella immunisation with measles, mumps and rubella (MMR) vaccination, thus minimising circulating virus
* Ensuring all women entering pregnancy are seroimmune.

Vaccination

A live attenuated vaccine has been available for many years. In the UK it was previously given to 13-year-old girls and women of childbearing age who were found to be susceptible. Since October 1988, it has also been given as part of the MMR vaccine to all children at 13 months of age. In November 1994 a mass campaign to immunise with MR all schoolchildren aged under 16 years took place. Since then, rubella vaccine is no longer given to schoolgirls. In most people the vaccine is thought to provide lifelong protection. However, there is a small proportion of people where there is a primary or secondary failure of the vaccine to protect. Congenital rubella has occurred in the babies of mothers known to have been immune in the past. Exactly the same situation applies to protection after the disease. The vaccine should not knowingly be given to a pregnant woman; however, there is a large body of evidence that while it may infect the fetus it does no harm. Inadvertent vaccination in pregnancy is therefore not a reason for termination.

CONGENITAL RUBELLA

The risk of congenital rubella (congenital rubella syndrome or CRS) is maximal in nonimmune pregnant women acquiring infection in the first 8–10 weeks of pregnancy. At that stage the probability of some degree of damage, frequently severe, is considered to be 90%. Beyond 13 weeks' gestation the risk of any abnormality apart from deafness is extremely low and by 16 weeks of pregnancy the risk has fallen to 10–20%. Infection beyond 16 weeks' gestation is not thought to cause deafness. Between January 1991 and June 1994 in the UK 14 infants were notified to the National Congenital Rubella Surveillance Programme, including one set of triplets. Nine of the 12 mothers were immigrants, indicating the importance of these groups being immunised after their arrival. However in 1996 there was a resurgence in rubella in the community in the UK, especially in unimmunised adolescents and adults, leading to 12 reported births with CRS and nine terminations, few of which were in immigrants.

There were no further cases in 1997 and 1998. In 1999, there was a small outbreak of rubella among university students. This could be traced to students from Greece. One case of CRS was associated with one of these outbreaks. Severe clinical manifestations that have been described include fetal death and stillbirth, growth retardation, cardiac anomalies (septal defects, patent ductus arteriosus and pulmonary artery stenosis), eye involvement (cataract, blindness, micro-ophthalmia), neurological damage (nerve deafness, meningoencephalitis, microcephaly), thrombocytopenia and jaundice. However, milder cases do occur and congenital rubella is worth considering as a differential diagnosis in any growth-retarded newborn or child with idiopathic nerve deafness.

Notification of cases of congenital rubella

Cases of suspected congenital rubella detected in the UK must be notified to the National Congenital Rubella Surveillance Programme, Department of Epidemiology and Biostatistics, Institute of Child Health, 30 Guilford St, London WC1E 7HT, tel. 020 7242 9789. Paediatricians may do this by ticking the box on the British Paediatric Surveillance Unit 'orange card'. Reporting by laboratories, audiologists, etc. also reveals significant numbers of cases.

Pregnancy and rubella

Pregnant women exposed to rubella should all be investigated serologically irrespective of a history of immunisation, clinical rubella or previous positive rubella serology. As soon as possible after exposure maternal blood should be tested for antirubella IgG or IgM. There should be close consultation between the clinician managing the woman and the virologist to ensure prompt taking of further samples and correct interpretation of results. A high likelihood of congenital rubella infection having occurred is an indication for offering the woman termination of pregnancy.

Screening pregnant women and women contemplating pregnancy

All pregnant women should be screened for antirubella IgG in every pregnancy and on request when pregnancy is contemplated irrespective of a previous positive serology. Serological testing of nonpregnant women should be performed whenever possible before immunisation but need not be undertaken where this might interfere with the acceptance or delivery of vaccine.

Girls and women migrating to the UK from countries where rubella vaccination is not routine are at particular risk of being nonimmune and should be tested for antirubella IgG or given MMR.

Women found to be seronegative on antenatal screening should not be immunised during the pregnancy but should receive immunisation after delivery before discharge from the maternity unit. If anti-D immunoglobulin is required the two may be given at the same time at different sites.

Health-care staff

All health-care staff, both male and female, should be screened and those who are seronegative should be immunised (some occupational health departments may choose to immunise without prior serology).

95 Salmonellosis

> See also Chapter 106. Food poisoning through whatever cause is a notifiable condition

ORGANISM

Salmonellas are Gram-negative bacilli with a number of species and many serovars (more than 2200). Important species include *Salmonella enteritidis* and *S. typhimurium*. These two produce most of the cases in the UK.

EPIDEMIOLOGY

Salmonellas are present worldwide with animals considered to be the reservoir of infection for nontyphoidal salmonellas. The species seemingly the source of most infections in human are poultry and cattle and the major vehicles are poultry, meat and eggs. Circulation of infection may occur through spreading of human and animal faecal waste on farmland. Occasional infections in children have occurred though spread from reptiles (e.g. turtles and terrapins) kept as pets. Poultry eggs remain a potent source of human infection because they are often used uncooked, e.g. in mayonnaise, and outbreaks have also been reported due to contamination of artificial baby milk and infant snacks. Cases occur at all ages and outbreaks occur in families through contamination of food in day-care facilities and schools. Most cases are sporadic but outbreaks receive the most publicity. The infection is more apparent in children and the elderly because they experience the highest attack rates. Only a small proportion of infections are diagnosed and reported. Invasive infections occur with typhoid and paratyphoid infection, in infants under 6 months and in children with certain chronic conditions, notably sickle-cell disease and other haemoglobinopathies, HIV infection, constitutional immunodeficiencies and malignancies and chronic gastrointestinal disease such as Crohn's disease or colitis. *Salmonella* species occasionally cause meningitis in neonates (see Chapter 4).

Transmission

Most cases are transmitted in food products, water and by faecal–oral spread. Large outbreaks have occurred through infectious food handlers or contamination of food products used for catering. Infectivity continues while symptoms persist and for up to several weeks, although risk of transmission decreases considerably as the diarrhoea subsides. Asymptomatic infection occurs and rarely carriers are found who remain infectious for months. Babies seem more likely to develop this state. Antibiotic treatment is usually ineffective in rendering carriers uninfectious and may even prolong carriage.

Incubation period

This varies from 6 hours to 3 days (usually 12–36 hours) depending on the infecting dose.

NATURAL HISTORY AND CLINICAL FEATURES

Salmonella infections cause a number of clinical syndromes including asymptomatic infection, gastroenteritis, focal infections, bacteraemia and enteric fever, although the commonest are asymptomatic infection and gastroenteritis and the severe manifestations are more often seen in infection with *S. typhi* and *S. paratyphi* (see Chapter 106). Constitutional illness and bacteraemia may occur without any apparent gastrointestinal illness. Systemic signs can include headache and general malaise; fever is uncommon. Alternatively there may only be diarrhoea and vomiting with abdominal cramps. Diarrhoea rarely contains pus (dysentery) and may be watery, although it rarely contains blood. Focal signs can be caused by invasive disease in immunocompromised patients.

Diagnosis

Usually by culture of stool or urine. Culture of blood will be useful during fever or material from foci of infection.

MANAGEMENT

Normal management of a child with an infective diarrhoeal disease applies (see Chapter 18). Treatment with antibiotics is not recommended unless there is severe systemic illness or the child is one of the groups of children with conditions that make them susceptible to *Salmonella* disease (see Epidemiology, above). It will not shorten the duration of disease or excretion of infective organisms. Ampicillin, chloramphenicol, co-trimoxazole, ceftriaxone or ciprofloxacin may be used for invasive disease, and the choice may be guided by the sensitivity of the organism as well as the age and clinical condition of the child. Antidiarrhoeal agents should not be used as they may prolong the period of infectivity.

PREVENTION OF FURTHER CASES (see also Chapter 33)

Important measures include good hygiene and proper methods for food production, preparation and cooking. Uncooked eggs should not be used in food and all poultry should be well cooked. Reptiles are a potent source of infection and are not suitable pets for young children. Infected children should be excluded from day-care facilities until the risk of infection is minimal. In schools the provision of well-maintained and provisioned toilet facilities is essential. A long course of ciprofloxacin has been shown to clear carriage in adult carriers but evidence is lacking in children where the use of this unlicensed drug may not be appropriate in this setting. Food handlers need to be excluded from work until they are shown to be noninfectious by three negative stools. Referral of positive isolates to the central reference laboratory is important for detecting common source outbreaks and contamination. The PHLS laboratory in England and Wales with special diagnostic services for *Salmonella* and other food-borne infections is the Laboratory for Enteric Pathogens, Central Public Health Laboratory, Colindale, tel. 020 8200 4400. With CDSC, this coordinates a multicountry surveillance network for gastrointestinal pathogens (ENTERNET) to detect international outbreaks across the European Union.

96 Scabies

ORGANISM

Sarcoptes scabiei is a mite.

EPIDEMIOLOGY

Transmission

Transmission is by prolonged skin-to-skin contact. Scabies can be a sexually transmitted disease.

Incubation period

In the first infestation this may be several weeks. It is shorter in subsequent infections.

NATURAL HISTORY AND CLINICAL FEATURES

After mating, the female mite burrows into the skin and lays one to three eggs daily along a linear track. She dies after 4–5 weeks in the burrow. After 3–5 days the eggs hatch into larvae, which grow and become nymphs on the surface. They reach maturity in 2–3 weeks, mate and repeat the cycle. Outside infancy the areas most affected tend to be the interdigital spaces, wrists, elbows, ankles, buttocks, groins, genitalia and areola. The rash consists of vesicles, weals, papules, the burrows themselves and a superimposed dermatitis. In infancy the palms, soles, head and neck are often infected. Bullae and pustules may be present, while there may be no burrows. Because the pruritus is so extreme, the skin changes resulting from scratching may obscure the underlying lesions.

Diagnosis

The presence of burrows is almost diagnostic. Mites and ova can be seen in scrapings from burrows, eczematous lesions and fresh papules. In immunosuppressed patients, there may be a generalised dermatitis with scaling and even vesiculation and crusting ('Norwegian scabies').

MANAGEMENT

Malathion or permethrin, as an aqueous preparation, should be applied to the whole body and left for a day without rinsing. A second application may be necessary after 3 days.

PREVENTION OF FURTHER CASES

Careful laundering of clothes and bedding is important. Treatment of family members and sexual contacts is recommended.

97 Shigellosis

Dysentery (diarrhoea with pus) is a notifiable condition

ORGANISM

Shigellas are Gram-negative bacilli in the family Enterobacteriaceae with a number of species: *Shigella sonnei*, *S. flexneri*, *S. dysenteriae* and *S. boydii*. *S. sonnei* and *S. flexneri* provide most of the cases in the UK.

EPIDEMIOLOGY

Shigella spp. are present worldwide with humans as the reservoir of infection. Most cases are in children, although cases are uncommon under 6 months of age. In the early 1990s there was an increase in the numbers of cases in the UK. Outbreaks occur particularly in families, day-care facilities and primary schools. Children and adults with severe learning difficulties are at particular risk of involvement in transmission because of the difficulty of maintaining hygiene. Cases also occur in adults where hygiene is poor. Worldwide it is thought that shigellas are responsible for around half a million child deaths.

Transmission

Shigella spp. are some of the most highly infectious organisms known and only a few organisms may result in transmission. It is thought that as few as 10 organisms can result in disease. Faeces are the source of infection through faecal–oral transmission. Occasionally, transmission occurs through food or drink when they are faecally contaminated. The period of infectivity is during symptoms and up to 4 weeks in the untreated patient, although risk of transmission decreases considerably as the diarrhoea subsides. Asymptomatic infection occurs and rarely carriers are found who seem to remain infectious for months. However if they are asymptomatic and able to apply simple hygiene precautions they can be regarded as noninfectious. Appropriate antibiotic treatment (see below) renders the patient uninfectious in 5 days.

Incubation period

1–3 days (longer for some *Shigella* species).

NATURAL HISTORY AND CLINICAL FEATURES

The infection may be mild with only gastrointestinal symptoms or it may extend to constitutional involvement. Consequently there may only be diarrhoea, perhaps with abdominal cramps (vomiting is unusual) or abdominal tenderness. Diarrhoea may contain pus (dysentery) or it may be watery or contain blood. Constitutional signs include fever, headache and general malaise. Fever may cause febrile convulsions. Unusual complications include gut perforation and, with *S. flexneri*, Reiter's syndrome.

Diagnosis

Stool specimens or rectal swabs will normally be sufficient for culture diagnosis. However, routine laboratory methods are relatively insensitive and may miss a significant proportion of asymptomatic cases. The PHLS laboratory with special diagnostic service for *Shigella* is at the Laboratory for Enteric Pathogens, Central Public Health Laboratory, Colindale, tel. 020 8200 4400.

MANAGEMENT

Normal management of a child with an infective diarrhoeal disease applies (see Chapter 18). Treatment with antibiotics is recommended if there is systemic illness and may be of some value in shortening the length of the illness and making the case noninfectious to others. A 5-day course of oral ampicillin is usually sufficient, although ampicillin resistance occurs and co-trimoxazole is an alternative. Hospitalisation is usually avoided because of the risk of infecting other patients. If cases have to go into hospital they should be isolated and enteric precautions applied (see Chapter 32). Antidiarrhoeal agents should not be used as they may prolong the period of infectivity.

PREVENTION OF FURTHER CASES (see also Chapter 33)

Good hygiene is essential, with hand-washing an important feature. The most important control features are the provision of toilet facilities (including toilet paper) and thorough hand-washing after use of toilets and before meals, using soap and warm water. Where at all practical, children should be excluded from day-care facilities until the risk of infection is minimal. In schools the provision of well-maintained and provisioned toilet facilities are essential (shigellosis is one of the few infections that can be acquired from toilet seats). Very occasionally, in families where hygiene cannot be guaranteed, it is necessary to issue antibiotic therapy to all members so as to break cycles of reinfection but this should be a last resort. Food handlers need to be excluded from work until noninfectious. Consultants in Communicable Disease Control or their equivalents will advise.

98 Staphylococcal infections

ORGANISM

Staphylococci are Gram-positive bacteria.

Staphylococcus aureus produces a coagulase enzyme (coagulase-positive staphylococcus). Coagulase-negative staphylococci include a number of species including *S. epidermidis*. Methicillin-resistant *S. aureus* (MRSA) mainly causes nosocomial infection.

EPIDEMIOLOGY

Staphylococci are common surface colonisers of humans. *S. aureus* is found in the nares or on the skin in up to 50% of individuals and in nearly all children with atopic eczema. *S. epidermidis* is part of the normal 'resident' skin flora in all individuals and is also found on mucosal surfaces.

Compromised defences, either local or generalised, lead to infection with these organisms. The proportion of *S. aureus* isolates that are MRSA has been rising in the UK in recent years. MRSA particularly affects surgical patients and the elderly. Recent reports record the emergence of vancomycin-resistant *S. aureus* (VRSA), a worrying development. Coagulase-negative staphylococci are the commonest cause of infections associated with implanted foreign materials – central venous lines, cerebrospinal fluid shunts, orthopaedic or cardiac prostheses – see Chapter 13.

Outbreaks of *S. aureus* infection may be caused by particularly virulent strains such as those producing toxins, as in toxic epidermolysis of infants (scalded skin syndrome).

Enterotoxins produced by *S. aureus* are among the commonest agents causing food poisoning.

Transmission

Many staphylococcal infections are caused by the body's own endogenous bacteria. Transmission between individuals can occur by close contact especially via the hands.

Incubation period

1–10 days for scalded skin syndrome and impetigo.

NATURAL HISTORY AND CLINICAL FEATURES

S. aureus most commonly causes superficial infection in the form of boils, paronychia, impetigo or wound infections. Skin disorders such as eczema predispose to such infections. Invasion beyond the skin, which is relatively rare, may result in suppurative localised lymphadenitis and further invasion leads to deep infection such as septicaemia, pneumonia, osteomyelitis, septic arthritis, endocarditis or deep organ abscess. Staphylococcal pneumonia produces characteristic cavitating lesions and empyema. Deep-seated infections are more common in immunocompromised patients but are not exclusive to this group.

Toxin-producing *S. aureus* may result in scalded skin syndrome (Ritter's disease) through release of an epidermolysin, which produces general effects though the initiating infection may be very localised and minor. Other toxin-producing *S. aureus* strains can lead to toxic shock syndrome (see Chapter 9). Staphylococcal food poisoning results from the ingestion of food contaminated with preformed enterotoxins elaborated by toxigenic strains of *S. aureus*. It has a very short incubation period (30 minutes to 6 hours) and typically causes profuse vomiting and abdominal cramps with or without diarrhoea.

Coagulase-negative staphylococci are of relatively low pathogenicity. However in those with implanted foreign materials (prostheses, central lines, etc.) they may cause deep infections, including septicaemia and endocarditis. Slime-producing species result in indolent infections that are extremely difficult to eliminate with antibiotic therapy and can only be cured by the removal of the foreign body. Coagulase-negative staphylococci are the commonest cause of sepsis in premature newborns (see Chapter 4) and in immunocompromised individuals.

S. saprophyticus can cause urinary tract infections, mainly in those with urological problems.

Diagnosis

Gram stain and culture are the standard tests. Cultured staphylococci are then further identified by the coagulase test. Anti-staphylococcal-antibody tests for both *S. aureus* and coagulase-negative staphylococci are available but have relatively low sensitivity for detecting invasive disease in children.

Phage typing and toxin identification are useful in suspected toxic shock or scalded skin syndrome.

MANAGEMENT

Localised *S. aureus* infection often requires surgical drainage of the abscess. In systemic infection antibiotic therapy is required. Most (95%) *S. aureus* strains are β-lactamase producers and therefore penicillin-resistant. Flucloxacillin is the treatment of choice but other useful agents include sodium fusidate, gentamicin, clindamycin, rifampicin and the glycopeptides vancomycin and teicoplanin. In deep-seated infection prolonged courses (several weeks) are required. The glycopeptides are the treatment of choice for MRSA.

Coagulase-negative staphylococcal infections require intravenous antibiotic therapy with or without removal of any infected foreign body. Multiple antibiotic resistance is common and so glycopeptides should be used as first-line treatment.

PREVENTION OF FURTHER CASES

Strict hand-washing procedures in newborn nurseries and in the care of surgical patients should be routine. In outbreaks of staphylococcal disease, e.g. of scalded skin syndrome, isolation and cohorting is necessary.

Screening for MRSA carriage is advisable on transferring patients between hospitals. Those identified as positive, particularly if they have desquamative skin disease or discharging wounds, should be isolated. Elimination of MRSA carriage may be attempted in selected patients/staff members using topical antistaphylococcal agents such as mupirocin.

Patients with recurrent furunculosis should be treated with topical anti-staphylococcal agents such as chlorhexidine soap and shampoo and nasal carrier cream (chlorhexidine or mupirocin).

Meticulous attention to aseptic technique during insertion and subsequent handling of central venous lines and during surgical implant procedures reduces coagulase-negative staphylococcal infection. Short courses of prophylactic glycopeptides to cover insertion of foreign bodies, although widely used, are of unproven value. There are concerns that such practices might encourage the emergence of vancomycin-resistant enterococci (VRE) in hospitals. In future, impregnation of implants with combinations of antimicrobials at the time of manufacture is a likely development and will hopefully reduce the incidence of colonisation and infection.

Avoidance of food handling by individuals with active staphylococcal infections and the rapid refrigeration of foods after cooking are measures that reduce the risk of staphylococcal food poisoning.

If there is an outbreak of MRSA or a hospital has high levels, expert advice should be sought, starting with the infection control team (hospital) or the Consultant in Communicable Disease Control (community).

99 Streptococcal infection

STREPTOCOCCUS PYOGENES

ORGANISM

Streptococcus pyogenes (group A), is a Gram-positive coccus and β-haemolytic. There are about 80 different types characterised by different M proteins in the cell wall, which act to stick the bacteria to host cells. Certain types are associated with rheumatic fever (1, 3, 5, 6, 12, 14, 17, 18) and others with acute glomerulonephritis (1, 4, 12, 49).

EPIDEMIOLOGY

Infections occur worldwide, although impetigo is more common in tropical countries and in the northern hemisphere. Streptococcal pharyngitis and scarlet fever are more common in the autumn and winter months. During outbreaks of streptococcal pharyngitis asymptomatic carriage may occur in up to 50% of children. Toxic shock syndrome (see Chapter 9) may be a result of streptococcal infection.

Transmission

Pharyngitis and scarlet fever result from contact with a person who has active streptococcal pharyngitis; carriers do not appear to transmit infection.

There is no evidence that fomites are a source of infection. Occasionally, food-borne spread can occur. Impetigo results from skin-to-skin transmission of streptococci. When untreated, infectivity lasts for 7–21 days. With antibiotics this is less, 1–2 days, but some children have pharyngeal colonisation for weeks or months and may be contagious for much of this time.

Incubation period

This is 12 h–5 days for streptococcal pharyngitis and ?7–10 days for impetigo.

NATURAL HISTORY AND CLINICAL FEATURES

The most common manifestation is a purulent tonsillitis or pharyngitis. Complications of this include suppurative cervical lymphadenopathy. In young children under the age of 3, infection may result in a low-grade fever with anorexia and cervical lymphadenopathy. In the older child scarlet fever may develop with pharyngitis and a characteristic rash produced by an erythrogenic toxin. The rash develops during the first day of fever, is a deep red in colour and quickly becomes generalised. Lesions are punctate – the size of pinheads, and give the skin a sandpaper like texture. There is a generalised erythema of the face and forehead but the area around the mouth is spared (circumoral pallor). Fever peaks on the second day and in untreated infection persists for another 3–4 days. The tonsils are enlarged and covered with exudate (if present). There are characteristic changes to the tongue: for 1–2 days the dorsum is covered in a white fur; the papillae become red and thickened, protruding through the coat to produce the white strawberry tongue. By the fourth or fifth day the white coat disappears, leaving a red strawberry tongue (see Plate 6). Petechiae can be seen on the palate during the illness.

Impetigo is seen in children with eczema. Streptococcal cellulitis, characterised by a dark red induration of the skin, occurs when *S. pyogenes* enters via a break in the skin following trauma or frequently through open varicella lesions. Lymphatic spread of infection in streptococcal cellulitis results in the characteristic red streaks of lymphangitis.

In children who develop rheumatic fever, which is very rare, there is usually a history of tonsillitis or pharyngitis in the previous few weeks. Glomerulonephritis may follow skin sepsis, cellulitis or impetigo. This may present with haematuria, oliguria, oedema and hypertension. In most children this recovers spontaneously.

Diagnosis

A throat swab culture is the most useful indicator of streptococcal infection in tonsillitis and suspected scarlet fever. Streptococcal throat infections cannot be distinguished from viral infections on clinical grounds. An important disease to be considered in the differential diagnosis of scarlet fever is Kawasaki disease. Skin swab culture may be indicated for impetigo. Antigen detection tests are available but many are of high sensitivity and low specificity. Antistreptococcal antibody tests may be useful in the diagnosis of post-streptococcal glomerulonephritis.

MANAGEMENT

Penicillin V is the treatment of choice for children with streptococcal infection. Erythromycin or a cephalosporin are acceptable in the presence of penicillin allergy. Research in the 1950s showed that the risk of rheumatic fever was reduced if penicillin treatment was given for 14 days but shorter courses were not evaluated and a 5-day course may well be sufficient. Although it is recommended that streptococcal tonsillitis is treated with antibiotics, the need for this in areas where rheumatic fever does not occur is questionable.

Treatment of streptococcal impetigo and cellulitis is with penicillin; prolonged intravenous courses (up to 14 days) may be needed in cases of cellulitis.

Treatment of acute glomerulonephritis includes penicillin during the illness, with symptomatic treatment – fluid restriction, bed rest and antihypertensive drugs if necessary.

STREPTOCOCCUS AGALACTIAE (GROUP B STREPTO-COCCUS, GBS) (See also Chapter 4)

ORGANISM

This is a Gram-positive coccus and is β-haemolytic.

EPIDEMIOLOGY

This organism colonises the genital tract of up to 15% of pregnant women in the UK and may be a cause of chorioamnionitis. Early-onset streptococcal infection in the newborn occurs in about 1% of colonised women. There are five main serotypes, I–V; serotype III is the commonest cause of neonatal infection.

Infections caused by group B streptococci are the commonest cause of bacterial pneumonia and meningitis in the newborn. Disease is generally classified into early (first week of birth) and late (more than one week) GBS disease. The epidemiology is poorly described in the UK but combining estimates from small studies gives a range of 0.60–0.85/1000 births.

Transmission

Transmission to the newborn occurs in utero or during delivery. Nosocomial infection also occurs.

Incubation period

About 3 days, although it may be shorter.

NATURAL HISTORY AND CLINICAL FEATURES

Infection presents in a number of different ways; early-onset infection (during the first few days) may be associated with pneumonia, which produces tachypnoea and respiratory distress. It is often accompanied by septicaemia with hypothermia, or pyrexia and hypotension. In the preterm infant there may be little to distinguish streptococcal pneumonia from respiratory distress syndrome from surfactant deficiency. Meningitis may be a feature of early-onset infection but when it occurs after the first few days of life the illness has a more insidious onset and is less likely to be associated with septicaemia. Features of meningitis have been discussed in the section on neonatal infection. Other types of late-onset disease include arthritis, osteomyelitis and abscess formation. Although most infections occur in the first month, they may occur at any time during infancy.

Diagnosis

By culture or antigen-detection tests.

MANAGEMENT

Treatment is with benzylpenicillin, ampicillin or a cephalosporin. It is difficult to exclude a diagnosis of this infection on clinical grounds in the newborn, and so antibiotic treatment should be considered for any baby with respiratory distress. Studies in the USA have shown that the risk of streptococcal infection in the newborn is reduced when mothers with risk factors for such infection (spontaneous preterm onset of labour, prolonged rupture of membranes, maternal fever and a previously infected baby) are given high-dose ampicillin before delivery (2 g 4-hourly) – see Further reading in Chapter 4, p. 30. Although there may be indications for maternal screening in some populations, this is not yet generally recommended in the British population, where the overall prevalence of GBS, and therefore the cost-effectiveness of screening or a risk factor approach, are unclear. One consensus view at this stage is that intrapartum antibiotics should be given to women with risk factors and a Best Practice Guide has been issued by a broad-based PHLS Working Group on GBS. There is no indication for the administration of antibiotics to well infants colonised at birth.

VIRIDANS STREPTOCOCCI

ORGANISM

These Gram-positive cocci are named viridans because they are α-haemolytic (i.e. turn blood agar green). There are at least 21 different species but five have an animal host and can spread to humans (e.g. *S. bovis*). All are part of the normal flora (usually of the mouth and upper airways) and are subdivided into the *mitis* group (e.g. *S. oralis*, *S. pneumoniae*, *S. mitis*), the *salivarius* group (e.g. *S. salivarius*), the *mutans* group (e.g. *S. mutans*, *S. sobrinus*), the *bovis* group (e.g. *S. bovis*, *S. equinus*) and the *milleri* group (e.g. *S. anginosus*, *S. intermedius*).

EPIDEMIOLOGY

The *mutans* group of streptococci is implicated in the development of dental caries. This results from their saccharolytic activities, which release acid and cause demineralisation of the teeth.

The viridans streptococci most frequently isolated from cases of subacute endocarditis are *S. sanguis* (32% of isolates), *S. oralis* (30%) and *S. gordonii* (13%). They are particularly associated with pre-existing valvular damage (congenital or rheumatic fever). Surgical procedures in the mouth such as tooth extraction, apicectomy, teeth scaling or periodontal surgery cause transient bacteraemia. The viridans streptococci have a particular ability to adhere to platelets, fibronectin, fibrinogen and laminin, which are present on damaged cardiac tissue. If adults and children are considered together it is estimated that there are 20 cases of infective endocarditis per 10^6 population of England and Wales, with a mortality rate of about 20%.

Transmission

These streptococci are derived from the patient's own normal flora.

NATURAL HISTORY, CLINICAL FEATURES, MANAGEMENT AND PREVENTION

See Chapter 17.

STREPTOCOCCUS PNEUMONIAE (PNEUMOCOCCUS)

ORGANISM

Streptococcus pneumoniae, a capsulate α-haemolytic Gram-positive coccus also known as the pneumococcus.

EPIDEMIOLOGY

This is the usual cause of lobar pneumonia and common cause of acute pleural effusion in childhood. It is a cause of meningitis from the neonatal period into adulthood. Many individuals are carriers of the organism in the upper respiratory tract; disease occurs in association with a viral upper respiratory tract infection or in the presence of a particularly virulent strain (e.g. capsular serogroups 1, 6, 14). Certain groups of children are at high risk of severe infection. These include those with nephrotic syndrome, varicella, sickle-cell anaemia or after splenectomy. Patients with congenital or acquired immunodeficiency are also at risk.

Transmission

Transmission is from droplets of respiratory-tract secretions or recently soiled handkerchiefs and is associated with acute otitis media. Infectivity is low in most cases and isolation is not required.

Incubation period

1–3 days.

NATURAL HISTORY AND CLINICAL FEATURES

Pneumococcal pneumonia is normally lobar. Infection in the right upper lobe may be associated with meningism and lower-lobe infection with abdominal pain. Meningitis caused by *S. pneumoniae* cannot be distinguished on clinical grounds from that caused by *Neisseria meningitidis* or *Haemophilus influenzae*, although the onset may be more gradual than with the other two agents. Long-term complications (physical handicap and sensorineural deafness) occur more commonly following pneumococcal meningitis.

Recurrent episodes of meningitis suggest immunodeficiency or a defect in the coverings of the central nervous system, which may or may not be associated with chronic leakage of cerebrospinal fluid. Septicaemia may occur in the immunodepressed and in children with functional asplenia. Occult bacteraemia may be associated with febrile convulsions. Pneumococci are also an important cause of otitis media, mastoiditis, osteomyelitis and arthritis.

Diagnosis

This is by identification of Gram-positive diplococci on Gram stain or following culture. Blood cultures may be helpful and a polymorphonuclear leukocytosis is characteristic. Rapid diagnostic antigen-detection tests are available (latex agglutination) but there is no evidence that they are any more sensitive than culture methods.

MANAGEMENT

Benzylpenicillin (150 mg/kg/day, 4-hourly) is the drug of choice for severe infections in childhood, with a minimum of 10 days recommended for meningitis and longer courses in the presence of effusions or in high-risk groups. Penicillin-resistant pneumococci are present with varying prevalences in many parts of the world. Those of intermediate resistance (minimum inhibitory concentration 0.1–1.0 mg/L) causing meningitis will not respond to penicillin therapy. Treatment should be with a third-generation cephalosporin such as cefotaxime or ceftriaxone, or vancomycin if the organisms is also cephalosporin-resistant (see Chapter 10).

Intravenous penicillin or oral amoxycillin are recommended for lobar pneumonia in childhood. So close is the association with *S. pneumoniae* that treatment should be started before identification of the organism, although a blood culture should be done first. When there is a clear history of penicillin allergy (rare in children) erythromycin can be given. Penicillin resistance has been described but is very unusual in the UK (5% of isolates) and there is little evidence of a poor response to therapy in infection with intermediate resistant pneumococci.

PREVENTION

Children in the risk groups should be given pneumococcal vaccine and prophylactic penicillin. These include children with nephrotic syndrome, sickle cell disease, post-splenectomy and with HIV infection.

The current vaccine contains 25 of the most frequently isolated capsular serotypes but these are T-cell-independent antigens and the vaccine is poorly protective in young children. A conjugate vaccine incorporating the seven most frequent disease-causing capsular serotypes has recently become available in the USA.

STREPTOCOCCUS MILLERI

ORGANISM

This is a group of usually α-haemolytic Gram-positive cocci associated with purulent infections. The group comprises *S. anginosus*, *S. constellatus* and *S. intermedius*.

EPIDEMIOLOGY

All are part of the normal oral flora and cause disease when they move from their colonisation sites to deeper tissues. *S. intermedius* is particularly associated with brain and liver abscesses and *S. anginosus* with abscesses of genitourinary and gastrointestinal origin.

NATURAL HISTORY AND CLINICAL FEATURES

These streptococci, either alone or with other bacteria, cause dental, brain, liver, abdominal and pelvic abscesses. There are no particular clinical features that distinguish such abscesses caused by *S. milleri* from those due to other bacteria. The presentation and course of infection depend upon the site of the abscess.

Diagnosis

Diagnosis of the abscess will depend upon clinical suspicion and demonstration of the site by imaging techniques such as magnetic resonance imaging, computed tomography or radionuclide-tagged neutrophils. Bacteriological diagnosis will require examination of the pus by microscopy and culture.

MANAGEMENT AND PREVENTION

The *milleri* group streptococci are still penicillin-sensitive and this should be the treatment of choice. For blind empirical therapy prior to results of culture and sensitivity metronidazole should be added, since mixed infection with anaerobes is not uncommon. The abscess must be drained.

There are no specific preventative measures.

ENTEROCOCCUS FAECALIS AND E. FAECIUM

These organisms may be the cause of invasive disease in the newborn and in childhood, producing infections in the urinary tract as well as meningitis and endocarditis. The organisms show reduced sensitivity to penicillin and are inherently resistant to cephalosporins. Vancomycin-resistant enterococci (VRE) are an increasing and worrying cause of infections in hospitalised (often immunocompromised) patients. Combination therapy guided by in-vitro sensitivity testing may be required, with either ampicillin, vancomycin or teicoplanin and an aminoglycoside. The new combination agent quinupristin/dalfopristin can be used for treating invasive disease due to *E. faecium* (but not *E. faecalis*).

100 Syphilis (congenital and acquired) and nonvenereal treponematoses

SYPHILIS

ORGANISM

Treponema pallidum ssp. *pallidum*, a spirochaetal bacterium.

EPIDEMIOLOGY

These infections occur only in humans. Syphilis is endemic in many low-income countries. Serological studies in Africa suggest infection in 2–20% of pregnant women. A resurgence of adult and congenital infection in the USA began in the 1980s, particularly in blacks in large cities and more recently in rural areas in the south-eastern USA. The risk factor for adult infection was drug use. The major reason for congenital infection is lack of screening of the mother during antenatal care (syphilis screening), usually because of failure of the mother to receive any antenatal care. Levels of infection in the UK are considered to be low for adult infection (300–400 cases per annum, although numbers of adult cases rose in 1997 and 1999) and very low for congenital infection.

Transmission

Vertical transmission occurs in later pregnancy from mothers with untreated or inadequately treated syphilis. Infection in children is otherwise very unusual until they become sexually active. Vertical transmission rate varies with the stage of maternal infection. If the mother is untreated, it is 40–50% in primary, secondary or early latent syphilis and 10% in late latent syphilis. Acquired syphilis occurs through sexual intercourse and transmission can take place through blood transfusions.

Incubation period

Unknown. Congenital disease often commences in utero.

NATURAL HISTORY AND CLINICAL FEATURES

If the mother's infection is untreated, there is a considerable probability of any pregnancy resulting in a miscarriage or stillbirth and the infant death rate is doubled (Table 100.1). Untreated congenital syphilis can be a severe disease affecting many organs. Infected infants may present nonspecifically with hepatosplenomegaly, lymphadenopathy, skeletal abnormalities, skin rash, anaemia, jaundice, low birth weight, premature birth or neonatal death. However, approximately two-thirds of live-born infected infants do not have any signs or symptoms at birth but present over the following weeks, months or years. Because of this, the infection is usually subdivided into early congenital syphilis, presenting in children under 2 years old, and late congenital syphilis, which presents in older children or adulthood. Late congenital syphilis may result in neurological disease, skeletal abnormalities or, more rarely, cardiac disease. Because of these multiple presentations a serological test is appropriate for a variety of presentations.

Women with syphilis	Premature, neonatal death or stillbirth (%)	Syphilitic infant (%)	Nonsyphilitic infant (%)
Primary or secondary syphilis	50	50	0
Early latent syphilis	40	40	20
Late latent syphilis	20	10	70

Table 100.1 Effect of untreated syphilis on pregnancy outcomes (Source: PHLS *Report on Syphilis in Pregnancy*, 1998)

Diagnosis

The definitive positive test is dark field microscopy of exudate showing treponemes. However, usually the first test will be a specific serological test such as a *Treponema pallidum* haemagglutination assay (TPHA) or an IgG or IgM enzyme-linked immunosorbent assay (ELISA) or fluorescent treponemal antigen. Reagin test (e.g. VDRL) or IgM ELISAs will suggest recent infection.

Interpretation of test data in children is difficult and for adults is even more complex and specialist advice should be taken. Colleagues in genitourinary medicine should be involved and in England a laboratory reference service is provided free by the PHLS by the laboratories in Birmingham, Bristol (lead), Manchester, Newcastle and Sheffield.

MANAGEMENT

Treponemes remain sensitive to parenteral penicillin. For infants, aqueous penicillin is recommended – 100 000 units/kg/day given every 8–12 hours for 10 days. Mothers with primary, secondary or early latent syphilis should receive a prolonged course of parenteral penicillin, although for mothers where there are difficulties in follow-up an alternative is a single dose of 2.4 million units of benzathine (long-acting penicillin). However, this use is not licensed in the UK (although it is standard in the USA) and mothers have to receive treatment with benzathine penicillin on a named patient basis.

PREVENTION

Routine antenatal syphilis screening of each pregnancy has been recommended by the Public Health Laboratory Service and will probably be supported by the National Screening Committee.

NONVENEREAL TREPONEMATOSES – YAWS, BEJEL AND PINTA

These are a group of treponemal infections endemic among rural populations in tropical countries (the Amazon Basin, west and central Africa, south-east Asia and Indonesia). They are much less prevalent than in the past as a result of mass treatment campaigns that took place in the 1960s and 1970s and the widespread use of antibiotics in the tropics. The causative organism is indistinguishable from *Treponema pallidum* causing syphilis and includes the same serological response. Transmission is primarily thought to be by direct physical contact between children. Characteristically, yaws and pinta initially show papillomatous skin lesions while with bejel the first lesions are in the mouth. Yaws and bejel can occasionally proceed to destructive gummas of the bones and skin. Treatment is as for acquired syphilis.

101 Tetanus

Notifiable disease

ORGANISM

Clostridium tetani, a spore-forming anaerobic Gram-positive bacillus. In its spore form it is to be found ubiquitously in soils. It produces a potent exotoxin, which acts on the nervous system.

EPIDEMIOLOGY

In the UK and most European countries almost all women of childbearing age are immune, so that antitoxin antibodies are transmitted to the fetus by the transplacental route. Neonatal tetanus has been eliminated from the UK and elsewhere in western Europe. In 1998 only nine cases were reported in England and Wales. Apart from one 20-year-old man, all were men over 40. Most such cases are in older persons who would not have been immunised.

The picture is very different in many low-income countries, where tetanus immunisation is not routinely performed and so there is no maternal protection for newborns. Neonatal tetanus is a relatively important cause of infant mortality in less developed countries, because of unhygienic birth practices and inadequate care of the umbilical cord stump. In 1997 an estimated 355 000 cases of neonatal tetanus occurred worldwide, with 248 000 deaths, a mortality rate of under 3 per 1000 live births. However 20 countries (all in south or south-east Asia and Africa) account for 90% of these cases. The World Health Organization's global goal (adopted in 1993) is to reduce the incidence of neonatal tetanus to less than 1 death per 1000 births.

Transmission

This is by the direct transfer of spores of *C. tetani*, which can be found in soil, and the excreta of animals and humans.

Incubation period

This can range from 4 days to 3 weeks: the length is dependent on the infecting dose and the severity of the injury, with more severe injuries resulting in a shorter period.

NATURAL HISTORY AND CLINICAL FEATURES

Following contamination of traumatised tissue, burns or the umbilical stump, spores multiply in anaerobic conditions and produce tetanus toxin, which causes powerful muscle contractions, extreme irritability and death. Case fatality rates in neonates are high.

Diagnosis

This is on clinical grounds. Although infection is more possible in extensive wounds, the wound/site of entry may be trivial. Bacterial culture is positive only in a small proportion of cases.

MANAGEMENT

Exposed patient

If a wound is minor and clean and a full immunisation course for age has been given (see below), no further action is needed. If the wound is more serious and tetanus-prone (contaminated with dirt, puncture wound, containing substantial amounts of dead tissue or with evidence of sepsis) a tetanus toxoid booster should be considered even if the last booster was within 10 years. The wound will also require surgical attention and antibiotic treatment should be considered if there is sepsis. Human tetanus immune globulin (HTIG) is not indicated unless the wound is tetanus-prone and it is known that an exposed patient is unimmunised, or if they are underimmunised (last tetanus toxoid more than 10 years previously) or their immunisation status is uncertain, in which case a dose of HTIG is given in the contralateral limb to the toxoid.* Patients known to be suffering from impaired immunity are also given a dose of HTIG.

Patient with tetanus

If a diagnosis of tetanus is made specialist help should be sought. This includes tetanus immune globulin (150 IU/kg given in multiple sites), benzylpenicillin (100 000 units/kg/day) for 10–14 days, surgical-wound debridement where indicated and supportive medical management. Diazepam has proved beneficial in treating neonatal tetanus.

PREVENTION OF FURTHER CASES

This is achieved in high-income countries by ensuring adequate tetanus immunity through immunisation. By 1 year, every child should have had three doses of toxoid within diphtheria, tetanus and pertussis vaccine (DTP). A booster of DT is given at or around school entry (age 4) and a reinforcing booster of tetanus toxoid (T) or tetanus and adult-dose diphtheria (Td) before leaving school. These five doses are sufficient for travel abroad. It is considered that two further boosters at 10-year intervals will give full protection (i.e. the maximum tetanus vaccination is seven).

---

* **A guide for older patients is that, since immunisation began routinely in 1961, patients born before that date are unlikely to have been immunised as infants. Men will have been immunised if they were in the armed forces.**

Thayaparan B, Nicoll A (1998) Prevention and control of tetanus in childhood. Curr Opin Pediatr 10: 4–8.

102 Threadworms

ORGANISM

Enterobius vermicularis, also called pinworm, is a small (circumference 1 mm), white worm.

EPIDEMIOLOGY

Threadworms affect all ages throughout the world, especially preschool children. Infection is common in the UK.

Transmission is predominantly faecal–oral. Eggs may be carried under fingernails and on clothing, bedding or house dust.

Incubation period

The life cycle is 2–6 weeks.

NATURAL HISTORY AND CLINICAL FEATURES

Ingested ova hatch in the stomach and the larvae migrate to the caecum where they mature. The gravid female adult worms lay their eggs at night in the perianal area. This gives rise to the most common symptom, perianal itching, especially at night. Scratching can result in the transfer of eggs to the mouth and hence a cycle of autoinfection. Vulvovaginitis may occur in young girls, giving rise to a vaginal discharge. Tissue invasion does not occur.

Diagnosis

Occasionally the worms may be seen around the anus. The diagnosis is best made by pressing a piece of adhesive over the anus and then examining it with a magnifying glass for the presence of eggs. This test may be negative in the presence of highly suggestive symptoms – in this case treatment should be given.

MANAGEMENT

Treatment consists of a single dose of mebendazole (not to be given to children under 2 years old) or two doses of piperazine 2 weeks apart. Preparations of the latter often contain a laxative, senna, to aid the expulsion of the adult worms. There is a high incidence of reinfection. This can be reduced by keeping the fingernails short and wearing close fitting pants at night to prevent scratching.

PREVENTION OF FURTHER CASES

Strict attention to hygiene will prevent infection. Chemoprophylaxis is also necessary for all family members of the index case; although asymptomatic, they may be infected.

103 Toxocariasis

ORGANISM

Toxocara canis and *T. cati* are nematode worms.

EPIDEMIOLOGY

T. canis and *T. cati* are common gut parasites of dogs and cats respectively and occur worldwide. The parasite can be transmitted transplacentally in dogs and therefore puppies as young as 3 weeks old can be infectious. Soil from parks has been shown to contain *Toxocara* eggs in up to 25% of samples. Human disease is predominantly caused by *T. canis* and affects children mainly in the age group 1–6 years old. The prevalence of symptomatic infection is unknown but seroepidemiological studies suggest that 3% or more of children have been exposed to the parasite.

Transmission

Disease is caused by tissue invasion with parasite larvae after ingestion of *Toxocara* eggs. The eggs may be swallowed when a child eats soil (pica) contaminated with infective dog or cat faeces. Other potential sources include play-pit sand and unwashed vegetables contaminated with faeces. The eggs require a 1–3 week incubation period before becoming infective and the infection therefore cannot be transmitted by eating faeces that are fresh.

Incubation period

The acute illness (visceral larva migrans) can occur within a matter of a few weeks or as long as several months after exposure. The form presenting with an ocular granuloma may take up to 10 years to develop.

NATURAL HISTORY AND CLINICAL FEATURES

There are two relatively distinct forms of disease and it is rare for children to progress from one to the other.

Visceral larva migrans (VLM) is a syndrome of fever, hepatomegaly, pulmonary symptoms (wheezing) and signs and eosinophilia, which is often very marked, caused by migrating helminth larvae and the ensuing immune response they provoke. A minority of children also develop splenomegaly and lymphadenopathy. It is most common in children aged 1–3 years old and symptoms can persist for up to a year.

Eye infection (**ocular larva migrans**) is detected in older children, most commonly about the ages of 6–8 when the child's optic fundus is examined because of strabismus or problems with visual acuity. The dead larva causes a granulomatous reaction in the retina, which is most damaging when close to the macula but is fortunately unilateral in most cases.

Diagnosis

VLM is diagnosed clinically on the basis of a multisystem disease accompanied by an eosinophilia, especially in a child who has not been out of northern Europe, although other parasites such as *Fasciola hepatica*, *Gnathostoma spinigerum*, *Ascaris lumbricoides* and *Clonorchis* spp. should also be considered after foreign travel (see Chapter 62). Serum *Toxocara* antibodies may be detected, although not reliably so in the acute infection. Occasionally, *Toxocara* larvae may be found if a liver biopsy is performed.

Ocular toxocariasis is diagnosed clinically from the appearance of the inflammatory mass in the retina, although it may be difficult to distinguish from other retinal problems. Serum antibodies are not always detected in this form of the disease.

MANAGEMENT

Toxocariasis presenting with VLM can be treated with diethylcarbamazine or thiabendazole, although with limited success, and in mild cases it is probably best to treat the child symptomatically only. There may be some benefit in giving steroids to children with severe disease. Antihelminthic drugs are not effective in the ocular form of disease but local or systemic steroids may be of benefit.

PREVENTION

Toxocara infection could be largely prevented if pet owners regularly dewormed cats and dogs and prevented them from defecating in public places. Children's sandpits should be covered after use to prevent cats defecating in them. There is no advantage in giving prophylactic antibiotics if a child has ingested dog or cat faeces.

104 Toxoplasmosis

ORGANISM

Toxoplasma gondii – a protozoon.

EPIDEMIOLOGY

Toxoplasmosis is a common infection. Usually asymptomatic or without serious symptoms, it has serious consequences if it is acquired by pregnant women or immunocompromised patients. Incidence varies considerably between populations. For example, incidence is considered to be high among adults in France, resulting from culturally preferred consumption of uncooked and undercooked meat products. A significant proportion of most communities have usually acquired infection by middle age. However, serological evidence suggest that incidence has been falling recently in a number of industrialised countries.

When the first infection occurs in pregnancy transplacental transmission occurs in around 30% of cases although the risk varies with the stage of pregnancy (see Transmission, below). The incidence of congenital infection is harder to determine, because diagnosis is difficult and because most cases present with choroiditis, which may not become apparent until late childhood. Some of these cases may have resulted from postnatal infection. Every year around 100–300 cases of choroidoretinitis are reported in British patients with *Toxoplasma* antibodies; it is not clear how many of these are caused by *Toxoplasma* infection or at what stage.

A total of 423 reports of toxoplasmosis in pregnancy were received by the Public Health Laboratory Service between 1981 and 1992. The annual rate of toxoplasmosis reported in pregnancy rose in the late 1980s but it is thought that this is due to increased professional awareness rather than increased incidence and that the rate of congenital toxoplasmosis changed little over this period. A survey conducted through the British Paediatric Surveillance Unit survey (1989/90), confirmed and validated by laboratory reports, found an estimated maternal infection rate in pregnancy of 2 per 1000 live births. This indicated a low burden of congenital infection, insufficient to justify routine screening in pregnancy.

Transmission

Acquisition from the environment – toxoplasmosis is a zoonosis. The organism is found worldwide in many mammals. Members of the cat family are the only known definitive host, acquiring the organism from infected prey such as mice. The parasite replicates in the cat intestine and for 2–4 weeks after a primary infection oocysts are excreted in the stool. They then mature for 24–48 hours outside the cat before becoming infective by the oral route. Many other animals – sheep, pigs and cows – also become infected as intermediary hosts. Infected animals develop tissue cysts in muscle and brain, which remain viable for long periods. Humans often become infected from ingestion of poorly cooked meat or milk containing tissue cysts or sporulated oocysts excreted by cats. Transmission from organ transplantation has also occurred but otherwise human-to-human transmission does not occur.

Congenital infection

The risk of mother-to-child transmission has been estimated at around 30% with about 30% of infected infants showing signs or symptoms by age 5 years. However, the risk of transmission and of significant damage to the fetus varies inversely with the stage of pregnancy. Early in pregnancy (the first trimester) the risk of infection is low but infected infants are more commonly affected. Maternal infection late in pregnancy more commonly results in infection of the fetus but signs or symptoms are rare.

The risk of an infected and affected infant is highest (around 10%) between 24 and 30 weeks of pregnancy.

428

Incubation period
7–21 days.

NATURAL HISTORY AND CLINICAL FEATURES

Congenital toxoplasmosis
Many congenital infections are without any signs of symptoms, especially if infection occurs near term. Symptomatic infection is most likely when infection occurs in the first trimester. The classic triad of congenital toxoplasmosis comprises choroidoretinitis, hydrocephalus from aqueduct stenosis and intracranial calcification. It is unusual for the components of the triad to be present together. Other features include rashes, generalised lymphadenopathy, hepatomegaly, splenomegaly, jaundice and thrombocytopenia. There is a high mortality in the most severely affected infants but those surviving may develop epilepsy and mental retardation. Those children with choroidoretinitis may not develop visual impairment until later in childhood or early adulthood.

Acquired toxoplasmosis
Acquired toxoplasmosis may be asymptomatic, although nonspecific symptoms such as fever, sore throat, lymphadenopathy and myalgia may occur. Cervical lymphadenopathy may be a feature of infection. The most serious outcome is in the immunocompromised. In children with severe HIV disease, reactivation of infection may result in cerebral toxoplasmosis.

Diagnosis

Infection in pregnancy (see also Chapter 3)
Diagnosis is generally by serology. A number of specific enzyme-linked immunosorbent assay (ELISA) IgM assays are available that when positive indicate infection over the previous 6 months. In addition, IgA and IgG avidity tests may be used. The *Toxoplasma* dye test and a number of other IgG tests are in use but are now considered to of less value. When there is serological evidence of maternal infection, fetal blood sampling may be used for both serology and culture of *T. gondii*. However, there is a small but definite risk of an adverse outcome from this procedure. Products of conception can also be investigated by parasite isolation or detection using tissue culture, mouse isolation or polymerase chain reaction (PCR).

Congenital infection
This can be detected by serology on blood from the infant. If there is strong suspicion of maternal infection, then serology should be performed for the first year at 3-monthly intervals as antibodies may be slow to rise. When infection is suspected, then cerebral ultrasound should be performed to exclude hydrocephalus and intracranial calcification, and an ophthalmological examination performed.

MANAGEMENT

Infection in pregnancy

Three antibiotics are used in management: spiramycin, pyrimethamine and sulphadiazine. When a diagnosis of recent maternal infection is made, spiramycin should be given, which is thought to reduce the risk of transmission of infection to the fetus. If fetal serology is positive, pyrimethamine, sulphadiazine and folinic acid can be given daily for 3 weeks and then alternated with spiramycin, also for 3 weeks, until delivery. However, reviews of studies of treatment of women seroconverting in pregnancy have failed to show convincing evidence of benefit to the fetus. Because infection during the first trimester carries the highest risk of fetal morbidity, termination following fetal infection is sometimes considered as an option to be discussed with the mother in this situation.

Treatment of the newborn

Following maternal infection during pregnancy, if there is no evidence of infection in the infant either clinically or on serological grounds, spiramycin should be given until 6 months providing that serology remains negative. If the newborn infant is infected, alternating courses of pyrimethamine and sulphadiazine and spiramycin should be given until the age of 1 year.

Treatment of ocular toxoplasmosis with macular involvement in the older child

Pyrimethamine and sulphadiazine with corticosteroids.

Treatment of the immunocompromised child

Specialist advice should be taken if an immunocompromised child is suspected or found to have acquired or reactivated toxoplasmosis. Treatment is generally similar to that of the infected newborn, based on using oral pyrimethamine, sulphadiazine and spiramycin. Clindamycin is sometimes substituted for sulphadiazine, especially for ocular toxoplasmosis. If *Toxoplasma* infection has been confirmed in HIV-infected children some clinicians use maintenance treatment after initial therapy.

PREVENTION

Pregnant women can reduce the risk of infection by cooking meat products thoroughly. They should avoid or exercise caution in contact with cats. By changing cat litter daily, the risk of infection is thought to be reduced.

Screening to prevent congenital disease

Although it has been suggested that pregnant women should be screened for toxoplasmosis in the UK, a Royal College of Obstetricians and Gynaecologists committee concluded in 1992 that this was not appropriate. Screening is, however, routine in other European countries such as France and Austria. An alternative approach has been suggested of screening and treating infected newborns using dried blood spots and comparing the results of these with the result of maternal dried blood spots in pregnancy.

105 Tuberculosis

> **Notifiable disease**

ORGANISM

Tuberculosis is caused by *Mycobacterium tuberculosis* and occasionally *M. bovis* (around 1.5% of isolates). These pleomorphic, weakly Gram-positive bacilli grow slowly in vitro and in vivo. They form stable (fast) complexes with dyes resistant even to the presence of acid and alcohol to show a characteristic red colour when stained with Ziehl–Neelsen stain.

EPIDEMIOLOGY

M. tuberculosis and *M. bovis* are only found in mammalian hosts, unlike nontuberculous mycobacteria, which are commonly found in soil and water. Up to 35% of the world's population are infected, 95% of whom live in low-income countries. It has been estimated that in 1990 7.5 million people developed tuberculosis and 2.5 million people died from the disease. There is no evidence that the burden has diminished since then and it was estimated that, unless control improved, 90 million new cases and 30 million deaths would occur between 1990 and the end of 1999. The incidence of tuberculosis in England and Wales in 1998 was higher (10.9/100 000) than in 1993 (10.1/100 000) and 1988 (9.4/100 000 (adults and children combined). White and Indian subcontinent ethnic groups each accounted for 38% of cases and the black African ethnic group for 13%. Most of the UK rise is accounted for by an increase in London, where numbers rose especially among black Africans.

The incidence varies considerably from one ethnic group to another among children as it does in adults. In the last survey 365 children with tuberculosis were notified during 1998 in England and Wales, a rate of $3.6/10^5$; however, incidence rates ranged from $1.1/10^5$ among white children to $70.6/10^5$ among children whose families originated in the Indian subcontinent (India/Pakistan/Bangladesh). West Indian and all other children showed an intermediate incidence of between $9.0/10^5$ and $23.1/10^5$. The highest rate of $193.4/10^5$ was in children born abroad. Despite these high rates in black African children the most numerous groups were Asian (33%) followed by white (27%) children. Ethnic minority children born in the UK generally seem to be at a relatively lower risk than those born in their country of origin. Tuberculosis is associated with poverty as well as country of origin.

The decline in incidence in the UK this century (see Fig. I.13, p 453) has been attributed largely to rising living standards. The HIV epidemic has contributed to the rising number of cases of tuberculosis in sub-Saharan Africa and has contributed to some of the UK rise. Antimicrobial resistance is a growing problem internationally, although levels are low as yet in the UK.

Transmission

The tubercle bacillus is usually inhaled in small droplets. Young children with the disease are almost always noninfectious. Communicability is highest from untreated pulmonary tuberculosis; however, prolonged close (most often household) contact with an infected adult is usually necessary for transmission. Such adults will nearly always have 'open' tuberculosis (i.e. they are expectorating large numbers of tubercle bacilli from a cavity in the lung). Such cases are usually smear-positive.

Incubation period

The time from exposure to development of the primary complex is 1–3 months. However, because of dormancy and reactivation the period from initial infection to appearance of significant disease can be far longer.

NATURAL HISTORY AND CLINICAL FEATURES

Tuberculous disease progression depends on the balance between bacterial multiplication and host immune responsiveness. On entering the respiratory tract the bacilli settle in peripheral alveoli and are ingested by pulmonary macrophages, which may completely eliminate the mycobacteria with no sign of infection or immune response. In other cases multiplication within macrophages occurs both in the distal site (primary or Ghon focus) and the regional lymph nodes. Activated T lymphocytes surround the infected macrophages, releasing cytokines that should enable the macrophages to kill the organisms in both the primary focus and the regional lymph node, a reaction often associated with the development of fever and tuberculin hypersensitivity. A chest X-ray taken at this stage may show a peripheral lung lesion together with hilar lymphadenopathy, the primary complex. In most cases resolution now occurs, sometimes leaving a calcified Ghon focus and regional lymph nodes, although viable organisms may lie dormant ready to reactivate many years later. Alternatively there is sufficient immunity to prevent distant infection but the disease progresses in the lung with clinical sequelae resulting from destructive immune responses to the organism.

Pulmonary disease is commonest, accounting for 66% of cases in children, of whom about half will have parenchymal lung lesions (with or without enlarged intrathoracic nodes). Progressive hilar lymphadenopathy may obstruct bronchi, leading to collapse or consolidation of the affected lobes; if this obstruction is incomplete and air enters the affected segment more easily than it can leave the segment becomes hyperinflated (ball-valve effect); sometimes, lymph nodes rupture causing a segmental pneumonia or pericarditis. In other children there may be progressive primary tuberculosis resulting in bronchopneumonia from extension of the pulmonary focus, or the disease may progress around a peripheral focus leading to the development of a large pleural effusion.

Alternatively, the disease may spread only in the lymphoid system leading to cervical, supraclavicular or axillary node involvement. During this initial phase of infection haematogenous spread probably occurs but only rarely leads to disease at a distant site. However in 0.5–3% of cases haematogenous spread produces multiple foci of infection, usually within 3–6 months, leading to miliary shadowing seen on chest X-ray and/or tuberculous meningitis. For these reasons young children should be investigated carefully and given early prophylaxis to prevent the potentially catastrophic consequences of disseminated disease. Tuberculosis can affect virtually any part of the body with 20% of affected children developing extrapulmonary lymphadenitis and 5–10 % metastatic lesions in bones or joints, which often do not become apparent until a year or more after infection. Renal disease may not be apparent until 5 or even 20 years after the initial infection.

The spectrum of immunopathological responses to tuberculous infection accounts for its protean clinical manifestations. The slow growth of the organism leads to an insidious onset of symptoms and these features, together with its relatively low incidence, mean that diagnosis is often delayed. Tuberculosis is still surrounded by social stigma and so a positive family or contact history is not often volunteered. Thus a high index of suspicion and direct questions concerning contact with tuberculosis are imperative.

There is a great spectrum of clinical presentation but in pulmonary tuberculosis there is typically fever, weight loss, unilateral hilar lymphadenopathy with or without segmental lung changes or overinflation of a segment. Phlyctenular conjunctivitis, erythema nodosum or pleural effusions in children should be considered to be tuberculous until proven otherwise. Small children with miliary tuberculosis present with nonspecific features such as weight loss, apathy and poor feeding. They may have hepatosplenomegaly and a chest X-ray will show miliary shadowing. Alternative diagnoses such as Langerhans cell histiocytosis or atypical pneumonia are usually considered first. The signs and symptoms of tuberculous meningitis usually evolve over a few weeks with a history of a low-grade fever, headache, vomiting and increasing drowsiness. The chest X-ray may be normal and all too often the diagnosis is not made until there are frank neurological signs, which are unfortunately associated with a very poor long-term outlook.

The finding of choroidal tubercles is a very helpful diagnostic sign in both tuberculous meningitis and miliary tuberculosis, and so careful fundoscopy is essential. In tuberculosis meningitis the cerebrospinal fluid is usually clear and contains 50–410 WBC/mm^3, most of which are lymphocytes; the protein content is raised and the glucose low. Computed tomography often shows a degree of hydrocephalus with contrast enhancement of the brain stem. Focal disease forming tuberculomas may be evident. Bone and joint tuberculosis usually presents with swelling or loss of function, often without signs of acute inflammation and toxicity; X-rays reveal lytic lesions with a sclerotic margin (the spine being affected in over half of cases).

Diagnosis

In adults a previously healed Ghon focus or a new infective lesion in the lung breaks down and forms a cavity containing a large number of acid-fast bacilli that are expectorated (so called postprimary disease). This process is rare before adolescence and so childhood tuberculosis is rarely diagnosed by identifying acid-fast bacilli in a smear of fresh sputum, making diagnosis much more difficult than in adults. Greater reliance has to be placed on clinical and X-ray findings together with the results of tuberculin testing. A culture of *M. tuberculosis* on biopsy will confirm the diagnosis and positive histology is highly suggestive, but if these are not available a suggested set of criteria for making the diagnosis in a child is the presence of two or more of the following:

- A positive tuberculin test
- Clinical findings suggestive of tuberculosis
- A history of contact
- A suggestive chest X-ray.

Tuberculin testing

Two forms of the tuberculin test are commonly used in the UK. The Heaf test is usually used for screening but should not be used for diagnostic purposes.

The Mantoux test is performed by giving an intradermal injection of purified protein derivative of tuberculin, either 10 units (0.1 mL of 1:1000) or 1 unit (0.1 mL of 1:10 000). 10 units should always be used except where there is a likelihood of a very strong hypersensitivity reaction to tuberculin (which includes children with phlyctenular conjunctivitis, erythema nodosum or BCG immunisation within the preceding 12 months). The test should be performed on the volar aspect of the forearm and has only been properly carried out if a bleb has been raised in the skin. It should be read after 48–72 hours by measuring the diameter of induration in millimetres. Only the diameter of the indurated area that can be palpated should be recorded. The area of redness should not be recorded. A reaction of 5 mm or greater is considered positive. Severe reactions should be treated with topical corticosteroids. Mantoux tests are less easy to interpret in children who have had a previous BCG. A 10 mm or greater response can be suggestive of infection in children who have had a previous BCG while a reaction of 15 mm is more indicative. However, some children may give a response of over 15 mm due to BCG alone. A grade II–IV Heaf test is indicative of infection where there is no history of BCG.

Culture and histology

Isolation of *M. tuberculosis* from culture remains the diagnostic gold standard. It is also important to perform antibiotic susceptibility tests. Unfortunately, as infected children usually harbour a small number of organisms, specimens are often negative and in only about 30% of children is the diagnosis confirmed either by culture or if positive histology is available. Early morning gastric washings taken on three successive days remains the best way to obtain specimens from which mycobacteria can be cultured. Bronchoalveolar lavage is less effective, probably because only those mycobacteria that are in one bronchial segment at one time will be found whereas gastric washing specimens contain all the mycobacteria that have been coughed and swallowed overnight. Early morning urine specimens are less useful but may be positive in disseminated tuberculosis. Microscopy is often negative and it can take 6–8 weeks for *M. tuberculosis* to grow on culture (although new liquid culture methods are more rapid). Newer culture techniques that employ DNA hybridisation on cultured material offer the promise of much quicker results in less than 1 week but are not yet generally available. Histological examination of lymph nodes will reveal caseating granulomata and acid-fast bacilli may be demonstrated but such results must be interpreted in the clinical context as it is not possible to distinguish infection with *M. tuberculosis* from atypical mycobacterial infection on histological grounds.

Radiology

Tuberculous infection is suggested by the presence of hilar or mediastinal lymphadenopathy, particularly when it is unilateral. Pulmonary, cervical or abdominal calcification may be a further clue and in children who have disseminated disease the characteristic expanded lucent lesions may be present in many bones even when there is no clinical evidence of disease at that site.

Other diagnostic techniques

There is a great need for quick, reliable and specific diagnostic tests that will detect tuberculosis in children. Detecting mycobacterial DNA by polymerase chain reaction, or mycobacterial lipids by gas liquid chromatography, as well as changes in humoral or cell-mediated responses, may eventually offer useful tests but none is yet available for general clinical use.

MANAGEMENT

Children should be managed by a paediatrician with special experience and training in tuberculosis or by a general paediatrician in conjunction with a suitably trained physician. Children with TB are rarely infectious as cavitating disease is very unusual, and they thus pose no direct risk to other patients. However, in hospital it is wise to nurse them in a cubicle until contact tracing is completed because of the possibility of a relative having smear-positive pulmonary tuberculosis. Older children and adolescents may have smear-positive disease and should be regarded as infectious and isolated in a single room. If the organism is fully sensitive they will normally become noninfectious after 2 weeks of appropriate treatment.

Antituberculous chemotherapy is generally well tolerated in children. Although the present regimens were derived from adult studies, more recent work suggests that the 6-month 'short course chemotherapy' regimen is equally effective in children. This comprises rifampicin and isoniazid for 6 months, supplemented by pyrazinamide for the first 2 months. To cover the possibility of drug resistance, ethambutol should be included in the first 2 months if the child or index case are immigrants, refugees or noncaucasian, have previously been treated for TB, are at risk of being HIV-positive or are contacts of a case with known drug resistance. Treatment should always be directly observed. When adherence is poor or likely to be poor. Directly observed therapy given three times a week is equally effective.

All children should have liver function tests performed at the commencement of therapy; however, even though liver function test abnormalities can sometimes complicate treatment with rifampicin, isoniazid or pyrazinamide, regular monitoring of liver function is not necessary in those with no evidence of pre-existing liver disease. If liver dysfunction does occur, expert advice should be sought and all the drugs should be stopped and then reintroduced sequentially. Peripheral neuropathy complicating isoniazid therapy is rare and pyridoxine supplementation is recommended only in malnourished children and breastfed infants. Skin rashes and (in the case of pyrazinamide treatment) photosensitivity can occasionally occur. The risk of toxic effects of ethambutol in the eye is very low; visual acuity and colour vision should be checked in children of 5 years of age or older and parents should be told to report immediately visual symptoms or changes in vision. Streptomycin is too ototoxic and nephrotoxic for routine use but may be considered along with other 'second-line agents' – cycloserine, capreomycin, amikacin and ciprofloxacin – when there is resistance to front-line agents.

Pulmonary and glandular tuberculosis

In uncomplicated cases the standard regimen is used. Steroid therapy is added when a hilar lymph node is obstructing a bronchus. Expert advice should be sought and it may be necessary to give steroids for 6–8 weeks.

In glandular disease the affected nodes may initially enlarge after commencement of therapy. Persistent failure of cervical lymph node disease to respond may suggest atypical mycobacterial infection (see Chapter 80).

Extrapulmonary tuberculosis, including tuberculous meningitis

There have been few studies of the best treatment for extrapulmonary tuberculosis, particularly tuberculous meningitis. Experience from centres treating many cases suggest good results from the same drug regimen as for pulmonary disease but given for longer, namely rifampicin and isoniazid given for 12 months supplemented by pyrazinamide and a fourth drug, usually ethambutol, for at least the first 2 months. Concomitant steroid therapy is recommended for tuberculous meningitis and tuberculous pericarditis.

Infants born to mothers with tuberculosis

There is rarely a need to separate mothers with tuberculosis from their infants but such infants should be investigated carefully as there is a high risk of damaging disseminated disease. Babies born to mothers with infectious pulmonary tuberculosis should receive isoniazid chemoprophylaxis for 3 months and then be tuberculin tested; if they are tuberculin-negative and the mother has become smear-negative, BCG should be given; if the tuberculin test is strongly positive a further 3 months isoniazid should be given. Babies may be breastfed. Isoniazid-resistant BCG is no longer used.

Congenital tuberculosis

Congenital tuberculosis, caused by genital tract tuberculosis in the mother, is rare and difficult to diagnose. Infants present with nonspecific features of congenital infection such as hepatosplenomegaly, fever, leukopenia and jaundice. A high index of suspicion is vital and these children should be treated as for extrapulmonary tuberculosis.

Drug-resistant tuberculosis

Initial drug resistance is uncommon in previously untreated patients born in the UK, although alarmingly more common in other parts of the world. Patterns of drug resistance in children tend to mirror those found in adults from the same populations. Resistance is most common to streptomycin and isoniazid and is still rare for rifampicin. Multidrug resistance is still uncommon in the UK.

Outcome

The prognosis for most forms of childhood tuberculosis in non-immune-deficient hosts is good. In tuberculous meningitis the outcome is dependent on the stage of the disease at which treatment is initiated. If treated early the results are generally good. In the more advanced cases there is a high likelihood of permanent neurodevelopmental sequelae. Postinfective hydrocephalus may occur and require shunting.

PREVENTION OF FURTHER CASES

Prompt treatment of infectious cases of tuberculosis and thorough contact tracing are the most important preventive measures. BCG vaccination and the screening of entrants to the UK from high-incidence countries* make supplementary contributions to the prevention of tuberculosis in the UK.

BCG vaccination

Bacillus Calmette–Guérin (BCG) vaccine has been used routinely in the UK since the 1950s. Its effectiveness is disputed as studies in different populations have given varying results but there is a consensus that it does protect against disseminated disease and tuberculous meningitis in particular. Studies in the UK suggest around 75% protection against all forms of disease. It is recommended for all infants born into a household where there is a recent history of tuberculosis or whose families are Asian or African in origin, for immigrants from countries with a high incidence of tuberculosis, tuberculin-negative contacts of open TB cases, health-care workers at risk and all tuberculin-negative schoolchildren (the Schools Programme).

BCG vaccination is contraindicated in tuberculin-positive individuals and in children with potentially impaired immunity (see Chapter 21). The vaccination is given intradermally. Percutaneous (multiple puncture) injec-

---

* **Tuberculosis incidence more than 40 per 10^5 population per annum.**

tion may also be used for infants and neonates but the strength of BCG is different for the two methods and must not be confused. In most individuals a papule forms 2–6 weeks after immunisation. This sometimes discharges but usually needs no treatment. More severe reactions, including prolonged deep ulceration, lymphadenitis and osteomyelitis, are rare and usually caused by faulty technique resulting in subcutaneous rather than intradermal injection. Treatment with isoniazid for 6 weeks is often helpful. Specialist advice should be sought in these circumstances.

The school BCG programme

BCG vaccination is recommended for tuberculin-negative schoolchildren between the ages of 10 and 14 years. The Heaf test is used for prior screening in the UK. This is a multiple puncture test, which is easy to perform. The result should be read 3–10 days later and graded on a scale of 0–IV with a grade II response considered positive (grade III or greater in a child who has had a previous BCG). Heaf testing and BCG are not necessary for children with a definitive BCG scar. Heaf grades 0 and I receive BCG, no action is taken for those with grade II unless there are other signs, symptoms or a suspicious history. Children with grade III and IV reactions should be referred for specialist examination. Even if the children are normal to examination chemoprophylaxis may be indicated if they have been in contact with tuberculosis or resident in a high-prevalence country in the preceding 2 years. The school programme is under review as, with the decline of tuberculosis in the 1980s, BCG vaccination was considered barely cost-effective and some districts with very low incidence have stopped the programme prior to a national decision.

Screening of immigrants

All immigrants from Asia, Africa, South and Central America and the Caribbean and other countries where tuberculosis is common and all refugees should be screened. Initial screening may take place at the port of entry but it is important that information on new immigrants is passed to the Consultant in Communicable Disease Control in the district of intended residence so that comprehensive screening can be arranged. Screening consists of an interview about health status, current symptoms and previous BCG vaccination. Screening by tuberculin testing is not needed in asymptomatic individuals with a definite BCG scar. Individuals with suggestive symptoms or positive Heaf tests (grades II, III and IV in children, III and IV in adults) must be referred for specialist opinion. Heaf-negative (grade 0 and I) children should receive BCG.

Contact tracing and chemoprophylaxis for contacts

Up to a third of children with tuberculosis are diagnosed by contact tracing. Thorough and effective tracing of all children exposed to tuberculosis is vital if they are not to develop potentially life-threatening disease. Children under the age of 5 years who are close contacts of a smear-positive adult are particularly at risk and should be evaluated promptly following their contact history being established. Children should be examined for evidence of disease, a chest X-ray should be performed and a Heaf or Mantoux test. If there is clinical evidence of disease then full chemotherapy should be given (see British Thoracic Society Guidelines, 2000). If the findings are negative, children under the age of 5 years should in any case be given a 6-month prophylactic course of isoniazid while those over the age of 5 years* should be re-evaluated after 6 weeks (as screening tests performed during the incubation period may have given a false-negative result). If they remain tuberculin-negative and have a normal chest X-ray then BCG vaccination is given. If they are tuberculin-positive but have a normal chest X-ray and no clinical signs of disease, isoniazid prophylaxis is given for 6 months. If the source case has been smear-positive it is probably wise to review the children after 6 months and 1 year even if initial screening was negative.

Most children are infected by an adult in the same household. Those who are felt to be close contacts of a child with tuberculosis should also be screened, not to identify individuals infected by the child (as children are rarely infective) but rather to identify the source case from whom the child was infected.

Protection of staff at risk

All health-care workers should report symptoms suggestive of tuberculosis and they should also be protected by Heaf testing and BCG vaccination if nonimmune (Heaf grade 0 or I). Evidence of infectious tuberculosis should be sought among prospective NHS staff and students, teachers and nursery staff.

FURTHER READING

Joint Tuberculosis Committee of the British Thoracic Society (2000) Control and prevention of tuberculosis in the UK: code of practice 2000. Thorax 55: 887–901.

Starke JR, Smith MHD (1998) Tuberculosis. In: Feigin RD, Cherry JD (eds) Textbook of paediatric infectious disease, 4th edn. WB Saunders, Philadelphia, PA, pp. 1321–1362.

---

* **Age varies in different sets of recommendations – 2 years in the latest BTS guidelines.**

106 Typhoid and paratyphoid fever

See also Chapter 95. Typhoid and paratyphoid are notifiable diseases

ORGANISM

Typhoid – *Salmonella typhi*; paratyphoid – *S. paratyphi* A, B and C. Salmonellas are Gram-negative bacilli. The main reservoir for *S. typhi* and *S. paratyphi* is man, although rarely domestic animals are found to be infected with *S. paratyphi* and, as both organisms can exist for some time outside the body, sewage, water and food contaminated by sewage can act as environmental reservoirs.

EPIDEMIOLOGY

Typhoid and paratyphoid occur worldwide and are endemic in low-income countries. It has been estimated that there are over 15 million cases worldwide with nearly half a million deaths, mostly among children. Most cases reported in industrialised countries such as the UK and other parts of western Europe are imported. In the UK most imported cases of typhoid come from India and Africa, while paratyphoid is indigenous in the UK. In 1998 there were 134 cases of typhoid reported by laboratories in England and Wales and 188 cases of paratyphoid.

Transmission

Transmission of both infections is usually by food or water contaminated by faeces or urine from an infected person. Because heat destroys the bacteria, uncooked foods, salads, cold drinks and milk products are the commonest vehicles. Typhoid infection can be long-term and symptomless with the organism reproducing in the biliary tree and being excreted with faeces.

Incubation period

For both infections 1–3 weeks depending on the size of the infecting dose. Shorter periods have been reported for paratyphoid gastroenteritis.

NATURAL HISTORY AND CLINICAL FEATURES

The presentations of both infections are similar, although paratyphoid fever is rarely as severe as typhoid and if there is fever the onset may be more abrupt and the outcome is rarely fatal. Both infections are systemic bacterial diseases that can range from being totally asymptomatic to severe enteric fever with systemic spread and intestinal perforation. Enteric fever is characterised by slow onset of a sustained fever, malaise, headache and constipation rather than diarrhoea. Physical findings can include splenomegaly, bradycardia and rose-coloured spots on the trunk. The organisms can be isolated from the blood early in the diseases and from faeces and urine after the first week.

Diagnosis

Isolation of organisms from cultures of stool, rectal swabs, blood cultures. Paired serology specimens may confirm a diagnosis but are rarely useful clinically.

MANAGEMENT

Antibiotic therapy is indicated for these invasive infections. The drugs of first choice for typhoid and paratyphoid are ampicillin, co-trimoxazole and chloramphenicol, although many organisms acquired in low-income countries (especially in the Indian subcontinent and south-east Asia) are often resistant to the more common antibiotics. Cefotaxime or ciprofloxacin may need to be considered for those infected abroad and sensitivity testing should help guide the choice. There is a worrying increase in multiple resistance in the organisms. Treatment for enteric fever is for a minimum of 2 weeks, or for 10 days after the fever has completely settled. If there are foci in abscesses or osteomyelitis, treatment may need to be parenteral and prolonged for up to 6 weeks, especially in the immunocompromised patient.

PREVENTION OF FURTHER CASES

Cases must be formally notified by the doctor providing care to the local Consultant in Communicable Disease Control or the Director of Public Health. For both infections enteric precautions must be applied. Family and close contacts need to be screened by stool specimens. Infected food handlers cannot work until their infection is demonstrated to have cleared by three negative stool specimens. Long-term carriers may have their infection cleared by a course of high-dose ampicillin in children or ciprofloxacin in adults. Occasionally, persistent carriers have been cured by cholecystectomy.

Immunisation

Vaccination against typhoid is not recommended for children under 1 year. Three typhoid vaccines are available:

- A monovalent whole-cell killed vaccine given as one or two doses separated by 4–6 weeks giving respectively 1 or 3 years' protection at a level of 70–80%
- A typhoid Vi polysaccharide antigen vaccine giving the same level of protection from a single dose for about 3 years; this is not considered effective in children under 18 months old
- An oral live attenuated vaccine based on *S. typhi* (strain Ty21) taken as three doses of a single capsule every alternate day so that a course is completed in 5 days; this is thought only to give protection for a year and is not considered suitable for children before their sixth birthday.

All three vaccines are only partially effective. Hence, while they are widely employed, especially for travellers going to low-income countries, it is important to also emphasise the importance of general enteric precautions to avoid gastrointestinal infections in general (see Chapter 26).

107 Warts and verrucae

ORGANISM

The human papilloma virus (HPV) belongs to the papovavirus group of DNA viruses. At least 80 types have been recognised as pathogenic in humans. Types 1–5 tend to be associated with cutaneous warts whereas types 6, 11, 16, 18, 31 and 33 are more likely to be associated with anogenital warts. Sometimes two types may coexist at the same site in the same person.

EPIDEMIOLOGY

Warts occur worldwide and in all ages, with different types having a predilection for different age groups. The overall prevalence rises with increasing age throughout childhood but studies show widely different figures. A survey of children born in 1958 showed that 3.9% had visible warts at 11 years and 4.9% at 16 years old. In an Australian study the overall prevalence rose from 12.5% at 4–6 years old to 21.6% at 7–9 years old and 24.4% at 16–18 years old. Whereas common warts showed an increasing prevalence with rising age, especially in boys, there was no significant age effect for plane and plantar warts (verrucae). Genital warts occur mainly in the sexually active. Planar and common warts are more frequently found on the upper limb than at any other site, whereas plantar warts are most commonly found on the sole of the foot. The only reservoir for human warts is humans.

Transmission

Infectivity is low and spread occurs with direct contact. Genital warts can be acquired during delivery if the mother is infected (see Chapter 3, p. 12). They may not become apparent for up to 2 years. Genital warts in children should always raise the possibility of sexual abuse. The proportion reported due to sexual abuse varies markedly from study to study depending on how thoroughly the possibility of sexual abuse is investigated. Some may be due to self-inoculation from other parts of the body. Laryngeal papillomas are most probably transmitted from the mother's cervix at birth. The infectivity of plantar warts is uncertain but there is some evidence of spread in communal showers and similar facilities.

Incubation period

From 1 month to 2 years.

NATURAL HISTORY AND CLINICAL FEATURES

Plantar warts are flat hyperkeratotic lesions on the soles of the feet. They are frequently painful. Laryngeal papillomas occur on the vocal cords and epiglottis in young children. Skin warts may be flat or raised, smooth or rough, varying in size from a pinhead to over a centimetre. Genital warts (condylomata acuminata) are fleshy growths seen most commonly in moist areas in and around the genitalia and anus.

Diagnosis

Clinical. Earlier hopes that typing of papilloma virus isolates from genital warts might distinguish those with a sexual mode of spread have not been confirmed.

MANAGEMENT

Most warts are self-limiting within months, although it may take a year or more for a minority to regress. Where treatment is needed, a number of paints containing salicylic acid, glutaraldehyde, formaldehyde or podophyllum are available. They should be applied daily after removing superficial dead skin. Cryotherapy can be used, except on those in the genital region. For these, podophyllin paint is more appropriate. It is applied weekly. Curettage, cryotherapy and/or salicylic acid plasters are often used for verrucae. Laryngeal warts are removed by laser therapy or surgery.

108 Yersiniosis

ORGANISM

Yersinia enterocolitica and Y. pseudotuberculosis are Gram-negative bacilli.

EPIDEMIOLOGY

The main reservoir of these organisms is in farm animals, especially pigs, and rats. Infections occur following ingestion of contaminated food. Infection is more common and more serious in individuals with iron overload such as thalassaemics on long-term transfusion programmes.

Transmission

From contaminated food, especially undercooked pork, or directly from farm animals.

Incubation period

4–16 days (range 1–16 days).

NATURAL HISTORY AND CLINICAL FEATURES

Y. enterocolitica causes acute diarrhoea, often with blood and mucus in the stools and associated with fever and pain. The pain may be so severe as to mimic appendicitis or other acute surgical problem. Bacteraemia and nonintestinal disease such as osteomyelitis may occur. Erythema nodosum and reactive arthritis may complicate the infection, most commonly in adults.

Y. pseudotuberculosis causes abdominal pain, usually with diarrhoea. This results from an acute ileitis and mesenteric adenitis. There is fever (often prolonged) and frequently a blotchy red rash. Erythema nodosum can occur.

Bacteraemic illness with either organism is most likely to occur in iron-overloaded patients, particularly those on desferrioxamine treatment.

Diagnosis

Both organisms can be identified in the stool and blood early in the illness. Stool isolation requires prolonged culture under special conditions and the laboratory has to be made aware of the suspected diagnosis in order to set these up.

Serological tests looking for agglutinating antibodies are also available through reference laboratories but false-positive results can occur as a result of cross-reactivity with a number of other microbes.

MANAGEMENT

Co-trimoxazole, aminoglycosides, ciprofloxacin, cefotaxime and, in those over 12 years old, tetracycline are all useful in systemic (blood-culture-positive) infection. Their benefits in disease confined to the intestine is unproven but it is reasonable to treat if symptoms are severe or prolonged.

PREVENTION OF FURTHER CASES

Strict food hygiene should be observed. Pork dishes should be thoroughly cooked. Children visiting farms and handling animals should always be made to wash their hands before eating (see Chapter 33).

Part Three: Appendices

Appendix I Mortality and morbidity from infectious disease in the United Kingdom

Numbers and rates of deaths among children in the UK from selected causes during the years 1992–96 are shown for infants (children under age 1 year) in Table I.1 and for all children (14 years and under) in Table I.2. These show a relatively constant number of deaths from infectious and parasitic disease and from combined infections. In contrast, the numbers and rates for 'all causes' have been steadily declining. The rise in deaths for combined infections in both age groups from 1992 to 1993 resulted from changes in coding procedures between those two years. It should be noted that in 1992 the introduction of Hib vaccination reduced deaths from invasive *Haemophilus* disease. Just before 1992 there was a sharp fall in deaths from sudden infant death syndrome, which is attributed to the advice given to parents to place infants on their backs when sleeping.

Morbidity and immunisation data are shown graphically for the vaccine-preventable diseases, selected gastrointestinal infections, vertically acquired HIV, meningococcal disease and respiratory syncytial virus using notifications, clinical and laboratory reports variously for England and Wales, England, Wales and Northern Ireland and the UK as they are available.

Diphtheria notifications (Fig. I.1) shows the dramatic effect of immunisation, which began after 1940, while the figure for tetanus notifications and deaths (Fig. I.2) lagged behind the introduction of routine childhood immunisation in the mid-1950s because of the large number of unimmunised adults who remained unprotected. The graph for polio (Fig. I.3) demonstrates the large-scale epidemics that took place after the Second World War and the protective effect of the introduction of the Salk and Sabin vaccines. Laboratory reports of *Haemophilus influenzae* type b (Fig. I.4) have fallen dramatically since the introduction of Hib vaccine in 1992. Measles from 1950–93 show (Fig. I.5a) the characteristic two yearly epidemic subsiding after immunisation began in 1968 and (Fig. I.5b) the effect of the measles/rubella ('MR') campaign of the autumn of 1994. Meningococcal infections have shown slow rises and falls apart from the dramatic epidemic that took place during the Second World War and an increase in type C disease most recently, particularly in older children and adolescents (Fig. I.6a). Since the introduction of meningococcal C conjugate vaccine in November 1999 there has been a fall in type C disease. Figure 1.6b shows a fall after late 1999 in infants (under 1 year). Infants and teenagers were immunised first in the programme and initially the fall was confined to this group. The pattern for whooping cough demonstrates what can happen when confidence and use of vaccine falls. It was largely controlled in the 1950s but experienced a resurgence in the late 1970s and early 1980s (Fig. I.7) following a controversy over vaccine safety and it took a decade to make up the lost ground. Vaccine coverage data (Fig. I.8) show a steadily improving picture over the period 1988–97 but these national data conceal poor coverage in a number of districts and there was a small decline in MMR in 1997/8 following unwarranted concern over vaccine safety issues.

Table I.1 Selected causes of death in children under 1 year old in the UK 1992–96 (rates per 1000 live births)

ICD9 code	Disease	1992	1993	1994	1995	1996
001–009	Intestinal infectious disease	10 (0.01)	22 (0.03)	19 (0.03)	25 (0.03)	14 (0.02)
036	Meningococcal infection	36 (0.05)	4 (0.05)	30 (0.04)	39 (0.05)	34 (0.05)
038	Septicaemia	19 (0.05)	20 (0.03)	20 (0.03)	35 (0.05)	25 (0.03)
030–041	Other bacterial disease*	59 (0.07)	70 (0.09)	56 (0.07)	79 (0.11)	67 (0.09)
045–079	Viral disease	6 (0.01)	12 (0.02)	12 (0.02)	11 (0.02)	10 (0.01)
001–139	All infectious and parasitic diseases	81 (0.10)	17 (0.05)	98 (0.13)	129 (0.18)	105 (0.14)
320–322	Meningitis	27 (0.03)	38 (0.05)	21 (0.03)	30 (0.04)	35 (0.05)
466	Acute bronchitis and bronchiolitis	20 (0.03)	33 (0.04)	29 (0.04)	18 (0.02)	21 (0.03)
480–486	Pneumonia	60 (0.08)	102 (0.13)	96 (0.13)	83 (0.11)	91 (0.12)
	Combined infections*†	188 (0.24)	290 (0.38)	244 (0.33)	260 (0.36)	252 (0.34)
798	Sudden death, cause unknown	504 (0.64)	491 (0.65)	463 (0.62)	412 (0.56)	453 (0.62)
	Live births (× 1000)	787.4	759.5	750.2	731.9	733.4

* Includes totals for meningococcal infection and septicaemia.
† All infections and parasitic disease, plus meningitis, acute bronchitis and pneumonia.

Table I.2 Selected causes of death in children aged 14 years and under in the UK 1992–96 (rates per 100 000 child population)

ICD9 code	Disease	1992		1993		1994		1995		1996	
001–009	Intestinal infectious disease	15	(0.13)	24	(0.21)	23	(0.20)	29	(0.26)	17	(0.15)
036	Meningococcal infection	100	(0.89)	115	(1.02)	89	(0.78)	120	(1.06)	119	(1.05)
038	Septicaemia	20	(0.18)	32	(0.28)	35	(0.31)	54	(0.48)	49	(0.43)
030–041	Other bacterial disease*	140	(1.25)	163	(1.44)	136	(1.20)	183	(1.61)	180	(1.58)
045–079	Viral disease	20	(0.18)	33	(0.29)	33	(0.29)	30	(0.26)	31	(0.27)
001–139	All infectious and parasitic diseases	192	(1.72)	254	(2.25)	218	(1.92)	273	(2.40)	257	(2.26)
320–322	Meningitis	58	(0.52)	67	(0.59)	32	(0.28)	48	(0.42)	52	(0.46)
466	Acute bronchitis and bronchiolitis	35	(0.31)	50	(0.44)	41	(0.36)	28	(0.25)	35	(0.31)
480–486	Pneumonia	92	(0.82)	185	(1.64)	189	(1.66)	153	(1.35)	160	(1.41)
	Combined infections*†	337	(3.37)	556	(4.92)	480	(4.23)	502	(4.42)	504	(4.44)
798	Sudden death, cause unknown	531	(4.75)	511	(4.52)	485	(4.27)	430	(3.78)	476	(4.19)
	All causes	7180	(64.16)	7096	(62.77)	6712	(59.09)	6519	(57.38)	6367	(56.06)
	Child population (× 100 000)	111.9		113.1		113.6		113.6		113.6	

* Includes totals for meningococcal infection and septicaemia.
† All infections and parasitic disease, plus meningitis, acute bronchitis and pneumonia.

I Mortality and morbidity

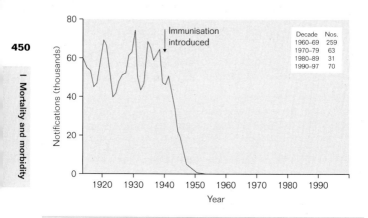

Fig. I.1 Diphtheria notifications, England and Wales 1914–97

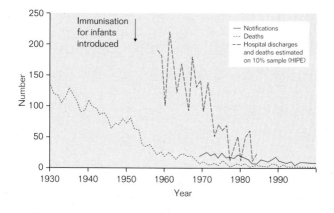

Fig. I.2 Tetanus notifications, deaths and hospital discharges and deaths, England and Wales 1930–97

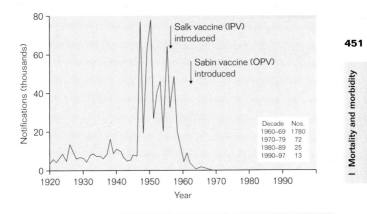

Fig. I.3 Poliomyelitis notifications, England and Wales 1920–97

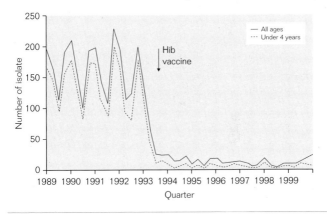

Fig. I.4 Quarterly laboratory reports of Hib cerebrospinal fluid and blood isolates, 1989–99. Figures for 1999 provisional (Source: PHLS Communicable Disease Surveillance Centre)

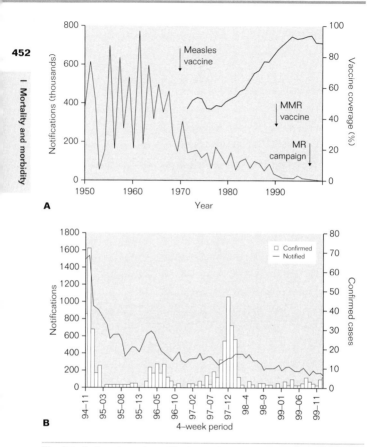

Fig. I.5 A. Annual measles notifications and vaccine coverage, England and Wales 1950–99. Figures for 1999 provisional (Source: Office for National Statistics and Department of Health) **B.** Notified and confirmed cases of measles, November 1994–December 1999. Figures for December 1999 provisional (Source: PHLS Communicable Disease Surveillance Centre, ERVL, ONS)

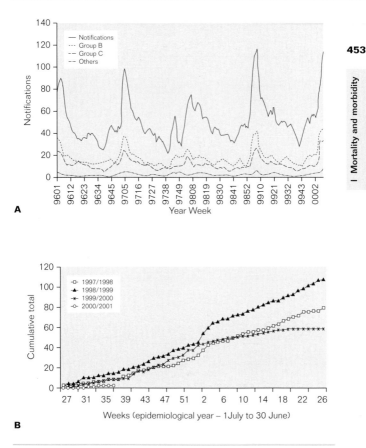

Fig. I.6 A. Meningococcal disease 5-week moving average, England and Wales 1996–99. Figures for 1999 provisional (Source: PHLS Communicable Diseases Surveillance Centre) **B.** Cumulative cases of meningococcal C disease in children aged under 1 year, England and Wales 1997–2000 (Source: PHLS Communicable Disease Surveillance Centre)

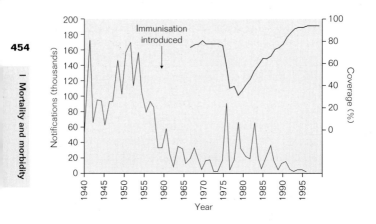

Fig. I.7 Whooping cough notifications and vaccine coverage, England and Wales 1940–99

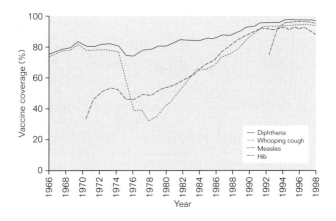

Fig. I.8 Vaccine coverage 1966–98: percentage coverage of third dose diphtheria, whooping cough and Hib, single-antigen measles or MMR vaccines as at 2 years old (Source: Department of Health Statistics Division and COVER/Körner programme)

In contrast to these vaccine-preventable diseases laboratory reports of gastrointestinal infections (shown for all ages in Fig. I.9) increased steadily for a number of infections with relentless steady rises in reports of rotavirus, *Salmonella* and *Campylobacter* species between 1980 and the early 1990s and a particular rise in *Shigella* dysentery in 1991 and

1992. Since the start of the 1990s there has been a relentless rise in reports of *Campylobacter* species, which have recently exceeded reports of *Salmonella* species. Prevalence of HIV-1 infection among pregnant women in Inner and Outer London also rose fivefold between 1988 and 1992. There was also an increase in prevalence in England outside London in 1996, which was sustained in 1997 and 1998, while prevalence in Scotland has declined (Fig. I.10). Because testing was not routinely offered to mothers in pregnancy until April 2000, vertically acquired AIDS infections in infants has not yet declined in the UK compared to other parts of Europe (Fig. I.11). Epidemics of respiratory syncytial virus infection occur every winter (Fig. I.12). Notifications of tuberculosis in children showed a rise in infections in children over age 2 years in the early 1990s but little change since (Fig. I.13).

Sources: Office for National Statistics; General Register Office Scotland; Department of Health and Social Services, Northern Ireland; reports to the Public Health Laboratory Service Communicable Disease Surveillance Centre and the Scottish Centre for Infection and Environmental Health.

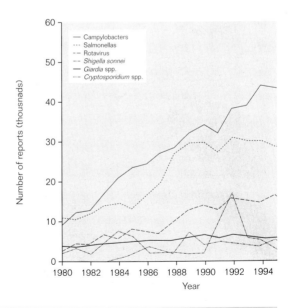

Fig. I.9 Laboratory reports of selected gastrointestinal infections, England and Wales 1980–98 (Source: PHLS Communicable Disease Surveillance Centre)

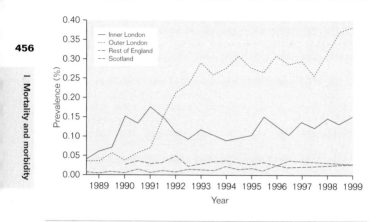

Fig. I.10 Trends in prevalence of HIV-1 infection among pregnant women by area of residence, 1988–June 1999 (newborn infant dried blood spots taken for metabolic screening) (Source: PHLS Communicable Disease Surveillance Centre/Institute of Child Health – London)

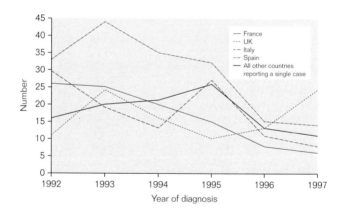

Fig. I.11 Mother-to-child HIV transmission in European countries, 1992–97: AIDS cases in children aged less than 1 year at diagnosis (Source: PHLS Communicable Disease Surveillance Centre; from European non-aggregate AIDS Dataset – EUROHIV Centre, IVRS, Paris)

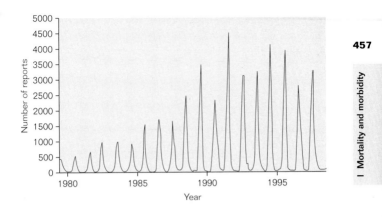

Fig. I.12 Laboratory reports to the Communicable Disease Surveillance Centre of RSV infections: 4-weekly totals 1980–98

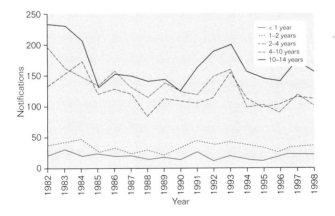

Fig. I.13 Notifications of tuberculosis (all forms) in children, England and Wales 1982–98

Appendix II Neonatal antibiotic dosages

Antibiotic	Single dose	Dose frequency	Postnatal age (days)	Weight/ gestation	Administration and notes
Aciclovir	i.v. 10–20 mg/kg	8-hourly	Any	> 33 weeks gestation	Administer over 1 hour in a max concentration of 25 mg/mL. 20 mg/kg dose used for H. simplex encephalitis and for disseminated disease.
		12-hourly		< 33 weeks gestation	Reduce dose frequency in renal failure SeCr: 70–100 µmol/L every 12 h 110–130 µmol/L every 24 h > 130 µmol/L 5 mg/kg every 24 h or urine output < 1 mL/kg/h
Amikacin	i.v. or i.m. Loading dose 10 mg/kg then 7.5 mg/kg	12-hourly	Any	Any	Slow i.v. bolus or infusion over 30 min. Levels at third dose: Peak 20–30 mg/L (1 h after dose) Trough < 8 mg/L (before dose)
Amoxycillin	Oral 30–50 mg/kg	12-hourly 8-hourly	< 7 > 7	Any Any	
Amphotericin B	i.v. infusion 100 µg/kg then 300 µg/kg increasing by 250 µg/kg/day to a maximum 1 mg/kg	Once only as a test dose given over 1 h 24-hourly	Any	Any	Maximum total dose 15 mg. Infuse over 4–6 h a) Administer only in pH-tested glucose 5% b) Avoid other nephrotoxic drugs c) Protect from light d) Do not filter e) Monitor renal function and treat hypokalaemia early with potassium supplement ± amiloride

Drug	Dose	Interval	Age (days)	Weight	Notes
Amphotericin, liposomal	i.v. infusion 1 mg/kg increasing to 3 mg/kg	24-hourly	Any	Any	For use in infants with moderate/severe renal impairment or if conventional amphotericin not tolerated
Ampicillin	i.v. or i.m. 50 mg/kg	12-hourly 6–8-hourly	0–7 >7	Any Any	
Azlocillin	i.v. or i.m. 50 mg/kg 100 mg/kg 100 mg/kg	12-hourly 12-hourly 8-hourly	0–7 0–7 >7	< 2 kg > 2 kg Any	
Aztreonam	i.v. 30 mg/kg	12-hourly 8-hourly 8-hourly 6-hourly	<7 <7 >7 >7	< 2 kg > 2 kg < 2 kg > 2 kg	i.v. infusion over 20–60 min at concentration ≤20 mg/mL. Reduce dose by 50% in severe renal impairment
Benzylpenicillin	i.v. or i.m. 25–50 mg/kg	12-hourly 8-hourly 8-hourly 6-hourly	<7 <7 >7 >7	< 2 kg > 2 kg < 2 kg > 2 kg	Reduce dose by 50% in severe renal impairment as may cause convulsions 50 mg/kg dose used for meningitis
Cefotaxime	i.v. 50 mg/kg	12-hourly 12-hourly 8-hourly	<7 >7 >7	Any < 2 kg > 2 kg	In severe infections up to 200 mg/kg/day. Reduce dose by 50% in severe renal impairment

Appendix II: Neonatal antibiotic dosages (continued)					
Antibiotic	Single dose	Dose frequency	Postnatal age (days)	Weight/ gestation	Administration and notes
Ceftazidime	i.v. 30–50 mg/kg	12-hourly 8-hourly	< 7 > 7	Any Any	Increase dose interval to 24-hourly in severe renal impairment 50 mg/kg dose used in meningitis
Cefuroxime	i.v. 30 mg/kg	12-hourly 8-hourly	< 7 > 7	Any Any	Reduce dose in severe renal impairment In severe infections can use up to 50 mg/kg per dose
Chloramphenicol	i.v. only 12.5–25 mg/kg	24-hourly 24-hourly 12-hourly	< 7 > 7 > 7	Any < 2 kg > 2 kg	Monitor blood levels and adjust dose. Levels at fifth dose: Peak 10–20 µg/mL 30 min after dose; trough < 10 µg/mL Levels decreased by phenobarbitone and phenytoin Beware grey baby syndrome Avoid using this drug in neonates if possible
Ciprofloxacin	i.v. 5 mg/kg Oral 7.5 mg/kg	12-hourly 12-hourly	Any Any	Any Any	Infuse over 30–60 min. Only use when benefit outweighs risk as may cause arthropathy
Clarithromycin	i.v. or oral 7.5 mg/kg	12-hourly	Any	Any	Avoid using with cisapride
Clindamycin	i.v. or oral 5 mg/kg	8-hourly	Any	Any	

Drug	Dose	Frequency	Age (days)	Weight	Notes
Co-amoxiclav	i.v. 30 mg/kg	12-hourly 8-hourly	<7 >7	Any Any	Dose expressed as the combination (5:1 ratio of amoxycillin to clavulanic acid)
Co-trimoxazole	i.v. or oral 24 mg/kg	12-hourly	>14 days	Any	Avoid if possible Contraindicated in the presence of hyperbilirubinaemia
Erythromycin	i.v. infusion or oral 10 mg/kg 15 mg/kg	12-hourly 8-hourly 8-hourly	>7 >7 >7	Any <2 kg >2 kg	Infuse over 30–60 min. Caution in jaundice as displaces bilirubin. May increase serum levels of digoxin, theophylline and carbamazepine Avoid using with cisapride
Flucloxacillin	i.v. or oral 30–50 mg/kg	12-hourly 8-hourly 6-hourly	<7 >7 >21	Any Any Any	Increase dose interval in severe renal impairment In severe deep seated infection, e.g. osteomyelitis, cerebral abscess, doses of up to 100 mg/kg can be used
Fluconazole	i.v. or oral 3 mg/kg 6–12 mg/kg	24-hourly	Any	Any	Reduce dosage in severe renal impairment Superficial candidiasis Invasive candidiasis
Flucytosine	i.v. or oral 25 mg/kg 50 mg/kg	6-hourly 6-hourly	<28 >28	Any Any	Infuse over 30 min. Monitor blood levels. Ideal trough level 25–50 mg/L. Increase dose interval in renal impairment. Monitor blood count Usually combined with amphotericin B

Appendix II: Neonatal antibiotic dosages (continued)

Antibiotic	Single dose	Dose frequency	Postnatal age (days)	Weight/gestation	Administration and notes
Fucidin (sodium fusidate)	i.v. 5 mg/kg Oral 10–15 mg/kg (0.3 mL/kg of suspension)	8-hourly 8-hourly	Any Any	Any Any	Infuse over 6 h, although possible over 3 h if via central line. Do not use alone as resistance likely to emerge – usually combined with flucloxacillin NB. All doses calculated as sodium fusidate
Ganciclovir	i.v. 5 mg/kg	12-hourly	Any	Reduce dose in VLBW infants	Monitor blood counts
Gentamicin	i.v. or i.m. 4 mg/kg 4 mg/kg then 24 h later 3 mg/kg 3 mg/kg 4 mg/kg then 18 h later 3 mg/kg 3 mg/kg 3 mg/kg	36-hourly Loading dose 24-hourly 24-hourly Loading dose 18-hourly 18-hourly 12-hourly	< 7 > 7 < 7 > 7 < 7 > 7	< 28 weeks 28–32 weeks 32–38 weeks	At all gestational ages, predose (trough) and 1 h postdose (peak) levels around fourth dose Levels: trough < 2 mg/L; peak 6–10 mg/L

	Dose	Interval	Age (days)	Weight	Comments
	3 mg/kg	12-hourly	< 7		
	3 mg/kg	8-hourly	> 7		
Meropenem	i.v. 20–40 mg/kg	12-hourly	< 7	Any	Reserved for severe infections with resistant Gram-negative bacilli
		12-hourly	> 7	< 2 kg	Use highest dose in meningitis
		8-hourly	> 7	> 2 kg	
Metronidazole	i.v. or oral 7.5 mg/kg	8-hourly	Any	Any	Infuse over 30 min. Increase dose interval to 12-hourly in severe renal impairment. Injection solution may be given rectally
Mupirocin	Topical	8-hourly	Any	Any	NB. Different preparations used for nasal and cutaneous application
Neomycin	Eye drops	6-hourly	Any	Any	
Netilmicin	i.v. 3 mg/kg	18-hourly	< 7	< 2 kg	Give as slow i.v. bolus over 3–5 min or i.v. infusion over 30 min.
		12-hourly	< 7	> 2 kg	Monitor blood levels around third dose and individualise dose.
		12-hourly	> 7	< 2 kg	Peak 5–12 mg/L (1 h post dose); trough < 3 mg/L
		8-hourly	> 7	> 2 kg	
Piperacillin	i.v. 75 mg/kg	12-hourly	< 7	< 2 kg	Give as an infusion over 30 min or bolus over 3–5 min.
	100 mg/kg	8-hourly	> 7	> 2 kg	Increase dose interval in severe renal impairment
		8-hourly	< 7	< 2 kg	Hypokalaemia may occur
		6-hourly	> 7	> 2 kg	

II Neonatal antibiotic dosages

Appendix II: Neonatal antibiotic dosages (continued)

Antibiotic	Single dose	Dose frequency	Postnatal age (days)	Weight/ gestation	Administration and notes
Rifampicin	i.v. or oral 10 mg/kg	24-hourly	Any	Any	Monitor liver function
	10 mg/kg	12-hourly	Any	Any	Tuberculosis
	5 mg/kg	12-hourly	Any	Any	Severe staphylococcal infection
					Prophylaxis against *Neisseria meningitidis*
					Avoid in infants with hepatic function impairment
Teicoplanin	i.v. infusion 16 mg/kg	Loading dose	Any	Any	Infuse over 30 min
	then 8 mg/kg	24-hourly			Dosage reduced in renal impairment and in extreme prematurity
Trimethoprim	i.v. 3 mg/kg	Loading dose	Any	Any	Reduce dose in severe renal failure. Give as a slow bolus or infusion
	then 2 mg/kg	12-hourly			
	Oral 2 mg/kg	12-hourly	Any	Any	
	2 mg/kg	At night	Any	Any	Prophylaxis against urinary tract infection
Vancomycin	i.v. 15 mg/kg	24-hourly	Any	Gestation:	Predose (trough) and 1 h after infusion completed (peak) levels around third dose. Monitor levels, aim for: Trough < 10 mg/L; peak 25–40 mg/L
		18-hourly	< 7	< 28 weeks	
		12-hourly	> 7	28–35 weeks	
		12-hourly	< 7	> 35 weeks	
		8-hourly	> 7		

15 mg/kg	Once	Any	Prior to central venous line or VP/VA shunt insertion
Oral 10 mg/kg	6-hourly	Any	To treat staphylococcal enterocolitis. Use parenteral preparation orally
Zidovudine	Oral 2 mg/kg i.v. 1.5 mg/kg	6-hourly	Any	Prevention of maternal–fetal HIV transmission

A number of drugs listed above are not licensed for use in neonates but are often used under specialist supervision.

Appendix III Antimicrobials for the infant and child (excludes neonates)

Drug	Route	Times daily	1 year	7 years	14 years	Indications and comments
Aciclovir	i.v.	3	250–500 mg/m²	250–500 mg/m²	250–500 mg/m²	Used for severe HSV infection – herpes encephalitis, eczema herpeticum, and varicella in immunocompromised children. Higher doses in herpes encephalitis and the immunocompromised
	Oral	4	20 mg/kg	20 mg/kg		
	Oral	5			800 mg	
	Oral	3–4	100 mg	200 mg	200–400 mg	Herpes simplex prophylaxis. Higher dose in severely immunocompromised
	Oral	4–5	200 mg	400 mg	800 mg	Varicella zoster prophylaxis after exposure in immunocompromised children
Albendazole	Oral	2	5–7.5 mg/kg	5–7.5 mg/kg	5–7.5 mg/kg	Broad-spectrum antihelminthic. Use in treatment of hydatid disease (use lower dose) and tapeworm (alternative to praziquantel)
Amantadine	Oral	1–2	5 mg/kg	5 mg/kg maximum of 150 mg	200 mg	Treatment of severe influenza A (usually in immunocompromised). Reduce dose in severe renal impairment
Amikacin	i.v.	2	7.5 mg/kg	7.5 mg/kg	7.5 mg/kg	Aminoglycoside used for severe Gram-negative infections and for atypical mycobacterial infection. Check renal function prior to use. In prolonged treatment need weekly drug levels and regular hearing checks even when drug levels are acceptable
	Single daily dose regimen	1	15–20 mg/kg	15–20 mg/kg	15–20 mg/kg	

	Route					Notes
Amoxycillin	Oral i.v.	3	62.5–125 mg 30 mg/kg	125–250 mg 30 mg/kg	250–500 mg 30 mg/kg	Treatment of otitis media, pneumonia, etc.: standard course 5 days. Maximum 4 g/day. Reduce dose in renal impairment
Amphotericin B	i.v. (infuse over 6 h)	1	Test dose of 100 µg/kg Max. 1 mg Then 300 µg/kg increasing by 250 µg/kg daily to maximum of 1000 µg/kg	Test dose of 100 µg/kg Max. 1 mg Then 300 µg/kg increasing by 250 µg/kg daily to maximum of 1000 µg/kg	Test dose of 100 µg/kg Max. 1 mg Then 300 µg/kg increasing by 250 µg/kg daily to maximum of 1000 µg/kg	Invasive fungal disease, usually in an immunocompromised child. Several weeks' therapy may be required Used for visceral leishmaniasis Watch renal function and plasma K^+ levels Amiloride may help treat hypokalaemia
Amphotericin B (liposomal)	i.v.	1	1 mg/kg starting, increasing to 3 mg/kg	1 mg/kg starting, increasing to 3 mg/kg	1 mg/kg starting, increasing to 3 mg/kg	Better tolerated than conventional amphotericin. Use in renal failure or failure to tolerate conventional amphotericin
Ampicillin	Oral i.v.	4	125 mg 50–100 mg/kg	250 mg 50–100 mg/kg	500 mg 50–100 mg/kg	Otitis media, pneumonia and meningitis
Azlocillin	i.v.	3	75–150 mg/kg to maximum of 3 g	75–150 mg/kg to maximum of 3 g	75–150 mg/kg to maximum of 3 g	Treatment of *Pseudomonas* infection in the immunocompromised child and in cystic fibrosis. Combine with an aminoglycoside
Azithromycin	Oral	1	10 mg/kg	10 mg/kg	500 mg	Macrolide persists in tissues. 3-day course equivalent to full course of other antibiotics Good *Haemophilus* cover Avoid using with terfenadine or cisapride

NB. Doses are individual and not daily dosages.

Appendix III: Antimicrobials for the infant and child (continued)

Drug	Route	Times daily	1 year	7 years	14 years	Indications and comments
Aztreonam	i.v.	3–4	30–50 mg/kg	30–50 mg/kg	30–50 mg/kg	Active against Gram-negative bacteria, including *Pseudomonas aeruginosa, Haemophilus influenzae* Low risk of hypersensitivity in children with penicillin allergy. Maximum dose 8 g/day
Benzylpenicillin, *see penicillin G*						
Cefaclor	Oral	3	125 mg	250 mg	250–500 mg	Respiratory tract infection
Cefixime	Oral	1	8 mg/kg	200 mg	400 mg	Respiratory tract and urinary infections
Cefotaxime	i.v.	3–4	25–50 mg/kg	25–50 mg/kg	25–50 mg/kg	Treatment of septicaemia, meningitis and life-threatening infections Reduce dose in renal failure Maximum doses in meningitis
Cefpodoxime	Oral	2	4 mg/kg	4 mg/kg	200 mg	Respiratory tract infection
Ceftazidime	i.v.	3	25–50 mg/kg	25–50 mg/kg	25–50 mg/kg	Broad spectrum. Particularly effective in *Pseudomonas aeruginosa* infections Use high dose in children with cystic fibrosis, meningitis and the immunocompromised. Reduce dose frequency in renal impairment
Ceftriaxone	i.v., i.m.	1	50–80 mg/kg	50–80 mg/kg	50–80 mg/kg	Once daily treatment for serious bacterial infections, including meningitis.

	i.v.	1	100 mg/kg	100 mg/kg	100 mg/kg	Reduce dosage in combined renal and hepatic impairment
						For *Borrelia* meningitis
Cefuroxime	i.v.	3	25–50 mg/kg	25–50 mg/kg	25–50 mg/kg	*H. influenzae* infections. Reduce dose in renal impairment
Cephradine	Oral, i.v., i.m.	4	25–50 mg/kg	25–50 mg/kg	25–50 mg/kg	Treatment of orthopaedic and urinary tract infections caused by resistant organisms Reduce dose in renal impairment
Chloramphenicol	Oral, i.v.	4	25 mg/kg for 48 h then 12.5 mg/kg	25 mg/kg for 48 h then 12.5 mg/kg	25 mg/kg for 48 h then 12.5 mg/kg	Only used for treatment of meningitis, epiglottitis, and some cases of typhoid. Monitor levels. Well absorbed orally
Chloroquine	Oral	1	Initially 10 mg/kg maximum 600 mg: 6 h later 5 mg/kg per day, for 2 days	Initially 10 mg/kg maximum 600 mg: 6 h later 5 mg/kg per day, for 2 days	Initially 10 mg/kg maximum 600 mg: 6 h later 5 mg/kg per day, for 2 days	Initial treatment of simple malaria when chloroquine resistance is not a problem
Ciprofloxacin	Oral i.v.	2 2	3.75–7.5 mg/kg 5 mg/kg	3.75–7.5 mg/kg 5 mg/kg	3.75–7.5 mg/kg 5 mg/kg	*Pseudomonas* infection in cystic fibrosis and immunocompromised. Invasive salmonellosis and typhoid
Clarithromycin	Oral	2	7.5 mg/kg	7.5 mg/kg	250–500 mg	Macrolide. Pyogenic bacterial infections. Atypical mycobacterial infection. *Mycoplasma pneumoniae*, *Bordetella pertussis* and chlamydial infections Avoid using with terfenadine or cisapride
	i.v.	2	7.5 mg/kg	7.5 mg/kg	500 mg	Give as an infusion

NB. Doses are individual and not daily dosages.

Appendix III: Antimicrobials for the infant and child (continued)							
Drug	Route	Times daily	1 year	7 years	14 years	Indications and comments	
Clindamycin	Oral	4	3–6 mg/kg	3–6 mg/kg	3–6 mg/kg	Staphylococcal bone and joint infection	
	i.v.	3–4	5–10 mg/kg	5–10 mg/kg	5–10 mg/kg	Watch for pseudomembranous colitis	
Clotrimazole	Topical	3	Use topically on skin			Fungal infection – tinea pedis (athlete's foot)	
Co-amoxiclav	Oral	3	125/31 mg	125/31–250/62 mg	250/62–500/125 mg	Oral dose expressed as amoxycillin/clavulanic acid:	
	i.v.	3	30 mg/kg	30 mg/kg	30 mg/kg	i.v. dose as the combination. Clavulanic acid is a β-lactamase inhibitor; broadens spectrum of amoxycillin to include most Staphylococcus aureus and other β-lactamase-producing strains	
Colistin	Nebulised	2	250–500 000 units	500 000 units	1 million units	Resistant Pseudomonas infection in cystic fibrosis	
	i.v.	3	16 666 U/kg	16 666 U/kg	16 666 U/kg (max. 2 million units)	Resistant Gram-negative bacillary sepsis	
Co-trimoxazole	Oral/i.v.	2	24 mg/kg	24 mg/kg	960 mg	Chest infections, typhoid, invasive salmonellosis. Dose given as combination (5:1 sulphamethoxazole:trimethoprim);	
	i.v.	4	30 mg/kg	30 mg/kg	30 mg/kg	For Pneumocystis carinii pneumonia	
	Oral	2 (3 days a week)	240 mg (body SA 0.5–0.75 m^2)	360 mg (body SA 0.75–1.0 m^2)	480 mg (body SA > 1.0 m^2)	Prophylaxis against Pneumocystis carinii	

Drug	Route	Frequency	Dose	Dose	Dose	Indication/Notes
	Oral	1	24–30 mg/kg	24 mg/kg	24 mg/kg	Prophylaxis against bacterial infection in immunodeficient states
	Oral	1 (at night)	12 mg/kg	12 mg/kg	12 mg/kg	Prophylaxis against urinary tract infections
						Drug is mixture of 5 parts sulphamethoxazole and 1 part trimethoprim (dose = sum of each, mg)
Diethyl-carbamazine	Oral	2	0.5–3 mg/kg	0.5–3 mg/kg	0.5–3 mg/kg	Filariasis
Doxycycline	Oral	2	1–2 mg/kg (maximum 100 mg)	1–2 mg/kg	100 mg	Only in children < 12 years for serious infections when no alternative. Avoid in hepatic impairment
Erythromycin	Oral / i.v.	4 / 4	125 mg / 12.5 mg/kg	250 mg / 12.5 mg/kg	500 mg / 12.5 mg/kg	Use when definite history of penicillin allergy for otitis, tonsillitis, pneumonia. Treatment of Chlamydia trachomatis, C. psittaci, Legionella and Mycoplasma pneumoniae infection. Empirical treatment in encephalitis. Gastrointestinal upset is a common side effect
Ethambutol	Oral	1	15 mg/kg	15 mg/kg	15 mg/kg	Treatment of tuberculosis. Used in conjunction with isoniazid and rifampicin. Reduce dose in renal impairment. Visual problems can result and if possible alternative drugs should be used in children < 6 years. Test colour vision before and during treatment

NB. Doses are individual and not daily dosages.

Appendix III: Antimicrobials for the infant and child (continued)							
Drug	Route	Times daily	1 year	7 years	14 years	Indications and comments
Flucloxacillin	Oral	4	125 mg	250 mg	500 mg	Staphylococcal infections, including septicaemia and osteomyelitis May be combined with another antibiotic Drain any abscess surgically
	i.v.	4	25–50 mg/kg	25–50 mg/kg	25–50 mg/kg	
Foscarnet	i.v.	3	60 mg/kg	60 mg/kg	60 mg/kg	Cytomegalovirus infection, especially retinitis Resistant herpes simplex infection Reduce dose in renal impairment. Monitor renal function and electrolytes
	i.v	1	90 mg/kg	90 mg/kg	90 mg/kg	Maintenance regimen
Fluconazole	Oral, i.v.	1	6–12 mg/kg	6–12 mg/kg	6–12 mg/kg	For systemic candidiasis and cryptococcal infection and persistent superficial candidiasis Reduce dose in renal impairment Avoid using with terfenadine or cisapride
	Oral	1	3 mg/kg	3 mg/kg	2–3 mg/kg	Prophylactic dose
Flucytosine	Oral	4	25–50 mg/kg	25–50 mg/kg	25–50 mg/kg	For systemic candidiasis and cryptococcosis Monitor levels (aim for trough 25–50 mg/L) and blood count
	i.v.	4	25–50 mg/kg	25–50 mg/kg	25–50 mg/kg	
Fucidin (sodium fusidate)	Oral	3	250 mg (as fusidic acid)	500 mg (as fusidic acid)	750 mg (as fusidic acid)	Staphylococcus aureus infection, including osteomyelitis and suppurative arthritis Should be combined with flucloxacillin or erythromycin
	i.v.	3	6 mg/kg (as sodium fusidate)	6 mg/kg (as sodium fusidate)	6 mg/kg (as sodium fusidate)	

Drug	Route	Doses				Notes
Ganciclovir	i.v.	2	5 mg/kg	5 mg/kg	5 mg/kg	Treatment regimen (14–21 days) for CMV disease in immunocompromise
		1	5 mg/kg	5 mg/kg	5 mg/kg	Maintenance regimen Neutropenia and thrombocytopenia common Reduce dose in renal impairment
Gentamicin	i.v. Single daily dose regimen	3 1	2.5 mg/kg 6 mg/kg	2.5 mg/kg 6 mg/kg	1.5–2 mg/kg 4–5 mg/kg	Gram-negative infections, especially cystic fibrosis and immunocompromised status Always monitor levels. Aim for peak < 10 mg/L and trough < 2 mg/L (or < 1 on single daily dose)
Griseofulvin	Oral	2	5 mg/kg	5 mg/kg	5 mg/kg	For ringworm of scalp (6 weeks); nails (6 months) May cause photosensitivity
Isoniazid	Oral, i.v.	1	10 mg/kg	200 mg	300 mg	Treatment of tuberculosis. Combined with other drugs unless for prophylaxis For TB meningitis use 10–20 mg/kg Give pyridoxine to prevent peripheral neuritis in malnourished or breast-fed infants
Itraconazole	Oral	1	3–5 mg/kg	3–5 mg/kg	3–5 mg/kg	Treatment or prophylaxis of fungal infection (including *Aspergillus* spp.) in immunocompromised Monitor liver function NB Unreliable absorption
Mebendazole	Oral	Single dose	Not used	100 mg	100 mg	For threadworm infections
Mebendazole	Oral	2	Not used	100 mg	100 mg	3-day course for hookworm, whipworm or roundworm

NB. Doses are individual and not daily dosages.

Appendix III: Antimicrobials for the infant and child (continued)

Drug	Route	Times daily	1 year	7 years	14 years	Indications and comments
Meropenem	i.v.	3	20–40 mg/kg	20–40 mg/kg	20–40 mg/kg	Treatment of severe infections with resistant organisms, especially in immunocompromised Use highest dose in meningitis
Metronidazole	Oral	1	40 mg/kg (max. 500 mg)	1 g	2 g	Giardiasis. 3 days treatment
	Oral	3	200 mg	400 mg	800 mg	Amoebiasis. Treat for 5 days
	Oral, rectal	3	250 mg	500 mg	1 g	Anaerobic infection
	i.v.	3	7.5 mg/kg	7.5 mg/kg	7.5 mg/kg	
Miconazole	Oral	4	62.5 mg	125 mg	125–250 mg	Fungal infections, especially *Candida*. Oral preparation for oral thrush. i.v. for systemic infection – need specialist advice
	i.v.	3	12–15 mg/kg	12–15 mg/kg	12–15 mg/kg	
Mupirocin	Topical	3	Use topically on skin and intranasally			Elimination of staphylococcal carriage, including MRSA. Superficial staphylococcal skin infections. NB. Different preparations for skin and nasal use
Netilmicin	i.v., i.m.	3	2.5 mg/kg	2.5 mg/kg	1.5–2 mg/kg	Gram-negative infections, especially in cystic fibrosis and immunocompromised state Monitor levels: peak 5–12 mg/L; trough < 3 mg/L

Drug	Route	Number				
Nitrofurantoin	Oral	4	0.75 mg/kg	0.75 mg/kg	0.75 mg/kg	For lower tract urinary infections with multiply resistant organisms. Not suitable for pyelonephritis. May cause nausea and vomiting
	Oral	1 (at night)	1 mg/kg	1 mg/kg	1 mg/kg	Prophylaxis of urinary tract infection
Nystatin	Oral, topical	4	100 000 U	100 000 U	100 000 U	Given for oral thrush or candidal napkin dermatitis
Paromomycin	Oral	3	10 mg/kg	10–16.5 mg/kg	10–16.5 mg/kg	Suppression of cryptosporidial infection in the immunocompromised host. Amoebiasis
	Topical		Apply to skin lesions			Cutaneous leishmaniasis
Penicillin G (benzylpenicillin)	i.m.	4	150 mg	300 mg	600 mg	1 megaunit = 600 mg. Tonsillitis, lobar pneumonia, erysipelas, endocarditis, meningococcal and pneumococcal meningitis
	i.v.	4–6	25–50 mg/kg	25–50 mg/kg	25–50 mg/kg	Higher dose 4-hourly in meningitis and endocarditis
	i.m., i.v.	Single dose	600 mg	1200 mg	1200 mg	Domiciliary use – emergency treatment of meningococcal infection
Penicillin G as procaine penicillin	i.m.	1	60 mg/kg to maximum of 2.4 g	60 mg/kg to maximum of 2.4 g	60 mg/kg to maximum of 2.4 g	For treatment of gonococcal infection in childhood. Therapeutic level maintained better with probenecid given 30 min before injection (20 mg/kg b.d. (maximum 1 g))
Penicillin V (phenoxymethyl-penicillin)	Oral	4	125 mg	250 mg	500 mg	Tonsillitis and minor infections, prophylaxis of rheumatic fever and septicaemia after splenectomy and in sickle cell anaemia. For prophylactic usage given twice daily in doses shown

NB. Doses are individual and not daily dosages.

Appendix III: Antimicrobials for the infant and child (continued)

Drug	Route	Times daily	1 year	7 years	14 years	Indications and comments
Pentamidine	i.v.	1	4 mg/kg	4 mg/kg	4 mg/kg	Treatment of PCP unresponsive to co-trimoxazole. Give as an infusion. Monitor for hypoglycaemia
	Nebulised	1 per month	Not suitable	300 mg	300 mg	Prophylaxis of PCP. Pretreat with a salbutamol nebuliser
Piperacillin	i.v.	3–4	50–75 mg/kg	50–75 mg/kg	50–75 mg/kg Max. 4 g	For treatment of *Pseudomonas aeruginosa* infection in children with cystic fibrosis or immunocompromised status. Combine with aminoglycoside. Empirical treatment of febrile neutropenia
Piperazine	Oral	Two doses 14 days apart	Two-thirds of a sachet	1 sachet	1 sachet	For treatment of threadworms. Sachets – Pripsen® (piperazine phosphate 4 g and sennosides 15.3 mg)
Piptazobactam	i.v.	4	80/100 mg/kg	80/100 mg/kg	80/100 mg/kg	Resistant Gram-negative bacillary sepsis. Dose expressed as piperacillin/tazobactam. Reduce dose in renal impairment
Pivampicillin	Oral	3	Avoid	175 mg	250 mg	175 mg in 5 mL. Similar antibacterial spectrum to ampicillin with better absorption. Contains sorbitol
Pyrazinamide	Oral	3	7–12 mg/kg	7–12 mg/kg	7–12 mg/kg	Used in tuberculosis, including TB meningitis.

	Route					
Pyrimethamine	Oral	1	1 mg/kg	1 mg/kg	1 mg/kg	In combination with sulphadiazine for congenital toxoplasmosis in 3-week course alternating with spiramycin. Give weekly folinic acid supplement. Monitor blood count
Pyrimethamine and sulfadoxine	Oral	Single dose	Half a tablet	One and a half tablets	2 tablets	Fansidar®. Single dose for completing treatment of falciparum malaria
Quinine	Oral i.v. (over 4 h)	3 3	125 mg 10 mg/kg	300 mg 10 mg/kg	600 mg 10 mg/kg	Oral doses given as quinine sulphate i.v. doses given as quinine dihydrochloride. NB. 122 mg of both salts is equivalent to 100 mg quinine base and to 169 mg quinine bisulphate. Treatment of malaria, especially if chloroquine resistance or cerebral malaria
	i.v.	Loading 20 mg/kg dose	20 mg/kg	20 mg/kg	20 mg/kg	In severe disease give by i.v. route but switch to oral therapy as soon as possible. Infuse over 4 h. Monitor for hypoglycaemia, arrhythmias, hypotension. i.v. route not used below 3 years of age. Always seek specialist advice. Followed by single dose of Fansidar®
Quinupristin/dalfopristin	i.v.	3	7.5 mg/kg	7.5 mg/kg	7.5 mg/kg	For treatment of proven vancomycin-resistant *Enterococcus faecium* (but not *faecalis*) infection
Rifabutin	Oral	1	5 mg/kg	5 mg/kg	5 mg/kg	Atypical mycobacterial infection. May cause uveitis. Drug levels increased by use of clarithromycin

NB. Doses are individual and not daily dosages.

Appendix III: Antimicrobials for the infant and child (continued)

Drug	Route	Times daily	1 year	7 years	14 years	Indications and comments
Rifampicin	Oral, i.v.	1	20 mg/kg (max. 600 mg)	600 mg (max. 600 mg)	600 mg	Treatment of tuberculosis Warn about orange secretions
	Oral, i.v.	2	150 mg	300 mg	600 mg	Treatment of severe staphylococcal infections, brucellosis
Rifampicin as prophylaxis	Oral	2	10 mg/kg	10 mg/kg	600 mg	Prophylaxis of *Neisseria meningitidis* infection for 2 days
	Oral	1	20 mg/kg	20 mg/kg (max. 600 mg)	20 mg/kg (max. 600 mg)	Prophylaxis of *Haemophilus influenzae* infection for 4 days Drug interaction with oral contraceptive
Spiramycin	Oral	2	50 mg/kg	50 mg/kg	50 mg/kg	For congenital toxoplasmosis – alternating with pyrimethamine and sulphadiazine in 3-weekly cycles
Streptomycin	i.m.	1	30 mg/kg	30 mg/kg	30 mg/kg (max. 1 g)	Treatment of tuberculous meningitis for up to 12 weeks. Other antituberculous drugs always given simultaneously
Sulphadiazine	Oral	2	50 mg/kg	50 mg/kg	50 mg/kg	Congenital toxoplasmosis in combination with pyrimethamine alternating with spiramycin in 3-weekly cycles
Teicoplanin	i.v.	1	10 mg/kg 12-hrly × 3 doses then 10 mg/kg daily	10 mg/kg 12-hrly × 3 doses then 10 mg/kg daily	10 mg/kg 12-hrly × 3 doses then 10 mg/kg daily	Gram-positive infections, especially coagulase-negative staphylococci

Terbinafine	Oral	1	Avoid	125 mg	250 mg	Dermatophyte infections
Thiabendazole	Oral	2	25 mg/kg	25 mg/kg (max. 1.5 g)	25 mg/kg (max. 1.5 g)	Treatment of refractory hookworm, threadworm, whipworm, roundworm, visceral larva migrans, strongyloidiasis Treatment given for 2–7 days – see literature
Tobramycin	i.v.	3	2.5 mg/kg	2.5 mg/kg	1.5–2 mg/kg	Treatment of Gram-negative infections Ototoxic Monitor levels (peak < 10 mg/L; trough < 2 mg/L)
Tribavirin	Nebulised	1	6 g in 300 mL saline	6 g in 300 mL saline	6 g in 300 mL saline	Severe respiratory viral infections in compromised children, including RSV, influenza, parainfluenza, adenovirus
	i.v.	3	8 mg/kg × 24 h then 5 mg/kg	8 mg/kg × 24 h then 5 mg/kg	8 mg/kg × 24 h then 5 mg/kg	Systemic viral infections, including Lassa fever, adenovirus in the immunocompromised host
Trimethoprim	Oral	2	50 mg	100 mg	200 mg	For urinary tract infections
	i.v.	2	4 mg/kg	4 mg/kg	4 mg/kg	
	Oral	1	1–2 mg/kg	1–2 mg/kg	1–2 mg/kg	Single evening dose as urinary tract prophylaxis
Vancomycin	i.v.	3–4	15 mg/kg then 10–15 mg/kg – total daily dose 40–45 mg/kg	15 mg/kg then 10–15 mg/kg – total daily dose 40–45 mg/kg	15 mg/kg then 10–15 mg/kg – total daily dose 40–45 mg/kg	Use in resistant staphylococcal infections, including coagulase-negative *Staphylococcus* Other Gram-positive infections, including enterococci Ototoxic and nephrotoxic. Check levels
	Oral	4				For pseudomembranous colitis use i.v. preparation orally

NB. Doses are individual and not daily dosages.
A number of drugs listed above are not licensed for use in children but nevertheless are often used under specialist supervision.

III Antimicrobials

Appendix IV Notifiable diseases 2000

	England and Wales	Northern Ireland	Scotland
Acute encephalitis	+	+*	0
Acute poliomyelitis	+	+	+
Anthrax	+	+	+
Chickenpox	0	+	+
Cholera	+	+	+
Continued fever	0	0	+
Diphtheria	+	+	+
Dysentery (amoebic or bacillary)	+	+	Bacillary dysentery
Erysipelas	0	0	+
Food poisoning (all sources)	+	+	+
Gastroenteritis (under 2 years of age)	0	+	0
Legionella/Legionnaires' disease	0	+	+
Leprosy	+†	0	0
Leptospirosis	+	+	+
Lyme disease	0	0	+
Malaria	+	+	+
Measles	+	+	+
Meningitis	+	+*	0
Meningococcal septicaemia (without meningitis)	+	+	Meningococcal infection
Mumps	+	+	+
Ophthalmia neonatorum (includes *Neisseria gonorrhoeae* and *Chlamydia trachomatis* infection)	+	0	0
Paratyphoid fever	+	+	+
Plague	+	+	+
Puerperal fever	0	0	+
Rabies	+	+	+
Relapsing fever (*Borrelia* infection)	+	+	+
Rubella	+	+	+
Scarlet fever	+	+	+
Smallpox	+	+	+
Tetanus	+	+	+
Toxoplasmosis	0	0	+
Tuberculosis (all forms)	+	+	+
Typhoid fever	+	+	+
Typhus	+	+	+
Viral haemorrhagic fever	+	+	+
Acute viral hepatitis	+‡	+‡	+‡
Whooping cough	+	+	+
Yellow fever	+	+	0

Notify: **England and Wales** Consultant in Communicable Disease Control (or officer function); **Northern Ireland** Director of Public Health of the appropriate Health and Social Services Board; **Scotland** Director of Public Health/Consultant in Public Health in the appropriate Health Board.

Appendix IV continued

Adult AIDS and HIV cases are voluntarily reported on a special AIDS Clinical Report Form in strict medical confidence to the Director, PHLS CDSC, 61 Colindale Avenue, London NW9 5EQ. Paediatric cases are reported to the Institute of Child Health in London (see Chapter 23).

= = notifiable; 0 = not notifiable.

* As acute encephalitis/meningitis (bacterial); or acute encephalitis/meningitis (viral). † Reported directly to the Chief Medical officer, Department of Health. ‡ Reported as hepatitis A, B, or other.

Appendix V Exclusion periods

This appendix details the characteristics of various infectious diseases so that decisions about exclusion from school, etc. can be rationally based. In the past, information has often been based on small studies and best practice. Much of the data here is based on a systematic review undertaken by Dr Martin Richardson. This is indicated in the table by an asterix (*); further details are available on the PHLS website at www.phls.co.uk/schools/advice (see also Further reading). Where conditions were not part of this review, the information is based on the best available at the time.

The exclusion periods stated here are only guidelines and may need to be modified depending on the circumstances. A child who is feelingly significantly unwell should not return to school even if no longer infectious. Where there is an immunocompromised child within a class, periods of exclusion may need to be adhered to strictly, whereas when all the other children are essentially well the periods can be shortened. In a nursery, where the standards of personal hygiene may not be as good as with older children, it is important to keep to the exclusion periods for enteric illness because spread within the nursery environment is much more likely.

Wherever there is any doubt, it is important to consult with the school health service and the local Consultant in Communicable Disease Control (CCDC). Each district should have its own guidelines, which will include details of the circumstances in which the CCDC should be informed of any episodes of infection.

FURTHER READING

Richardson M, Elliman D, Maguire H, Simpson J, Nicoll A (in press) An evidence base of incubation periods, periods of infectiousness, and exclusion periods for the control of communicable diseases in schools and preschools. Pediatr Infect Dis J.

Appendix V Exclusion periods for infectious disease

	Usual incubation period	Period of infectivity	Recommended exclusion period	Mode of spread
AIDS/HIV	Variable – may be years	Indefinite	None	Blood or sexual contact. Congenital/perinatal
Amoebiasis	4 weeks to several years	Can be years	Until 24 hours after last episode of diarrhoea	Contaminated food or water and faeces
Ascaris	4–8 weeks	Person-to-person spread does not occur		Faeces in soil or contaminated food
Aspergillosis	Unknown	Organism is ubiquitous in the environment. Person-to-person spread is not important		
Botulism infant food-borne	3–14 days 12 hours to 7 days	Person-to-person spread does not occur		Contaminated food
Brucellosis	1 week to several months	Person-to-person spread is rare. Infection is from infected animals and tissues (including placenta) through cuts/abrasions of the skin, aerosol, oral ingestion or contact with conjunctival mucosa		
*Campylobacter enteritis**	1–10 days (median 3 days)	Not known	Until 24 hours after last episode of diarrhoea	Faeces and contaminated food, water or milk
Candidiasis	2–5 days	While organism present	None	Person-to-person and environmental
Cat-scratch disease	3–10 days to appearance of primary lesion. Further 2–6 weeks to appearance of lymphadenopathy	Requires bite, scratch or other close contact from an animal vector (cat, dog or monkey)		

	Incubation period	Infectious period	Exclusion period	Transmission
Chickenpox*	11–20 days (median 15 days)	From −4 to +5 days (usually −1 to +2 days)	5 days from start of skin eruption	Physical contact and respiratory droplets
Chlamydia				
C. pneumoniae	More than 10 days			Respiratory droplets
C. psittaci	5–21 days	Person-to-person spread unheard of	None	From infected birds of the parrot family, turkeys, pigeons and ducks. See main text for ewe abortion agent
C. trachomatis conjunctivitis	5–14 days			Acquired at or around birth from infected mother
pneumonia	4–6 weeks			
Cholera	1–3 days (range few hours to 5 days)	Until stools are negative (may be months if untreated)	Until 24 hours after last episode of diarrhoea	Contaminated food and water
Conjunctivitis*	3–29 days (mean 11 days)	?up to 2 weeks	None	Data refers mainly to adenoviruses
Cryptosporidiosis*	1–14 days (median 7 days)	Unknown	Young children: 2 weeks from onset. Older children: until 24 hours after last episode of diarrhoea	Faeces, pets, farm animals, food and water
Cytomegalovirus	Unknown	While virus excreted	None	Saliva and sexual contact. Congenital

Appendix V Exclusion periods for infectious disease

	Usual incubation period	Period of infectivity	Recommended exclusion period	Mode of spread
Dermatophytoses Tinea capitis Tinea corporis Tinea pedis Tinea unguium	 2–4 weeks 2–38 weeks	Presumably indefinite unless treated	None	See entry in main text.
Diphtheria	2–5 days (range 2–7 days)	2–3 weeks unless treated, in which case 24 hours after treatment started	Until throat swab negative	Contact with discharge from nose, throat, eye and skin of infected person
Enterovirus infections (non-HFM and nonpolio)*	2–7 days	Not known	None (exclusion may be necessary in outbreaks of viral meningitis)	Faeces, fomites, airborne and waterborne
Escherichia coli enteritis*	*E. coli* 1–10 days (median 4 days) EPEC: 2–48 h EIEC: 1–156 h ETEC: 3–166 h	Not known	*E. coli* O157: negative stool × 2. Others: until 24 hours after last episode of diarrhoea	Faeces, animals, food and water
Gastroenteritis* Adenovirus	8–10 days	Unknown	Until 24 hours after resolution of diarrhoea	Faeces

Astrovirus	3 days	Unknown	Until 24 hours after resolution of diarrhoea	Faeces
Caliciviruses	? 1–3 days	Unknown	Until 24 hours after resolution of diarrhoea	Faeces, food and water
Norwalk virus	4–77 h (median 36 h)	For 2–3 days after recovery	For 3 days after recovery	Food and water; ?air-borne
Rotavirus	2–4 days	Unknown	Until 24 hours after resolution of diarrhoea	Faeces; ?respiratory droplets
Giardiasis*	5–20 days (median 7 days)	Unknown	Until 24 hours after resolution of diarrhoea	Faeces or contaminated water
Gonococcal infections see Chapter 55				
Haemolytic uraemic syndrome	Usually 1–10 days (median 4 days) to onset of diarrhoea. Another week to onset of HUS	See Chapter 56		Faeces contaminated food, unpasteurised milk and water
Haemophilus influenzae invasive infections*	Organism carried an unknown time before onset of disease: however, there are case reports of contacts developing 4–5 days postexposure	Unknown	48 hours after treatment started	Direct contact or respiratory droplet. Not very infectious
Haemorrhagic fevers	For yellow fever see below, for others see Chapter 58			

Appendix V Exclusion periods for infectious disease

	Usual incubation period	Period of infectivity	Recommended exclusion period	Mode of spread
Hand, foot and mouth disease*	Unclear, but thought to be 3–5 days	Probably less than 7 days	None	Unclear, but possibly respiratory droplets, faeces and direct contact
Head lice*	7–10 days from nits to lice	As long as lice remain alive	None	Direct head-to-head contact
Helicobacter infection	Unknown	Unknown	None	Unknown
Hepatitis A*	15–50 days (median 33 days)	From 1–2 weeks before to 1 week after onset of symptoms	< 5 years: 5 days from onset ≥ 5 years: none	Faeces, food, water and blood
Hepatitis B	60–90 days (range 45–160 days)	Indefinite in carriers	None	Blood and sexual contact. Congenital/perinatal
Hepatitis C	6–8 weeks (range 2–29 weeks)	Indefinite in carriers	None	Blood and sexual contact. Congenital/perinatal
Hepatitis E	2–9 weeks (mean 6 weeks)	Person-to-person spread is rare		Usually via contaminated water and, less commonly, food. Rarely from faeces
Herpes simplex*	1–6 days (mean 3.5 days)	Unknown	None	Oral secretions and physical contact

Impetigo staphylococcal*	No true incubation period	Unknown	Until lesions are healed or crusted	Direct physical contact
streptococcal*	2–33 days (median 8 days)	Unknown	Until lesions are healed or crusted	Direct physical contact. Broken skin usually required for disease to occur
Infectious mononucleosis (glandular fever)*	33–49 days	At least 2 months	None	Oral secretions, via kissing, and droplets
Influenza (influenza A)*	1–3 days (median 1.5 days)	Unknown	None	Airborne via respiratory droplets
Invasive helminths	For ascariasis see above, for toxocariasis see below, and for others see Chapter 62			
Kawasaki disease	Aetiology is not yet known			
Legionnaires' disease	2–10 days (pneumonia); 1–2 days (Pontiac fever). Figures are for adults – not clear in children	Person-to-person spread not recorded		Aerosolised contaminated water
Leishmaniasis cutaneous visceral	A few weeks A few weeks to 6 months	Person-to-person spread not recorded		Sandfly bite
Leptospirosis	2–21 days		None	Organisms are found in animal urine. Transmission is via broken skin, mucous membranes or aerosol
Listeriosis	See Chapter 74		See Chapter 74	

Appendix V Exclusion periods for infectious disease

	Usual incubation period	Period of infectivity	Recommended exclusion period	Mode of spread
Lyme disease*	3–20 days (median 12 days)	Person-to-person spread does not occur	None	Tick vector found on deer
Malaria	See Chapter 76			See Chapter 76
Measles*	6–19 days (median 13 days)	Unknown	5 days from onset of rash	Airborne respiratory droplets
Meningococcal disease*	Unknown. Invasive disease follows colonisation of variable duration	Unknown	48 hours from start of treatment	Airborne respiratory droplets
Molluscum contagiosum*	2 weeks–3 months, but see text	Unknown; probably duration of lesions	None	Direct contact
Mumps*	15–24 days (median 19 days)	Unknown	5 days from onset of parotitis	Respiratory droplets
Nontuberculous (atypical) myco-bacterial infection	Weeks to months	Person-to-person spread not recorded		Ubiquitous in the environment
Mycoplasma infections	3 weeks (6–23 days)	Unknown	None	Airborne respiratory droplets
Parainfluenza			None	

Paratyphoid*	2–3 weeks	Unknown	> 5 years old: until 24 hours after last episode of diarrhoea. < 5 years old: until negative stools obtained	Faeces, contaminated food and water
Parvovirus (fifth disease)*	13–18 days	Unknown	None, ineffective	Respiratory droplets
Pertussis*	5–21 days (rarely >10 days)	Unknown (treatment with erythromycin and exclusion for 5 days prevents transmission)	Treated: 5 days from onset. Untreated: at least 3 weeks	Respiratory droplets
Plague bubonic	2–6 days	Person-to-person spread only from content of bubo, otherwise spread by flea bite		
pneumonic	2–4 days	While ill	For 3 days after start of treatment	Respiratory droplets
Pneumocystis	Unknown	Unknown	Unknown	
Poliomyelitis	7–21 days (range 3–35 days)	While virus present in stool – usually a few days before onset to several weeks after	On advice of CCDC	Faeces and rarely by food and water
Prion disease (transmissible spongiform encephalopathy (TSE))	See Chapter 89	None	See Chapter 89	

Appendix V Exclusion periods for infectious disease

Rabies	2 months (range 5 days to over 1 year). Injuries closer to the brain have shorter incubation periods	No person-to-person spread has been recorded, but the virus has been found in the saliva of infected individuals. Isolation is indicated	Via saliva through bites, scratches or abrasions. Person-to-person via corneal transplant
Respiratory syncytial disease	4–6 days (range 2–8 days)	While symptomatic	Respiratory droplets and infected fomites
		Virus shedding may continue for 3–4 weeks	
Roseola infantum*	10–15 days	None	Probably oral secretions
		Unknown	
Rubella* Respiratory droplets	15–20 days (median 17 days)	Probably mostly infectious in prodrome	5 days from onset of rash
Salmonellosis*	4 h–5 days (median 16 hours) (14 days has been reported)	Unknown	< 5 years of age: at least one negative stool > 5 years of age: until 24 hours after last episode of diarrhoea	Faeces, and contaminated food and water. Possibly fomites
Scabies*	7–27 days (median 12 days) (primary infection)	Probably indefinite without treatment	Until treated	Direct contact

Shigellosis* (bacillary dysentery)	1–6 days (median 2 days)	Unknown	< 5 years of age: at least one negative stool > 5 years of age: until 24 hours after last episode of diarrhoea	Faeces, fomites and contaminated food and water
Staphylococcal infection	See Chapter 98			
Streptococcal pharyngitis and scarlet fever*	12 h–5 days (median 2 days)	Unknown	5 days if treated	Respiratory droplets. May be food-borne
Syphilis (acquired) and nonvenereal treponematoses	See Chapter 100			
Tetanus	4 days to 3 weeks (range 1 day to several months)	Person-to-person spread does not occur	None	Contaminated wound. May be minor
Threadworms* Faeces and fomites	2–4 weeks	Presumably indefinite unless treated	None	None
Toxic shock syndrome	2 days	Unknown	None	Tampons. Staphylococcal and streptococcal infections
Toxocariasis	A few weeks to several months (up to 10 years for ocular granuloma to develop)	Person-to-person spread does not occur	None	Ingestion of worm eggs from environment contaminated with infected animal faeces

Appendix V Exclusion periods for infectious disease

	Usual incubation period	Period of infectivity	Recommended exclusion period	Mode of spread
Toxoplasmosis	7–21 days	Person-to-person spread does not occur	None	Ingestion of poorly cooked contaminated meat or milk. Cat faeces
Tuberculosis*	1–12 months (median 2 months)	Smear positive on treatment; < 2 weeks Smear negative: negligible	Smear positive: 2 weeks after starting treatment Smear negative: none	Respiratory droplets
Typhoid*	5–34 days (median 15–21 days) (3–90 days quoted)	Presumably > 2 weeks. Carriers indefinite	> 5 years old: until 24 hours after last episode of diarrhoea < 5 years old: until negative stools obtained	Faeces, contaminated food and water
Typhus endemic epidemic	1–2 weeks 1–2 weeks	Person-to-person spread does not occur	None None	Rat flea bite Body louse
Warts and verrucae*	1–24 months (median 6 months)	Unknown; presumably duration of lesion	None	Direct contact and possibly fomites
Yellow fever	3–6 days	Person-to-person spread does not occur	None	Bite from infected mosquito
Yersiniosis	4–16 days (range 1–16 days)	For 6 weeks after development of symptoms	While symptomatic	Faeces, contaminated food or water

* Taken from the work of Dr Martin Richardson

Appendix VI Immunisation against infectious diseases

Immunisation is one of the most effective measures in the field of health promotion. The immunisation schedule current in the UK is followed throughout the whole country and has been responsible for a marked reduction in many diseases and the total elimination of polio.

Passive immunisation is used predominantly after exposure (hepatitis B, measles, rabies and tetanus), whereas active immunisation is given prior to exposure.

Active vaccines contain either live attenuated organisms, killed organisms, components or toxoids (Table VI.1). By dividing vaccines into live or other, the side-effects and contraindications can be predicted.

The current UK schedule is detailed in Table VI.2.

Full details of the vaccines, their indications, contraindications and side-effects are published at intervals by the Department of Health. In spite of very clear guidelines, there is still confusion in relation to some vaccines, e.g. pertussis and MMR, and so it is important that all health professionals involved in immunising are familiar with current recommendations.

Table VI.1 Vaccines currently available in the UK

Classification	Vaccine
Live attenuated	BCG
	Measles – only available as MMR (measles, mumps, rubella vaccine)
	Polio (oral – OPV)
	Rubella
	Typhoid (oral)
	Yellow fever
Toxoid	Diphtheria
	Tetanus
Component	*Haemophilus influenzae* type b
	Hepatitis B
	Influenza
	Neisseria meningitidis A, C, Y, W135
	Neisseria meningitidis C
	Pertussis – acellular
	Pneumococcal polysaccharide
	Typhoid
Killed whole organism 'whole cell'	Hepatitis A
	Japanese encephalitis
	Pertussis
	Polio (inactivated – IPV)
	Rabies
	Tick-borne encephalitis

Table VI.2 The routine childhood immunisation schedule in the UK

Vaccine	Recommended age of administration
Hepatitis B*	Birth
BCG†	Birth
Hepatitis B*	4 weeks
Oral polio vaccine (OPV) Triple vaccine – diphtheria, tetanus and pertussis (DTP) *Haemophilus influenzae* type b (Hib) Meningococcal C (Men C) Hepatitis B*	8 weeks
OPV & DTP/Hib & Men C	12 weeks
OPV & DTP/Hib & Men C	16 weeks
Hepatitis B*	6 months
Hepatitis B*	12 months
Measles, mumps and rubella (MMR) MMR – second dose	12–18 months Any time after first dose as long as at least 3 months have elapsed
Diphtheria and pertussis (DT) & OPV	Before starting primary school, i.e. about 3.5 years onwards
BCG (if tuberculin test negative)	10–14 years
DT & OPV	At or before time of leaving school

*Hepatitis B vaccine should be given at these ages if the mother is known to be hepatitis-surface-antigen-positive (either the standard schedule 0, 1, 6 months or accelerated schedule 0, 1, 2, 12 months). † Given when the infant is at high risk or, in some areas, to all neonates.

There are some children who miss out on immunisation because their parents/carers 'just don't get around to it' or 'they are always unwell'. For this reason it is essential that immunisations are carried out opportunistically as well as by appointment. Whenever children are seen by a health professional, including in a hospital setting, their immunisation status should be ascertained and, where possible, any overdue immunisations should be offered according to the schema in Chapter 28. Minor illnesses are not a contraindication. When, after an injury, it is considered necessary to give a child a tetanus booster, this should be combined with diphtheria.

Latterly, as vaccine-preventable diseases have become less common, concerns about side-effects have overshadowed the value of the vaccines. This has been particularly true for the MMR vaccine.

Unsubstantiated reports of bowel disease and autism following the vaccine have been given wide publicity and have gained credence in many quarters. When considering the validity of such concerns a number of principles should be considered:

- For live vaccines, all the proven side-effects (apart from anaphylaxis) are known effects of the disease(s)
- Many conditions occur at the same age as immunisations are given, e.g. febrile convulsions and MMR, autism and MMR, sudden infant death and pertussis
- For some conditions the aetiology is still unknown, e.g. most cases of autism, developmental delay, sudden infant death and inflammatory bowel disease
- The fact that one event follows another is not proof of causation
- Even if an adverse event is proven to be caused by a vaccine, this has to be weighed against the incidence and severity of the disease
- Many diseases are rare because of high rates of immunisation. If they fall, the diseases will return, with disastrous consequences.

When a health professional is in a position where s/he cannot answer parents' or carers' concerns, they should be referred to a senior paediatrician or the local District Immunisation Coordinator, rather than withhold immunisation.

FURTHER READING

Bedford H, Elliman D (1998) Childhood immunisation: a review for parents and carers. Health Education Authority, London.

Departments of Health (1995) Immunisation against infectious disease. HMSO, London.

Health Education Authority. Factsheets on various immunisations.

Further reading

Clinical paediatrics

Feigin RD, Cherry JD (eds) (1998) Textbook of paediatric infectious disease, 4th edn. WB Saunders, Philadelphia, PA.
Recognised as the main reference work in its field

Remington JS, Klein JO (1995) Infectious diseases of the fetus and newborn infant, 4th edn. WB Saunders, Philadelphia, PA.
The authoritative work on neonatal infection

Report of the Committee in Infectious Diseases (2000) The 'Red Book', 25th edn. American Academy of Pediatrics, Elk Grove Village, IL.

Public health and immunisation

Chin J (ed.) (2000) Control of communicable diseases manual, 17th edn. American Public Health Association, Washington, DC.
Comprehensive guide to public health management of infections

Departments of Health (1995) Immunisation against infectious disease. HMSO, London.
The authoritative guide to immunisation practice in the UK

Plotkin SA, Orenstein W (eds) (1999) Vaccines. WB Saunders, Philadelphia, PA.
A comprehensive textbook

Royal College of Paediatrics and Child Health (2001) Working party report on immunisation of the immunocompromised child. RCPCH, London.

Microbiology

Belshe, RB (ed.) (1990) A textbook of human virology. Mosby Year Book, St Louis, MO.

Collee JG, Fraser AG, Marmion BP (1996) Mackie & McCartney: practical medical microbiology, 14th edn. Churchill Livingstone, Edinburgh.

Fields BN, Knipe DM, Howley PM et al (eds) Field's virology, 3rd edn. Lippincott-Raven, Philadelphia, PA.

Forbes BA, Sahm DF, Weissfeld AS (eds) (1998) Bailey & Scott's diagnostic microbiology, 10th edn. Mosby, St Louis, MO.

Shanson DC (1999) Microbiology in clinical practice, 3rd edn. Butterworth-Heinemann, Oxford.

Immunology

Chapel H, Haeney M, Misbah S, Snowden N (1999) Essentials of clinical immunology, 4th edn. Blackwell Science, Oxford.

Janeway CA, Travers P (1994) Immunobiology: the human system in health and disease. Blackwell, Oxford.

Kaufman S, Kaselitz D (eds) (1998) Methods in microbiology, vol 25: Immunology and infection. Academic Press, San Diego, CA.

Ochs HD, Smith CIE, Puck JM (eds) (1999) Primary immunodeficiency diseases. Oxford University Press, New York, NY.

Roitt I, Brostoff J, Male D (1998) Immunology. Mosby, London.

Pharmacopoeia

British National Formulary (2000)
Updated twice each year

Medicines for children (1999) Royal College of Paediatrics and Child Health, London.

Index

Page references in bold type indicate major discussions, those in italic type indicate data in tables.

497

Index

Page references in bold type indicate major discussions, those in italic type indicate data in tables.

Page references in bold type indicate major discussions, those in italic type indicate data in tables.

Page references in bold type indicate major discussions, those in italic type indicate data in tables.